VACCINATIONS: TYPES, POTENTIAL COMPLICATIONS AND HEALTH EFFECTS

VACCINATIONS: TYPES, POTENTIAL COMPLICATIONS AND HEALTH EFFECTS

VACCINATIONS: TYPES, POTENTIAL COMPLICATIONS AND HEALTH EFFECTS

DAVID B. STEEN
AND
HOWARD L. DYSON
EDITORS

Nova Biomedical Books
New York

For permission to use material from this book please contact us:
Telephone 631-231-7269; Fax 631-231-8175
Web Site: http://www.novapublishers.com

Library of Congress Cataloging-in-Publication Data

Vaccinations : types, potential complications, and health effects / [edited by] David B. Steen and Howard L. Dyson.
p. ; cm.
Includes bibliographical references and index.
ISBN 978-1-60692-969-8 (hardcover)
1. Vaccination. 2. Vaccines. I. Steen, David B. II. Dyson, Howard L.
[DNLM: 1. Vaccination. 2. Vaccination--adverse effects. QW 806 V1169 2009]
RA638.V326 2009
614.4'7--dc22

2009011898

Published by Nova Science Publishers, Inc. ✝ New York

Contents

Preface

Vaccinations are the administration of antigenic materials to produce immunity to a disease. Vaccines can prevent or ameliorate the effects of infection by a pathogen. Vaccinations are considered to be the most effective and cost-effective method of preventing infectious diseases. This book presents current research on vaccinations to treat a variety of diseases including cancer, bacterial meningitis, multiple sclerosis, hepatitis B, and tuberculosis. This book also presents a comparative study about vaccination behavior in health care students from different countries. Also presented is research on vaccinations for aquacultured fish in order to control viral diseases.

Chapter 1 - The number of tuberculosis cases worldwide continues to increase. Progress towards conquering tuberculosis is severely hampered by the lack of an effective vaccine, and by the fact even the best drug regimens need to be administered for 6 months, preferably with supervision. The solution to these problems might lie in the development of improved prophylactic and therapeutic vaccines.

Chapter 2 - Infectious diseases are an increasing global health problem. Comparative studies about vaccination behavior in health care students from different countries are lacking. Due to working close to patients and infected specimens, they are in risk of contracting infectious diseases. The study analyzed vaccinations in health care students against tetanus, diphtheria, poliomyelitis, measles, mumps, rubella and hepatitis A+B. Furthermore, the study tried to investigate assessments on the importance of vaccinations and possible influences on the vaccination behavior. In an international multi-center-study, 182 German medical/dental students, 121 Iranian medical students, 70 Lithuanian medical students and 201 Spanish nursing students participated by working on an anonymous questionnaire related to demographic data and vaccinations. The response rates were between 76% and 100%.

Altogether, the investigated students were not sufficiently vaccinated, except in the case offull coverage against hepatitis B in Spanish students. In the Lithuanian and Spanish samples, 30-50% of the students did not know if they have been vaccinated, especially against diphtheria and poliomyelitis. Gender differences, with better immunizations in female students, were found in the German and in the Iranian sample. Nearly all investigated students regarded vaccinations as important to prevent infectious diseases.

It becomes obvious that medical training does not affect personal preventive behavior in health care students. Insufficient coverage by vaccinations and lack of professional skills endangers health care students to contract and transmit infectious diseases.

The education of health care students should focus more on infectious diseases and vaccinations to optimize immunization in future health professionals. This will protect them against preventable infections. Additionally, they will be better skilled to prevent infectious diseases by educating and vaccinating the general population.

Chapter 3 - Hepatitis B is a highly contagious viral infection. It can lead to chronic carrier state and the hepatocellular carcinoma in the worst case. To prevent is better than to treat athis infection. An effective tool for prevention and control of hepatitis B infection is the vaccination. In this article, topics on the hepatitis B vaccination will be presented. The new concepts on vaccination strategies will be discussed. Also, the new advances on hepatitis B vaccinology will be presented.

Chapter 4 - On June 20, 2002, an advisory panel to the U.S. Centers for Disease Control and Prevention (CDC) voted against mass smallpox vaccination and instead recommended that 10-20 thousand first responders receive the vaccine. The recommendations are currently under review by CDC and the Department of Health and Human Services (HHS). Congress addresses control of the vaccine stockpile in the Homeland Security legislation (H.R. 5005, S. 2452). Although there is little uneasiness over the safety of the only known samples of variola virus, held by the CDC in Atlanta and a laboratory near Novosibirsk in Russia, there is some concern that samples of the virus may have been acquired by terrorists or rogue governments, particularly because of the unrest that occurred during the break up of the Soviet Union. The Public Health Security and Bioterrorism Preparedness and Response Act of 2002 (P.L. 107-188), signed by the President on June 12, 2002, directs the Secretary of HHS to ensure that there is enough smallpox vaccine in the Strategic National Stockpile to meet health security needs and authorizes $509 million for FY2002 and such sums as may be necessary through FY2006 for this purpose. H.R. 5005, the Homeland Security Act of 2002 as passed by the House, would amend P.L. 107-188 by moving authority for the stockpile to the Department of Homeland Security (DHS); HHS would continue to manage the stockpile and determine its contents. S. 2452, the National Homeland Security and Combating Terrorism Act of 2002, as reported by the Governmental Affairs Committee on July 25, 2002, directs DHS to consult with CDC in the administration of the stockpile by CDC. An emergency supplemental appropriation (P.L. 107-117), signed by the President on January 10, 2002, provided $512 million for the purchase of smallpox vaccine by HHS.

Chapter 5 - Autoreactive T cells appear both in healthy individuals and in people suffering from a variety of autoimmune diseases. In Multiple Sclerosis (MS) these cells have been extensively studied and regulatory mechanisms that keep them in check in the healthy individual are the subjects of much current and past research. The dysregulation that brings on the symptoms of multiple sclerosis appears to include aspects of genetic, environmental, and other unknown factors. Much early work aimed toward understanding these mechanisms was done using the experimental allergic encephalomyelitis model (EAE) in rodents. Indeed, a great deal of work on molecular aspects of regulatory function utilizes this model today. The early animal work led to an explosion of research aimed at using immunoreactive T cells as a suppression device to achieve the depletion of autoreactive T cells in human MS. To this end, for over ten years, a number of investigators have been developing and perfecting the use of these cells in a T Cell Vaccination (TCV) paradigm. Not only has this research path shown extensive promise, giving rise to several sets of clinical trials now in progress, but investigation into the array of regulatory mechanisms at work in TCV has opened up several areas of exciting research. Anti-idiotypic and anti-ergotypic T cell responses were identified as being of paramount importance in achieving a favorable TCV response in vaccine recipients. Anti-idiotypic antibody activity was noted and studied. Recently, a great upsurge in research on a newly recognized population of "T-Regulatory" cells has brought to light a major force in TCV success and has opened doors to a further understanding of immune system regulation on a molecular level. Unraveling the mechanisms by which the inflammatory and demyelinating processes take place continues to give rise to additional measures by which these processes may be slowed or stopped, allowing a new lease on life for those looking forward formerly to nothing but increased levels of debilitation. Meanwhile, work continues to increase efficiency of vaccine elaboration, decrease cost to the patient, and provide ever more promising approaches to mastering the regulation of autoimmune attacks on the nervous system of the MS patient. This chapter will detail the ongoing research into the regulatory mechanisms operating in T cell vaccine function within the immune system and will discuss the technical challenges in development of such a vaccine.

Chapter 6 - Bacterial meningitis is a serious health risk to the newborn. No effective vaccines against the important causative agents *E. coli* K1 and *N. meningitidis* group B exist, apparently due to tolerance induced by host tissue glycans structurally similar to the bacterial capsular polysaccharides. Insufficient data on these cross-reactivities and poor understanding of the antibody interaction with the immunologically evasive capsular polysialic acid have hindered the development of polysaccharide vaccines against meningitis. Recent advance in analytical techniques and novel immonotherapeutic approaches have however, improved the situation significantly. The nature of polysialic acid–antibody interaction is now established and new promising therapeutical strategies have emerged. In this article, studies of immunological properties of polysialic acid and vaccine development spanning more than quarter of century are reviewed.

Chapter 7 - Recombinant viral vectors are being developed as vaccine carriers since they have been shown to induce strong antigen specific T-lymphocyte responses, which will likely prove important for effective vaccination against diseases such as HIV, malaria and tuberculosis. Of the many different viral vectors under development, replication-incompetent adenovirus vectors are particularly promising. These vectors have excellent safety records in vaccine and gene therapy trials, a mature production platform resulting in high yields, and excellent transgene-specific immune responses in both pre-clinical and early clinical studies. Of the 51 known human adenoviruses, adenovirus serotype 5 (Ad5) was first characterized and completely sequenced and therefore Ad5 has been used in the vast majority of gene therapy and vaccination studies. However, the high prevalence and neutralizing antibody titer against Ad5 in human populations worldwide, coupled to data from both pre-clinical and clinical studies demonstrating significant reduction of Ad5 based vaccination potency in presence of anti-Ad5 immunity, indicates a serious potential limitation for the clinical utility of Ad5 vectors. To overcome this limitation, the development of alternative adenoviral vectors with low seroprevalence is currently an area of active investigation. Alternative vectors under investigation generally group into three categories: (1) human adenovirus serotypes other than Ad5, (2) non-human adenoviruses, and (3) Ad5-based chimeric vectors. In this chapter, we will review recent advances in our understanding of adenoviral biology and progress in the development of alternative adenoviral vectors for vaccination.

Chapter 8 - The success of dendritic cell based cancer vaccination in animal models has resulted in a rapid transformation to human cancer trials. This has become possible by the development of methods to produce large numbers of human dendritic cells (DC) as well as protocols for antigen preparation, dendritic cell maturation and administration. Since the first clinical trial was published in 1996, more than 1000 cancer patients have received dendritic cell based cancer therapy. However, large variability of the protocols employed in the trials has made it difficult to draw firm conclusions from these studies. Here, various aspects of dendritic cell manufacturing are discussed and some of the latest clinical vaccination trials are reviewed. In addition, methods to evaluate the immunological outcome of dendritic cell based therapy are described and suggestions for future strategies will be outlined.

The immune system constantly recognizes and eliminates arising tumours based on their expression of tumour antigens (TA) (1;2). Despite this fact, effective vaccination against established cancers requires an intensive activation of the immune response to break down tolerance towards a given tumour antigen. Therefore, cancer vaccination needs to result in activation of the adaptive immune response by means of activating T cells, including tumour specific cytotoxic T lymphocytes (CTLs) and CD4+ T cells. This process is facilitated by professional antigen-presenting cells (APC), in particular dendritic cells (DCs) which express high levels of T cell costimulatory molecules and secrete relevant T cell polarizing cytokines (3). DCs can be generated *in vitro* and pulsed with tumour antigens in order to generate a tumour-specific immune response and therefore, DCs are obvious as adjuvant cells in cancer vaccination.

Chapter 9 - In the present work we have developed several models of cancer vaccines, employing a murine melanoma and nonviral procedures for gene transfer. Many efforts have been made in relation to cancer vaccines, attempting to elucidate the best way to induce correct activation of the immune system in order to achieve proper antitumor response. Engineered cells seem to be the most successful approach, since they better reproduce the processes that occur in real patients, including events that today still escape our understanding. However, purified antigens represent an easier approach in terms of their preparation, reproducibility and facility to become a commercial medicine. This is why they continue to center attention, though their results are still not particularly satisfactory. In an attempt to establish the best approach for stimulating the immune response and also securing the simplest treatment, we have tested different preventive vaccination models such as: a) purified antigens from irradiated B16 melanoma tumor cells (Tumor Membrane Proteins, TMP); b) such antigens encapsulated in liposomes; c) lipopolyplexes formed by cationic liposomes bearing antigens plus the cationic polymer polyethyleneimine (PEI), carrying DNA; d) freshly transfected and irradiated B16 cells, producing cytokines; and e) a very reduced number of transfected cells, selected by means of magnetic bead procedures. The results obtained show different rates of tumor growth inhibition - performance improving when adjusting the combinations of plasmid bearing the cytokine gene and TMP antigens in the lipopolyplexes. The best inhibition (total) was obtained with freshly transfected (not selected) cells, which allowed us to perform further experiments consisting of a vaccine with only the truly transfected (cytokine-producing) cells. On this occasion, reducing the cell number to only 20% that of the prior doses, we achieved about 80% of tumor growth inhibition. All these results encourage the conduction of further studies of this kind, with the purpose of increasing accuracy and optimizing cancer vaccine procedures.

Chapter 10 - Vaccination seems like the most adequate method to control viral diseases in aquacultured fish. Up to date, very few viral vaccines are commercialised, since it has been a difficult task to obtain effective vaccines in fish that are both safe and cost-effective. In the past years, DNA vaccination has been proven as a very effective method to control some rhabdoviral infections, such as those caused by infectious hematopoietic necrosis virus (IHNV) and viral hemorrhagic septicemia virus (VHSV), responsible for great losses in aquaculture production. These vaccines consisting in a plasmid in which the viral glycoprotein gene is expressed under the control of the citomegalovirus (CMV) promoter, are able to confer protection in fish after intramuscular injection. Even though the protection conferred is high and long-lasting, these vaccines are still not being used worldwide due to safety issues concerning the viral promoter, to difficulties in the administration of the vaccine at a large scale, and to high vaccination costs. Up to date, only an IHNV DNA vaccine has been licensed for use in Canada.

Moreover, the immune mechanism through which they confer protection is still unknown, and this is a major restriction for the optimisation of DNA vaccines for other viral pathogens also of great importance in fish, such as for example nodavirus, for which DNA vaccines as formulated for rhabdovirus are not effective.

In this chapter, we discuss the trends in research dealing with DNA vaccination in fish, that will hopefully allow the improvement and finally the routine use of these vaccines in aquaculture. These will include the possible use of molecular adjuvants; the use of attenuated mutant glycoprotein genes and studies dealing with conformation versus lineal epitopes; the substitution of the CMV promoter for promoters of a non-viral origin; the use of induced plasmids or fish transposons, the study of new mass vaccination methods, or the inclusion of specific siRNA sequences within the plasmid. As well, we will review the most recent advances in studies related to the immune response towards these vaccines, some of them based on microarray technologies, that may help elucidate the immune mechanisms responsible for protection.

In: Vaccinations: Types, Potential Complications… ISBN: 978-1-60692-969-8
Editors: D. B. Steen and H. L. Dyson

Chapter I

Immunology of Tuberculosis: Implications for the Development of New Therapies and Vaccines*

Graham A. W. Rook and Keertan Dheda
Centre for Infectious Diseases and International Health, Windeyer Institute for Medical Sciences, Royal Free and University College Medical School, London, U.K.

Introduction

The number of tuberculosis cases worldwide continues to increase. Progress towards conquering tuberculosis is severely hampered by the lack of an effective vaccine, and by the fact even the best drug regimens need to be administered for 6 months, preferably with supervision. The solution to these problems might lie in the development of improved prophylactic and therapeutic vaccines.

The current vaccine, Bacillus Calmette et Guérin (BCG) is widely used, and while probably protective in some countries such as the UK, provides little or no protection in countries close to the equator where a vaccine is most needed. Several new prophylactic vaccine candidates are entering Phase I clinical studies designed to test safety and to prove immunogenicity. However optimism might be premature. We do not know for certain why BCG fails in developing countries, so we cannot rule out the possibility that the new vaccines will fail for the same reasons. Therefore in this chapter we pay particular attention to clues that might help us to explain why BCG fails, and therefore to design vaccines that overcome the problem. At present there is the risk that vaccines are being designed that will, like BCG, be effective in northern Europe, but useless where they are really needed.

---

* A version of this chapter was also published in *Development of New Antituberculosis Drugs*, edited by W. W. Yew published by Nova Science Publishers, Inc. It was submitted for appropriate modifications in an effort to encourage wider dissemination of research.

We also need therapeutic vaccines. Perhaps improved drugs will lead to shorter treatment regimens, but this is by no means certain. An alternative approach is to exploit our knowledge of the immune system, to develop immunotherapies that enhance the immune system's ability to destroy *M. tuberculosis.* This can be done in laboratory models of tuberculosis, and there are claims of success in the human disease. Interestingly, the vaccines that have therapeutic potential are distinct from those that are most active as prophylactics in animal models.

Protective immunity to tuberculosis in man is known to require a Th1 response because genetic defects in signaling by IFN-γ or IL-12 lead to susceptibility [1, 2], and neutralisation of TNF-α reactivates latent disease [3]. Some of this Th1-like response is driven by CD1-restricted T cells that recognize lipid and glycolipid antigens, rather than protein [4]. However as our knowledge of this Th1 response advances, it is becoming increasingly evident that it is not the complete answer [5]. We show in detail below that the size of the Th1 response does not correlate with its protective efficacy, implying that other factors are involved [5, 6] We need to take into account the disease-causing strategy that *M. tuberculosis* has evolved. We conclude that *M. tuberculosis* does not cause disease by failing to evoke the potentially protective Th1 response, but rather by driving a large Th1 response that is then corrupted so that it kills human tissue rather than mycobacteria. The crucial factors are those involved in the immunopathology which is the central feature of tuberculosis, because it drives the formation of cavities that open into bronchi, and hence permit spread of the infection by coughing. Therefore successful vaccines may need to switch off the mechanisms that disable the Th1 response and those that drive the immunopathology, particularly in developing countries where a potentially adequate Th1 response is almost universally present.

Immunity to TB

Location of Primary Foci and of Reactivation

Recent reanalysis of the physiology of the respiratory tract and its vasculature, has confirmed predictions made decades ago by Bill Dock, and casts light on the fact that primary lesions can occur anywhere in the lungs, while progressive disease tends to be located at the apices, reviewed in [7]. Firstly, inspired air tends to flow preferentially to the lower parts of the lung due to gravitational effects on lung conformation. Secondly particles contained within the air tend to follow the straighter airways, which are those leading out to the periphery. These two factors explain the frequency of primary foci (Ghon foci) close to the pleura in the lower half of the lungs, reviewed in [7].

So why does progressive disease due to reactivation tend to occur in the apices? Pressure in the pulmonary circulation is low, so there is wide variation in blood flow to the apices and to the lung bases. Oxygen tensions are a product of the balance between ventilation and pulmonary blood flow. The apices, despite having lower ventilation (V) and perfusion (Q), have a higher V/Q ratio than the bases. Consequently, oxygen tensions are higher at the apices (132mm Hg) than at the bases of the lungs (89mm Hg). Interestingly, in conditions like valvular mitral stenosis where there is pulmonary congestion and accordingly a low V/Q ratio, tuberculosis is exceedingly rare. By contrast, in pulmonary stenosis in which blood flow to the lungs is reduced, while ventilation is unimpaired (high V/Q ratio), tuberculosis is common, reviewed in [7]. So the apex is susceptible to reactivation because there is more oxygen there, relative to delivery of the immune response. What is the nature of that response?

The Early Th1 Response to *M. Tuberculosis*, and Latent Infection

Following exposure to *M. tuberculosis* most humans or animals develop a Th1 response. Release of IFN-γ in response to ESAT-6 (a highly immunogenic protein secreted by *M. tuberculosis*) is often used as a test for exposure and becomes positive rapidly [8, 9]. In most individuals this early Th1 response is protective. Approximately one-third of the world's population is infected with *M. tuberculosis*, but in about 90% the organisms are controlled by the immune system, and only in about 10% does exposure to *M. tuberculosis* lead to disease. In the majority some bacilli remain in the tissues in a latent state for many years, perhaps permanently. Studies of the location of these latent organisms are illuminating. In 1927 Opie and Aronson reported that less than 10% of old primary lesions contained live bacilli, while they could be recovered from macroscopically normal lung tissue in almost 50% of people who had died from causes other than tuberculosis [10]. This observation, dating from 1927, is rarely cited. However it was one of the pieces of evidence that led Balasubramanian *et al* to propose that rather than lying dormant in the primary complex, the latent bacilli lie dormant in sites that are seeded hematogenously during the early stages of the primary infection [11]. In the guinea pig model used by these authors this phase of haematogenous dissemination from the primary lesion occurred about 3 weeks after infection, and was manifested as widespread tiny granulomata that did not progress. This probably explains the widespread distribution of *M. tuberculosis* DNA that was subsequently demonstrated in a mouse model of latent infection following low dose challenge [12]. To establish the relevance of these observations to man, a study was undertaken using *in situ* PCR to locate the DNA of *M. tuberculosis* in human tissues taken from individuals who had died suddenly from accidents or heart attacks, and who showed no evidence of tuberculosis at post-mortem [13]. When these tissue samples were taken from individuals who had lived in endemic areas, DNA of *M. tuberculosis* was frequently found in histologically normal tissues from many different organs. By contrast, no DNA was detected in samples from Norwegians; there has been no community spread of tuberculosis within Norway for several decades. A striking aspect of the findings was the minimal cellular infiltration in the sites presumed to contain disseminated latent *M. tuberculosis* [13]. Thus not only do 90% of individuals control *M. tuberculosis* without developing disease, but close examination of the tissues suggests that in these individuals relatively little immunological activity is required to maintain this control.

Massive Production of IFN-γ in the Lungs of Tuberculosis Patients

The modest Th1 response required to control *M. tuberculosis* in most individuals contrasts with the powerful responses seen in many tuberculosis patients, particularly at the site of disease [14]. The poor expression of IFN-γ in peripheral blood lymphocytes that is sometimes observed seems to reflect the sequestration of Th1 cells in the lungs, rather than an immunological deficit. (An unusual subset of "anergic" patients with potent immunoregulation and IL-10 release is discussed later). In general massive quantities of IFN-γ can be demonstrated in the lungs by ELISA or RT-PCR [14].

The Koch Phenomenon

Many patients exhibit the necrotising response to tuberculin that forms part of the Koch phenomenon. Koch infected guinea pigs with *M. tuberculosis* intradermally. He then observed that after 6 to 12 weeks, injection of culture supernatant (Old Tuberculin) or live organisms at a distant site induced local necrosis both at that site, and in the existing tuberculosis lesion [15]. For a while he interpreted this as a protective reaction, because the lesion, being superficial, underwent necrosis and fell off. He therefore injected Old Tuberculin subcutaneously into tuberculosis patients. This resulted in the sloughing (and apparent cure) of the lesions of skin tuberculosis (*Lupus vulgaris;* a common consequence of infection with *M. bovis* at that time), but also caused necrosis in pulmonary and spinal lesions with disastrous consequences [16]. The Koch phenomenon causes necrosis of the host tissue, but is less effective at killing the bacteria than is the weaker response seen after successful BCG vaccination, or in people with latent disease. This was demonstrated in the early decades of the 20th century [17]. Wilson and colleagues used 400 out-bred guinea pigs that had undergone a variety of immunisation schedules with killed *M. tuberculosis.* The animals were then skin-tested with a range of doses of "Old Tuberculin", before they were challenged with about 12 virulent organisms by intramuscular injection. The crucial finding was that the animals exhibiting the Koch phenomenon, (manifested as exquisite sensitivity to intradermal injections of tiny quantities of tuberculin), were more susceptible to tuberculosis than were unimmunised controls. Only animals with moderate tuberculin sensitivity were protected [17]. We discuss the possible mechanism of the Koch phenomenon later, but at this stage it is sufficient to note that once again, the *size* of the response is not an indicator of protection.

Vaccine Efficacy and Induction of Th1 Effector Responses

The conclusion that the size of the Th1 response does not determine vaccine efficacy also emerges from recent studies of vaccine candidates. BCG, a predominantly Th1-inducing vaccine, has poor protective efficacy and possibly none at all (except against tuberculous meningitis in children) in most developing countries close to the equator [18]. Is it possible to enhance the protective efficacy by boosting BCG's ability to prime a Th1 response? In experimental animals, manipulations that increase the Th1 response still further than is achieved by BCG vaccine alone, do not provide any additional protection. An enhanced Th1 response was achieved in mice primed with a DNA vaccine expressing ESAT-6 and antigen 85A before boosting with BCG, but this did not increase protection from an aerosol challenge [19]. Similarly a recombinant BCG strain expressing IL-18 caused an enhanced IFN-γ response but nevertheless failed to increase protective efficacy beyond that seen with unmodified BCG [20] and C. Locht, personal communication.

The finding that more IFN-γ does not mean greater protective efficacy is not limited to experiments involving BCG. Recombinant human IL-6 and a monoclonal antibody specific for IFN-γ were evaluated as co-adjuvants in a subunit vaccine against tuberculosis consisting of the culture filtrate proteins of *Mycobacterium tuberculosis* (ST-CF) emulsified in the adjuvant dimethyldioctadecylammonium bromide (DDA). Both adjuvants enhanced IFN-γ production but this did not result in enhanced protection against either an intravenous or an aerosol challenge [21].

The Relationship between Infiltration of T Cells, Immunity and Immunopathology

Studies using genetically modified strains of *M. tuberculosis* have yielded a related finding. Relatively few of the T lymphocytes that enter a tuberculosis lesion are relevant to controlling the growth of the bacteria. Most are probably more concerned with immunopathology. Several mutations within transcription factors or associated components (*SigH, rpoV and WhiB3*) result in lack of control of regulated sets of genes [22, 23]. Strains containing these mutations proliferate normally in normal mice, but cause much less immunopathology. Thus while animals infected with the intact strain died with massive lung pathology, those infected with the *SigH* mutant strain remained healthy despite the presence in the lungs of exactly the same bacterial load. Moreover the virulence and rate of growth of the *SigH* mutant was indistinguishable from that of wild type strains in mice with severe combined immunodeficiency (SCID mice) which lack T cells [22]. So the pathology evoked by the intact organisms, but not by the *SigH* mutant, was dependent upon the T cell response. The *SigH* mutant evoked only about one-tenth of the T cell infiltrate seen during infection with the parent strain. The conclusion is that relatively few Th1 cells are sufficient to control proliferation, and that the remaining 90% may be more concerned with immunopathology. Immunopathology is probably essential for the life cycle of *M. tuberculosis* because cavities opening into bronchi allow the dissemination of massive numbers of bacilli by coughing. It is likely that there is a relationship between the Koch phenomenon, and this superfluous infiltration with T cells.

Immunity Versus Immunopathology; Faulty Immunoregulation, or Deliberate Sabotage?

These and other considerations have led several authors to postulate that something else is involved, in addition to the Th1 response and production of IL-12, IFN-γ, and TNF-α. There are two logical possibilities. Either immunity requires some *additional* Th1-associated activity such as an unidentified macrophage function with variable efficacy in different individuals [5], or immunity mediated by the Th1 response is only effective in the *absence* of another corrupting influence, which might, for instance, be faulty immunoregulation [24] or excessive Th2 activity [6]. These are not mutually incompatible concepts. For instance the "corrupting influence" might be incapacitating a crucial macrophage function. One way or another, this critical factor, whether an omission from the Th1 response, or a corrupting addition to it, might explain the immunopathology that is a critical part of the life cycle and disease-causing capacity of *M. tuberculosis.* It is reasonable to ask whether the pathogenicity of *M. tuberculosis* is due to a failure to evoke a protective Th1 response, or to deliberate sabotage of a deliberately large Th1 response, in order to drive immunopathology. In this section we discuss these possibilities, and candidate mechanisms.

Too Much Regulatory T Cell Activity?

One obvious candidate is the presence of excessive or inappropriate activity of regulatory T cells (Treg). These cells suppress immune responses and inflammation by poorly understood mechanisms involving cell-cell contact, and also by releasing the regulatory cytokines TGF-β and IL-10. There are several different types of Treg, though it is not yet clear how many [25]. This topic will not be reviewed here. It is clear that Treg can play crucial but complex roles in infections, because they can modulate both immunity and immunopathology [24]. For instance, excessive early Treg activity, that blocks the early Th1 response, can lead to susceptibility to malaria [26, 27]. By contrast, Treg activity can be beneficial after the first burst of Th1 activity, because it can damp down the otherwise fatal immunopathology [28]. Could similar arguments apply to tuberculosis?

There are "anergic" TB patients who are skin-test negative and whose T cells fail to proliferate in response to antigens of *M. tuberculosis* in vitro. These individuals' T cells include populations that secrete IL-10, but release little IL-2 or IFN-γ in response to *M. tuberculosis* [29, 30] There is also a report that many of the T cells that secrete IFN-γ in the lungs of tuberculosis patients also secrete IL-10 [31], in which case they might well be the recently discovered Th1-like regulatory T cells that express both t-bet (and so are Th1-like) and Foxp3 (and so are Treg) rather than true Th1 cells [32]. Similarly, a recent study using an ELISPOT assay for IL-10-secreting cells suggests that tuberculosis patients have as many circulating IL-10-producing PPD-specific CD4+ T cells as they have IFN-γ-secreting CD4+ T cells [33]. Neutralizing antibodies to IL-10 increased IFN-γ production by PBMNC from HIV-positive and HIV-negative tuberculosis patients by enhancing monocyte IL-12 production [34], and T cells from cured tuberculosis patients with negative tuberculin skin tests inhibit replication of HIV1 via a mechanism that involves IL-10 [35].

Clearly therefore some, perhaps all TB patients generate IL-10-secreting regulatory T cells, but their importance remains unclear. Although a few patients are certainly anergic, most have a powerful IFN-γ response at the site of disease [14], and the massive tissue-destructive reaction (Koch Phenomenon) described above. This suggests that in the chronic phase of progressive of tuberculosis, the extent of Treg activity is not the critical factor that determines outcome. Wherever the patients' immune systems lie on the Treg axis, they still have TB!

This argument does not apply to the possibility that excessive *early* Treg function might result in a delayed development of protective Th1 activity, as in some malaria models [26]. But the malaria parasite proliferates very fast, and a delay of a day or two might be critical. We do not know if the same is true for *M. tuberculosis.* There was a delay of 4-5 days in the expression of iNOS and IFN-γ in the lungs when C57Bl/6 mice lacking the chemokine receptor CCR2 were infected with low doses of *M. tuberculosis* [36]. These CCR2 -/- mice also had a severe and prolonged deficiency in the number of macrophages entering the lungs. Despite these deficiencies in cell migration, the CCR2 -/- mice did not have increased bacterial loads in the lungs compared to wild-type mice. Only when challenged with a high dose of *M. tuberculosis* did the CCR2-/- mice show increased susceptibility [36]. Although interesting, this experiment does not provide a definitive answer, and we need more data to find out whether a Treg-induced delay in the onset of the Th1 response could be important during the initiation of progressive tuberculosis. Such information as we have suggests that it is unlikely to be a critical factor.

Deliberate Sabotage?

If the problem does not lie in over-activity of Treg, is it possible that some other component of the immune system is "sabotaging" the Th1 effector response? Many authors have suggested that this corrupting influence might be a form of Th2-like response, because IL-4 downregulates iNOS [37], drives an inappropriate alternative form of macrophage activation [38], and in animal models can contribute to tissue damage and fibrosis which are neglected components of the human disease [39]. Studies of pulmonary infection in the BALB/c mouse have led to the observation that after an initial phase of relatively pure Th1 response, which temporarily stops replication of the organisms, the disease progresses again when IL-4 starts to be expressed above a certain threshold level [40]. Moreover TNF-α became toxic to the animals at the same time. Several other experimental models of infection have also revealed that immunopathology or toxicity of TNF-α can be associated with the simultaneous presence of IL-4 in a dominantly Th1-mediated site of inflammation [40-43]. We have reviewed these data, and the likely mechanisms elsewhere [6]. Subsequent reports noted that the presence of IL-4 is not merely a late consequence of progressive infection. In fact if a Th2 response to secreted antigenic components of *M. tuberculosis* [44], to cross-reactive antigens in environmental mycobacteria [40], or even to a single epitope expressed within a recombinant organism, is evoked before challenge with virulent organisms, the subsequent disease is enhanced, particularly immunopathology, weight loss and fibrosis [45]. Since these are important but neglected characteristics of the human disease, we investigated IL-4 KO BALB/c mice, and confirmed that in the absence of functional IL-4 genes, the infection was attenuated, the toxicity of TNF-α eliminated and fibrosis diminished [39]. The latter is interesting because there is a view that Th2 cytokines are needed for human pulmonary fibrosis, which is striking in TB, whereas IFN-γ downregulates fibrosis [46]. These effects will not be apparent in mouse strains where IL-4 is not a major feature of progressive disease, and most are probably not mediated via STAT-6 [47]. The "non-Th2" effects of IL-4 are signalled via IRS-1 and IRS-2.

IL-4 in Human Tuberculosis

Are these findings in BALB/c mice relevant to man, or is human tuberculosis more like that occurring in some other mouse strains in which IL-4 seems unimportant? Is IL-4 a feature of human tuberculosis?

Evidence for Increased Expression of IL-4 in Human Tuberculosis

We have summarised the mass of data elsewhere [6]. Before the year 2000, some authors reported that in addition to Th1 cytokines, there was also increased expression of IL-4 in TB [48-50]. However other authors failed to detect raised IL-4 and the issue remained controversial [51]. It is now clear that were two reasons for the discrepancies. First, IL-4 is produced at low concentrations and has a correspondingly low mRNA copy number, so it is difficult to measure. Secondly, there are striking differences in the quantity of IL-4 that accompanies tuberculosis in different parts of the world. (The last point is discussed in detail later). More recent studies, using sensitive methods such as RT-PCR, or flow cytometry have generated abundant evidence that in addition to Th1 cytokines, there is an IL-4 response in human TB, whether the patients are in Europe [52], Indonesia [53], Africa [54-56], South America [57-59], India [60, 61] or China [62]. Similarly, TB patients have a number of IL-4-dependent phenomena, including IgE antibody to *M. tuberculosis*, increased expression of DC-SIGN [63, 64], and antibody to cardiolipin [65]. It has been noted that both IL-4 mRNA, and T cells containing IL-4 correlate significantly with serum IgE, serum soluble CD30 and extent of cavitation [52-54, 66]. Interestingly, CD8+ T cells also make IL-4 in TB [53, 56], and CD8+ cells secreting IL-4 correlated with cavitation in van Crevel's work [53]. Expression of IL-4 can be detected in some pulmonary lesions by *in situ* hybridisation [67].

How Does *M. Tuberculosis* Drive Expression of IL-4 ?

Human monocytes infected with BCG and then matured with GMCSF and IL-4 develop into DC that drive IL-4 responses [68]. Similarly, mannosylated liporabinomannan from *M. tuberculosis* crosslinks mannose receptors and causes DC to release IL-10, IL-1R antagonist, IL-1R type II, while inhibiting IL-12. This pattern of DC maturation tends to favor development of Th2 responses [69]. The effects on human monocytes are even more striking when Beijing strains are used [70]. Exposure of monocytes to a Beijing strain previously shown to be hypervirulent in mice led to increased expression of IL-4 and IL-13. Thus some of the ability of *M. tuberculosis* to induce IL-4 in addition to the dominant Th1 response is likely to be attributable to adjuvant effects of bacterial components such as the lipids identified in the Beijing strains [70], acting via antigen-presenting cells. However there is also evidence that certain antigenic components such as the 16kDa heat shock protein (α-crystallin) contain specific sets of epitopes that are preferentially recognised by Th2 cells from tuberculosis patients [71]. This is reflected in the clear identification of IL-4-secreting T cells in cell lines driven with *M. tuberculosis* antigen *in vitro* [49, 54]

IL-4, Disrupted Protection, and Immunopathology

Why might IL-4 be critically important in human tuberculosis? IL-4 deactivates macrophages, switches off signalling via TLR-2 [72] and potently downregulates iNOS [37], which may play a crucial role in driving *M. tuberculosis* into latency [73]. A recent study has revealed that apparently healthy health-care workers whose CD8+ T cells made IL-4 in response to *M. tuberculosis,* went on to develop active disease within 2-4 years [74]. So IL-4 might undermine resistance in the early stages of disease. However it might also contribute to immunopathology, as in the BALB/c mouse. The presence of IL-4 in peripheral blood cells, whether assayed by quantitative RT-PCR, or detected by flow cytometry after stimulation with PMA and calcium ionophore, correlates with cavitary disease [52, 75]. Moreover, using bronchoalveolar lavage samples to look at the cytokine profile of lymphocytes infiltrating the lungs, the % of IL-4-secreting cells averaged 14% in samples from cavitary disease, but only 2-3 % in samples for non-cavitary disease [76]. This leads to the possibility that as in the mouse, the presence of IL-4 contributes to immunopathology within the dominantly Th1-mediated lesions. The IL-4 hypothesis therefore explains the well-known switch in the role of TNF-α from protective to toxic as the disease progresses [77], and the presence of fibrosis in dominantly Th1 lesions [39, 46].

IL-4 and the Recently Discovered Splice Variant, IL-4δ2

Our tenuous understanding of the role of IL-4 in human tuberculosis was recently undermined by the realisation that previous studies of this cytokine were simultaneously measuring the agonist, IL-4, and a recently discovered antagonist, IL-4δ2. The resulting data clearly cannot be interpreted [78]. IL-4δ2 resembles IL-4 but lacks the 16 amino acids encoded by exon 2. ELISA assays, flow cytometry, or immunohistochemistry that involve the use of antibodies might measure both or either cytokine. This is not yet known. Similarly RT-PCR using primers based on sequences within exon 1 and exon 3 or 4 measure both mRNAs simultaneously. IL-4δ2 seems to be present in most (perhaps all) species [79], including the mouse [80], and two groups have shown that the cloned molecule is a competitive antagonist of IL-4 [78, 81].

Since specific monoclonal antibodies have not yet been identified, the two forms can only be distinguished by RT-PCR, using appropriately re-designed primers. Using this method we previously established that in asthma there is a selective increase in expression of IL-4, indicating a "classical" Th2 response [82]. By contrast, in systemic sclerosis there is a selective increase in expression of IL-4δ2 [83]. In tuberculosis the situation is more complex, with increased expression of either or both forms [52].

Expression of IL-4δ2 mRNA is increased in unstimulated peripheral blood mononuclear cells from healthy donors who have latent TB, as defined by the presence of an IFN-γ response to ESAT-6. This has been shown by different methods in latently infected donors from Ethiopia and The Gambia [84, 85]. This might indicate that despite their healthy appearance, people with latent TB are involved in a "battle" between IL-4 and its inhibitor. We have hypothesised that this IL-4/IL-4δ2 ratio might be a factor that determines whether latent TB progresses or remains latent [6]. Similarly, during treatment mRNA encoding IL-4 very slowly decreases, whereas the IL-4δ2 mRNA is significantly *increased* by 6 months (Dheda, K. et al, unpublished results).

In conclusion, the potential detrimental effects of IL-4 listed above might be blocked if there is sufficient expression of IL-4δ2. Further studies will reveal whether a high IL-4δ2 contributes to protection from progressive disease following exposure to *M. tuberculosis.* Similarly it is theroretically possible that in patients with progressive disease, high IL-4δ2 helps to limit immunopathology.

Discordant Result of Attempts to Measure IL-4 in Tuberculosis Cases from Developed and Developing Countries

The levels of IL-4 detected in tuberculosis patients, or released by their lymphocytes when stimulated with mycobacterial antigen *in vitro,* differ markedly in different studies. At one extreme, free IL-4 may be detected easily by ELISA in the patients' serum or in supernatants of patients' peripheral blood mononuclear cells cultured with *M. tuberculosis* antigen *in vitro.* At the other extreme IL-4 is only detected using sensitive quantitative RT-PCR, or by flow cytometry after stimulating the cells in the presence of PMA, calcium ionophore and an inhibitor of cytokine export. Interestingly the studies that require the very sensitive methods are those based in Europe or the United States. In contrast, the studies where IL-4 was readily detected by ELISA in serum or in cell culture supernatants, tend to have taken place in developing countries, usually within 30° of the equator. This point has been reviewed and referenced in detail elsewhere reviewed in [86]. Clearly some of the patients studied in Europe or the USA will themselves have come initially from developing countries, but the distinction remains in the examples we have found, despite this potential dilution of the difference between the two environments.

Failure of BCG Vaccination in Developing Countries

It has been known for decades that the efficacy of BCG vaccination varies in different parts of the world. In general it is least effective in developing countries where it is most needed [18]. There has been no universally accepted explanation for this phenomenon. As outlined in the previous paragraph, in developing countries tuberculosis tends to be accompanied by particularly strong IL-4 production. But it might be more significant that in these environments even healthy individuals have a background of Th2 response to some components of *M. tuberculosis.* This was clearly demonstrated in blood samples from Malawians in which PPD induced IL-5 secretion, whereas little IL-5 was seen in samples from the UK run in parallel (Dockrell HM, Black GF, Weir RE, personal communication). BCG vaccination failed to down-regulate this IL-5 response (Dockrell HM, Black GF, Weir RE, personal communication). This Th2 activity might be attributable to the exposure of mother and child to helminths. BCG induced a Th2-biased response in babies that had been sensitised *in utero* to antigens of *Wuchereria bancrofti* or *Schistosoma haematobium* because their mothers were suffering from these infections [87]. Presumably contact with cross-reactive environmental mycobacteria would do the same thing in these babies. However these organisms also induce a Th1 response in Malawi that is demonstrably protective [88], and the possible interplay between the Th1 and Th2 components is crucial, and is discussed later.

High Fatality Rates Early During Treatment in Developing Countries

Death rates from tuberculosis during the first 2 months of treatment are said to be unusually high in many developing countries. If this is true (but see below), it is intriguing to speculate that in patients with a significant background of Th2 response to *M. tuberculosis,* release of antigen during therapy leads to a systemic Koch phenomenon mediated by IL-4 and TNF-α as outlined earlier. For instance a high mortality is claimed in Malawi [89], where a background of Th2 response to *M. tuberculosis* has been documented. However there is also a high rate of HIV in this country. Other confounding factors that affect death rates include distance from health-carecenters, and the severity of the disease at the time of diagnosis. Nevertheless death rates from tuberculosis are probably high in some developing countries even when these factors are taken into account [90, 91]. In an area of rural South Africa, with a TB control program and low sero-prevalence rates for HIV, the mortality in those diagnosed with tuberculosis was 13%[90]. Further studies will be needed to test the hypothesis that there are more deaths in developing countries, due to a systemic Koch phenomenon aggravated by IL-4.

Doses of *M. Tuberculosis* Required to Cause Infection in Developed and Developing Countries

Another aspect of tuberculosis that probably differs between developed and developing countries is the number of organisms required to establish infection. As discussed in the following sections, this too is likely to be attributable to the pre-existing state of immunity (naïve, or Th1+IL-4δ2, or Th1+ IL-4) before *M. tuberculosis* is encountered. The dose required to infect humans is often said to be 1-10 bacilli. The statement has its origin in experiments published in 1961 [11, 92]. Guinea pigs were housed in a penthouse above a tuberculosis ward consisting of 6 single rooms. The air from the ward was ducted through the guinea pig chamber on its way to the exterior. The animals were tuberculin-tested every month, and removed if positive. It was calculated that an animal had to breathe 12,000 cubic feet of air to become infected. Post-mortem examination revealed solitary lesions, suggesting infection with a single bacillus. We can assume this was progressive disease, because a single lesion will eventually kill a guinea pig. A similar calculation was then performed using historical data on the time it takes nurses to become tuberculin positive when working in tuberculosis wards (6-18 months). The result suggested that on average a nurse had to breathe 24,000 cu ft of air in a TB ward to become tuberculin positive, which seemed close to the volume that could infect guinea pigs with one bacillus [92]. This was interpreted as suggesting that humans (at least in Baltimore, USA), like guinea pigs, can be infected with 1 or 2 bacilli.

For a number of reasons this experiment is difficult to interpret. First, only small droplets would have passed via the ventilation ducts to the guinea pigs in the penthouse. By contrast, nurses working closely with patients are exposed in addition to larger droplets expelled by coughing, and larger infected dust particles, with limited life spans in the air. The number of CFU coughed out by different patients is very variable, but the authors suggested that some patients generate between 18 and 3,798 infectious units/hour [93]. Most particles coughed out that contain CFU are in the respirable size range [93]. So patients can be very infectious. These points suggest that nurses might have breathed in rather large numbers of bacilli before becoming tuberculin positive. But what do we mean by conversion to tuberculin positivity? This might indicate progressive disease (which is what was documented in the guinea pigs), but more often it would indicate latency, so a more important criticism is the drawing of a parallel between fatal disease in the guinea pigs, and tuberculin test positivity in the nurses.

Conclusions from More Recent Data

Recent data have cast light on these dilemmas, and suggest that the nurses were probably exposed to more bacilli than estimated by Riley [92]. Very brief exposure to a CFU-expelling case of tuberculosis can be sufficient to cause latent infection in some individuals, detected as release of IFN-□ in response to ESAT-6/CFP-10. Thus fifteen of 47 adults exposed over 4 days to a case of open tuberculosis in an Italian maternity unit were ELISPOT positive 11 weeks later, whereas only 4 were skin-test positive [9]. ELISPOT positivity correlated with hours of exposure to the patient, but exposures were inevitably short. Such brief exposures can also lead to progressive disease in certain very susceptible people. For instance progressive tuberculosis occurred following only three 15 minute exposures to an index case [94]. Work colleagues of the same patients showed 50% conversion to skin test positivity, but no disease [94]. We can conclude that some humans in Europe and the USA can indeed be “infected” by very low doses of M. tuberculosis, leading most often to ELISPOT positivity, more rarely to tuberculin skin-test positivity, and rarely to progressive disease.

However this may again be different in developing countries. Enormously heavy contact with TB cannot only fail to induce disease, but even fail to lead to tuberculin test positivity in developing countries [95, 96]. It is of course possible that in developing countries too there are a few individuals who can develop progressive disease following inhalation of single organism. If they exist, such individuals will quickly develop tuberculosis. However most cases in a high incidence country inevitably come from a population of relatively resistant individuals, already partially immunized by environmental organisms. Experimental evidence confirms that this variable resistance is likely to be at least partly due to the pre-existing state of immunity.

The Infectious Dose in Immunologically Naïve and Pre-Immunised Individuals

In most infectious disease models, the greater the degree of immunity, the greater the infectious challenge required to overcome it. Therefore the background Thl responses that exist in developing countries would be expected to increase the critical infectious dose. However Balasubramanian and colleagues postulated an interesting additional mechanism that will lead to the need for higher infecting doses in these countries. In areas of the world where there is a low incidence of vaccination or sensitization to environmental mycobacteria, *M. tuberculosis* reaches the vulnerable region (lung apices) via a bacillemia during the *first* infection. However prior exposure to environmental mycobacteria, TB strains of very low virulence, *M. avium* or BCG will block the phase of haematogenous spread. When there is a pre-existing immune response there is no hematogenous phase, and the tubercle bacilli must reach the vulnerable region (apex) via the airway, which requires repeated episodes of infection as the probability of a first implant occurring in the apical zones is low [11, 97]. In the Chingleput South India Trial 95% of those over 10 yrs old were skin-test positive to *M. avium*, so this is clearly a very common situation.

We suggest that mycobacterially naïve citizens of the USA resemble the immunologically naïve mice in a modern animal facility, and some will develop progressive infection following exposure to very low doses of *M. tuberculosis,* with little induction of IL-4. In contrast, most patients in developing countries rich in mycobacteria and helminths must have had pre-existing Th1 and Th2 responses induced by these organisms at the time that progressive tuberculosis developed. Under these conditions a high dose of *M. tuberculosis* is required for infection, which only progresses in those people in whom the TB is able to exploit the pre-existing Th2 component, and so induce an IL-4 response that is large enough to undermine the pre-existing Th1. Beijing strains should be particularly good at this [70]. In some individuals, for reasons that we do not yet understand, the effect of the IL-4 may be blocked by a disproportionate rise in IL-4δ2 [84, 85].

Conclusions and Implications

The overall conclusion is that despite rapid induction of a dominant Th1 response, *M. tuberculosis* may evoke a minor IL-4 response that is sufficient in some individuals to undermine the efficacy of Th1-mediated immunity and cause immunopathology (Fig) [6] This dual role of IL-4 (disarming of the Th1 response and induction of immunopathology) can explain many paradoxes (Table). Immunopathology is the crucial mechanism that allows tuberculosis to spread, because cavities open into bronchi, releasing organisms that are disseminated by coughing.

Table 1. Paradoxes in the Immunology of Tuberculosis that Can be Explained by the Ability of IL-4 to Undermine the Th1 Response and Enhance Immunopathology

Features of all tuberculosis patients

- Disease despite rapid development of Th1 response to *M. tuberculosis*
- Need for prolonged drug therapy because the response cannot eliminate the last few organisms
- Toxicity of TNF-α in progressive disease, despite its role in immunity
- The Koch Phenomenon
- Pulmonary fibrosis, despite the fact that IFN-γ inhibits fibrosis
- Correlation between IL-4 levels and cavitation and immunopathology

Additional features of tuberculosis within 30° of the equator

- Susceptibility to TB despite large cross-reactive IFN-γ responses evoked by environmental organisms
- Failure of BCG vaccine
- High levels of IL-4 in TB patients, measurable by ELISA
- High death rates early during treatment
- High exposure required to cause disease
- High expression of an antagonist of IL-4 (IL-4δ2) in healthy donors with latent TB that does not progress.

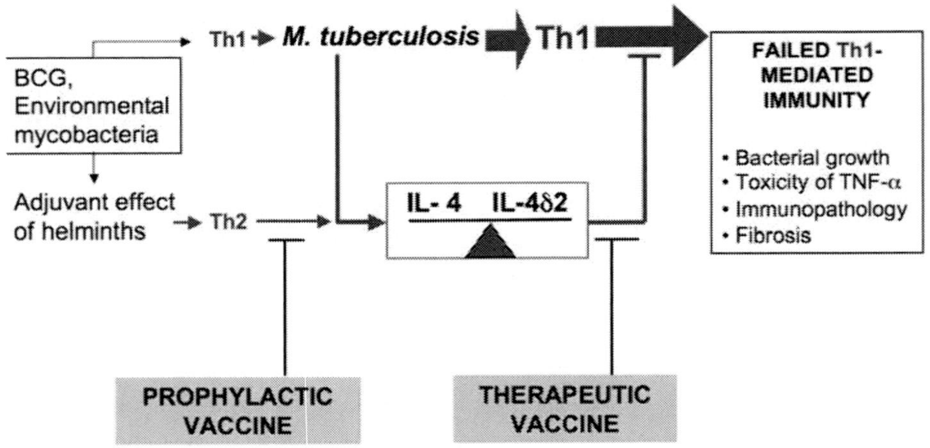

Figure 1. Probable Sequence of Immunological Events in the Development of Tuberculosis in Developing Countries. Early development of a mixed Th1 and Th2 response to a variety of antigens that cross-react with *M. tuberculosis* provides some protection [88]. However following exposure to large numbers of *M. tuberculosis*, the IL-4 component can increase [52-62] until it is easily measured in plasma or lymphocyte culture supernatants (reviewed in 86). The IL-4 may undermine the protective effect of the Th1 response, leading to disarming of macrophages [38], proliferation of *M. tuberculosis,* the Koch phenomenon, toxicity of TNF-α, and pulmonary fibrosis [37-39,77] (and reviewed in 6). Several mechanisms allow *M. tuberculosis* to drive IL-4 production [68-71], and this is a particular feature of virulent Beijing strains [70]. In some individuals levels of the antagonist IL-4δ2 increase, and the latent state can persist without progression [84,85].

The second conclusion is that environmental mycobacteria and helminths induce a mixed Th1+IL-4 response in the normal population in developing countries. This point explains a further set of paradoxes (Table), particularly the failure of BCG vaccination in these areas. Although the cross-reactive Th1 component can be protective, we suggest that at higher challenge doses *M. tuberculosis* exploits and enhances the pre-existing Th2 component, and progressive disease results, with the characteristically high IL-4 levels that are seen in patients close the equator [86].

These points do *not* suggest a classical Th1/Th2 "see-saw", such as that associated with *Leishmania* infection in BALB/c mice. In tuberculosis the IL-4 component is *superimposed* upon the larger Th1 response, and does not replace it. This mixed Th1+Th2 type of inflammatory response is associated with immunopathology in several infections [40-43].

Implications for Vaccine Design

Prophylactic Vaccines

It is estimated that there are now more than 260 vaccine candidates. These include attenuated *M. tuberculosis*, recombinant BCG or vaccinia over-expressing antigens from *M. tuberculosis*, DNA vaccines, and purified recombinant proteins with adjuvants. Some are, or are about to be, in Phase 1 clinical trials. Testing vaccines against TB is complex for a number of reasons. First, BCG does have some ability to protect against childhood forms of TB when given neonatally. Therefore BCG is widely used, and new vaccines may need to be given as booster vaccinations in people who previously received BCG. The evidence is that previous BCG vaccination will make live mycobacterial vaccines ineffective (whether recombinant BCG or attenuated MTB). Secondly, in countries where the vaccines are needed many adults will already have been exposed to *M. tuberculosis*. Thus a vaccine for use in adults will need to be able to function as a "post-exposure" vaccine. This might be difficult, because if the exposure to TB has already primed an immunopathological pattern of response, a post-exposure vaccine that merely enhances the Th1 response may not be protective, and could trigger disease.

The vaccines in Phase 1 clinical trials have all shown safety and efficacy in mouse, guinea pig and primate. The Phase I studies will test immunogenicity and safety.

(1) rBCG30: a recombinant BCG over-expressing the Ag85b, which is a secreted mycolyl transferase from MTB [98].
(2) Mtb72f: a fusion protein of two antigens from MTB, formulated in an adjuvant AS02A [99].
(3) MVA: a modified vaccinia virus Ankara, expressing MTB Ag 85A [100]

The Aeras foundation, with funding from Bill and Melinda Gates, is planning to test Mtb72f as a booster vaccine and rBCG30 as a potential substitute for BCG. Then the complete vaccine regimen might be rBCG30 given neonatally, followed by a boost with Mtb72f (or indeed, MVA).

Other vaccines that are expected to go into trials in the near future include a fusion protein of ESAT-6 and Ag85b [101], and a recombinant BCG expressing listeriolysin, which enables the organism to leave the phagosome, and so prime CD8+ cytotoxic T cells [102].

It will be a huge step forward if the problems of trial design can be overcome, and protection greater than that attributable BCG vaccination can be demonstrated following administration of these Th1-inducing vaccines, but this cannot be guaranteed. Alternative strategies ought to be considered. It might be important to devise vaccines that switch off the "subversive" Th2 component probably always present in developing countries as a consequence of interactions with helminths and environmental organisms. This might be feasible. Ways of switching off pre-existing Th2 responses by inducing appropriate types of regulatory T cell have been discovered in studies of allergic disorders, where much larger Th2 responses have been targeted [103]. *M. vaccae* is an environmental saprophyte which drives regulatory T cells that downregulate Th2 responses [103]. It is being given as 5 intradermal doses of 1 mg of heat-killed organisms [104], in what is effectively a Phase III trial for the prevention of TB in HIV+ individuals in Tanzania (http://www.dartmouth. edu/dms/dardar/).

Therapeutic Vaccines

This regulatory approach to vaccine design will be particularly relevant to therapeutic vaccination. Th1-inducing vaccines make ongoing disease worse [105, 106]. In other words they evoke local and distant Koch phenomena. (The findings of Robert Koch in the 1890's are rediscovered at regular intervals). Interestingly the only vaccine candidates shown to be effective therapeutically in the BALB/c mouse TB model both work at least in part by suppressing the IL-4 response [107, 108], which BCG, studied in parallel, failed to do [108]. The DNA vaccine based on the hsp65 gene from *M. leprae* is ready for trial in man [108], but progress has been hampered by a single observation, using a quite different construct, that led to immunopathology in a guinea pig model and fuelled fears of safety issues [109]. The other vaccine that is active therapeutically in mice is heat-killed *M. vaccae* [107], which activates regulatory T cells that suppress Th2 [103]. As a therapeutic in human disease *M. vaccae* was initially given as a single dose at the start of standard short-course chemotherapy in patients with fully drug-sensitive disease. Under GCP clinical trial conditions such patients rapidly recover, and the best that such studies could hope to show was increased sputum conversion early during treatment, compared to placebo controls (i.e. recipients of standard chemotherapy without immunotherapy). Results were inconclusive; at day 36 in the Ugandan study, p=0.01; [110] at 2 months in the Zambia/Malawi study, p=0.06 [111]. The same organism is claimed by Chinese workers to be active as a therapeutic vaccine in TB and MDR-TB, when given by multiple intramuscular injections [112, 113]. These studies not only used multiple injections, but also used patients who were difficult to treat, treatment failures, or infected with MDR strains [112, 113]. They also used a suboptimal chemotherapy regimen so that the results in the placebo (chemotherapy only) arm were poor. Under these conditions, which are prevalent in many countries, the beneficial effects of multiple *M. vaccae* injections were clear [112, 113], and further trials are warranted. Meanwhile *M. vaccae* has received regulatory approval in China and is marketed *(http://www.longcome.cn /longcome/english/contact.htm).*

Improved reagents for achieving these immunological changes are needed. One obvious approach would be the identification of the subsets of antigens that are targeted by the Th2 component of the response of tuberculosis patients, such as parts of the 16kDA hsp [71]. In the past such antigens have been discarded, because they failed to induce potent IFN-γ production. But were these antigens being ignored by the immune system, or were they driving IL-4? If there is a consistently IL-4-driving subset of antigens, they can be isolated and vaccines that downregulate the response to them can be devised.

In conclusion the time may have come for a radical reappraisal of the thinking behind the current wave of "rationally" designed vaccine candidates. There is more to designing vaccines for tuberculosis than merely causing as much release of IFN-γ as possible.

Acknowledgment

KD is grateful for support from the British Lung Foundation.

References

[1] Jouanguy E, Lamhamedi-Cherradi S, Altare F, et al. Partial interferon-gamma receptor 1 deficiency in a child with tuberculoid bacillus Calmette-Guerin infection and a sibling with clinical tuberculosis. *J. Clin. Invest.* 1997;100:2658-2664.

[2] de Jong R, Altare F, Haagen IA, et al. Severe mycobacterial and Salmonella infections in interleukin-12 receptor-deficient patients. *Science*. 1998;280:1435-1438.

[3] Keane J, Gershon S, Wise RP, et al. Tuberculosis associated with infliximab, a tumor necrosis factor alpha-neutralizing agent. *N. Engl. J. Med.* 2001;345:1098-1104.

[4] Dascher CC, Hiromatsu K, Xiong X, et al. Immunization with a mycobacterial lipid vaccine improves pulmonary pathology in the guinea pig model of tuberculosis. *Int Immunol.* 2003;15:915-925.

[5] North RJ, Jung YJ. Immunity to tuberculosis. *Annu Rev Immunol.* 2004;22:599-623.

[6] Rook GA, Hernandez-Pando R, Dheda K, Seah GT. IL-4 in tuberculosis: implications for vaccine design. *Trends Immunol.* 2004;25:483-488.

[7] Murray JF. Bill Dock and the location of pulmonary tuberculosis: how bed rest might have helped consumption. *Am J Respir Crit Care Med.* 2003;168:1029-1033.

[8] Pathan AA, Wilkinson KA, Wilkinson RJ, et al. High frequencies of circulating IFN-gamma-secreting CD8 cytotoxic T cells specific for a novel MHC class I-restricted Mycobacterium tuberculosis epitope in M. tuberculosis-infected subjects without disease. *Eur J Immunol.* 2000;30:2713-2721.

[9] Richeldi L, Ewer K, Losi M, et al. T cell-based tracking of multidrug resistant tuberculosis infection after brief exposure. *Am J Respir Crit Care Med.* 2004;170:288-295.

[10] Opie EL, Aronson JD. Tubercle bacilli in latent tuberculous lesions and in lung tissue without tuberculous lesions. *Arch. Pathol. Lab. Med.* 1927;4:1-21.

[11] Balasubramanian V, Wiegeshaus EH, Taylor BT, Smith DW. Pathogenesis of tuberculosis: pathway to apical localization. *Tuber. Lung. Dis.* 1994;75:168-178.

[12] Arriaga AK, Orozco EH, Aguilar LD, Rook GAW, Hernandez Pando R. Immunological and pathological comparative analysis between experimental latent tuberculous infection and progressive pulmonary tuberculosis. *Clin. Exp. Immunol.* 2002;128:229-237.

[13] Hernandez-Pando R, Jeyanathan M, Mengistu G, et al. Persistence of DNA from *M. tuberculosis* in superficially normal lung tissue during latent infection. *Lancet.* 2000;356:2133-2138.

[14] Ribeiro-Rodrigues R, Resende Co T, Johnson JL, et al. Sputum cytokine levels in patients with pulmonary tuberculosis as early markers of mycobacterial clearance. *Clin Diagn Lab Immunol.* 2002;9:818-823.

[15] Koch R. *Fortsetzung über ein Heilmittel gegen Tuberculose.* Deutsch. Med. Wochenschr. 1891;17:101-102.

[16] Anderson MC. On Koch's treatment. *Lancet.* 1891;i:651-652.

[17] Wilson GS, Schwabacher H, Maier I. The effect of the desensitisation of tuberculous guinea-pigs. *J. Path. Bact.* 1940;50:89-109.

[18] Wilson ME, Fineberg HV, Colditz GA. Geographic latitude and the efficacy of bacillus Calmette-Guerin vaccine. *Clin Infect Dis.* 1995;20:982-991.

[19] Skinner MA, Ramsay AJ, Buchan GS, et al. A DNA prime-live vaccine boost strategy in mice can augment IFN-gamma responses to mycobacterial antigens but does not increase the protective efficacy of two attenuated strains of Mycobacterium bovis against bovine tuberculosis. *Immunology.* 2003;108:548-555.

[20] Biet F, Kremer L, Wolowczuk I, Delacre M, Locht C. Mycobacterium bovis BCG producing interleukin-18 increases antigen-specific gamma interferon production in mice. *Infect Immun.* 2002;70:6549-6557.

[21] Leal IS, Smedegard B, Andersen P, Appelberg R. Failure to induce enhanced protection against tuberculosis by increasing T-cell-dependent interferon-gamma generation. *Immunology.* 2001;104:157-161.

[22] Kaushal D, Schroeder BG, Tyagi S, et al. Reduced immunopathology and mortality despite tissue persistence in a Mycobacterium tuberculosis mutant lacking alternative sigma factor, SigH. *Proc Natl Acad Sci U S A.* 2002;99:8330-8335.

[23] Steyn AJ, Collins DM, Hondalus MK, Jacobs WR, Jr., Kawakami RP, Bloom BR. Mycobacterium tuberculosis WhiB3 interacts with RpoV to affect host survival but is dispensable for in vivo growth. *Proc Natl Acad Sci U S A.* 2002;99:3147-3152.

[24] Mills KH. Regulatory T cells: friend or foe in immunity to infection? *Nat Rev Immunol.* 2004;4:841-855.

[25] O'Garra A, Vieira PL, Vieira P, Goldfeld AE. IL-10-producing and naturally occurring CD4+ Tregs: limiting collateral damage. *J Clin Invest.* 2004;114:1372-1378.

[26] Hisaeda H, Maekawa Y, Iwakawa D, et al. Escape of malaria parasites from host immunity requires CD4+ CD25+ regulatory T cells. *Nat Med.* 2004;10:29-30.

[27] Omer FM, de Souza JB, Riley EM. Differential induction of TGF-beta regulates proinflammatory cytokine production and determines the outcome of lethal and nonlethal Plasmodium yoelii infections. *J Immunol.* 2003;171:5430-5436.

[28] Jacobs T, Graefe SE, Niknafs S, Gaworski I, Fleischer B. Murine malaria is exacerbated by CTLA-4 blockade. *J Immunol.* 2002;169:2323-2329.

[29] Delgado JC, Tsai EY, Thim S, et al. Antigen-specific and persistent tuberculin anergy in a cohort of pulmonary tuberculosis patients from rural Cambodia. *Proc Natl Acad Sci U S A*. 2002;99:7576-7581.

[30] Boussiotis VA, Tsai EY, Yunis EJ, et al. IL-10-producing T cells suppress immune responses in anergic tuberculosis patients. *J Clin Invest*. 2000;105:1317-1325.

[31] Gerosa F, Nisii C, Righetti S, et al. CD4(+) T cell clones producing both interferon-gamma and interleukin-10 predominate in bronchoalveolar lavages of active pulmonary tuberculosis patients. *Clin. Immunol.* 1999;92:224-234.

[32] Stock P, Akbari O, Berry G, Freeman GJ, Dekruyff RH, Umetsu DT. Induction of T helper type 1-like regulatory cells that express Foxp3 and protect against airway hyper-reactivity. *Nat Immunol.* 2004;5:1149-1156.

[33] Guerkov RE, Targoni OS, Kreher CR, et al. Detection of low-frequency antigen-specific IL-10-producing CD4(+) T cells via ELISPOT in PBMC: cognate vs. nonspecific production of the cytokine. *J Immunol Methods*. 2003;279:111-121.

[34] Gong JH, Zhang M, Modlin RL, et al. Interleukin-10 downregulates Mycobacterium tuberculosis-induced Th1 responses and CTLA-4 expression. *Infect Immun.* 1996;64:913-918.

[35] Ranjbar S, Ly N, Thim S, Reynes JM, Goldfeld AE. Mycobacterium tuberculosis recall antigens suppress HIV-1 replication in anergic donor cells via CD8+ T cell expansion and increased IL-10 levels. *J Immunol*. 2004;172:1953-1959.

[36] Scott HM, Flynn JL. Mycobacterium tuberculosis in chemokine receptor 2-deficient mice: influence of dose on disease progression. *Infect Immun.* 2002;70:5946-5954.

[37] Bogdan C, Vodovotz Y, Paik J, Xie QW, Nathan C. Mechanism of suppression of nitric oxide synthase expression by interleukin-4 in primary mouse macrophages. *J. Leukoc. Biol.* 1994;55:227-233.

[38] Gordon S. Alternative activation of macrophages. *Nat Rev Immunol*. 2003;3:23-35.

[39] Hernandez-Pando R, Aguilar D, Garcia Hernandez ML, Orozco H, Rook GAW. Pulmonary tuberculosis in Balb/c mice with non-functional IL-4 genes; changes in the inflammatory effects of TNF-α and in the regulation of fibrosis. *Eur. J. Immunol.* 2004;34:174-183.

[40] Hernandez-Pando R, Pavon L, Arriaga K, Orozco H, Madrid-Marina V, Rook GAW. Pathogenesis of tuberculosis in mice exposed to low and high doses of an environmental mycobacterial saprophyte. *Infect. Immun.* 1997;65:3317-3327.

[41] Pina A, Valente-Ferreira RC, Molinari-Madlum EE, Vaz CA, Keller AC, Calich VL. Absence of interleukin-4 determines less severe pulmonary paracoccidioidomycosis associated with impaired Th2 response. *Infect Immun.* 2004;72:2369-2378.

[42] Lawrence CE, Paterson JC, Higgins LM, MacDonald TT, Kennedy MW, Garside P. IL-4-regulated enteropathy in an intestinal nematode infection. *Eur. J. Immunol.* 1998;28:2672-2684.

[43] Wynn TA, Cheever AW, Jankovic D, et al. An IL-12-based vaccination method for preventing fibrosis induced by schistosome infection. *Nature.* 1995;376:594-596.

[44] Lindblad EB, Elhay MJ, Silva R, Appelberg R, Andersen P. Adjuvant modulation of immune responses to tuberculosis subunit vaccines. *Infect. Immun*. 1997;65:623-629.

[45] Wangoo A, Sparer T, Brown IN, et al. Contribution of Th1 and Th2 Cells to Protection and Pathology in Experimental Models of Granulomatous Lung Disease. *J. Immunol.* 2001;166:3432-3439.

[46] Lee CG, Homer RJ, Zhu Z, et al. Interleukin-13 induces tissue fibrosis by selectively stimulating and activating transforming growth factor beta(1). *J. Exp. Med.* 2001;194:809-821.

[47] Jung YJ, LaCourse R, Ryan L, North RJ. Evidence inconsistent with a negative influence of T helper 2 cells on protection afforded by a dominant T helper 1 response against Mycobacterium tuberculosis lung infection in mice. *Infect Immun.* 2002;70:6436-6443.

[48] Schauf V, Rom WN, Smith KA, et al. Cytokine gene activation and modified responsiveness to interleukin-2 in the blood of tuberculosis patients. *J. Infect. Dis.* 1993;168:1056-1059.

[49] Surcel HM, Troye-Blomberg M, Paulie S, et al. Th1/Th2 profiles in tuberculosis based on proliferation and cytokine response of peripheral blood lymphocytes to mycobacterial antigens. *Immunology.* 1994;81:171-176.

[50] Sanchez FO, Rodriguez JI, Agudelo G, Garcia LF. Immune responsiveness and lymphokine production in patients with tuberculosis and healthy controls. *Infect. Immun.* 1994;62:5673-5678.

[51] Lin Y, Zhang M, Hofman FM, Gong J, Barnes PF. Absence of a prominent Th2 cytokine response in human tuberculosis. *Infect. Immun.* 1996;64:1351-1356.

[52] Seah GT, Scott GM, Rook GA. Type 2 Cytokine Gene Activation and Its Relationship to Extent of Disease in Patients with Tuberculosis. *J. Infect. Dis.* 2000;181:385-389.

[53] van Crevel R, Karyadi E, Preyers F, et al. Increased Production of Interleukin 4 by CD4+ and CD8+ T Cells from Patients with Tuberculosis Is Related to the Presence of Pulmonary Cavities. *J Infect Dis.* 2000;181:1194-1197.

[54] Marchant A, Amedei A, Azzurri A, et al. Polarization of PPD-Specific T-Cell Response of Patients with Tuberculosis from Th0 to Th1 Profile after Successful Antimycobacterial Therapy or In Vitro Conditioning with Interferon-alpha or Interleukin-12. *Am. J. Respir. Cell. Mol. Biol.* 2001;24:187-194.

[55] Lienhardt C, Azzurri A, Amedei A, et al. Active tuberculosis in Africas is associated with reduced Th1 and increased Th2 activity in vivo. *Eur. J. Immunol.* 2002;32:1605-1613.

[56] Smith SM, Klein MR, Malin AS, Sillah J, McAdam KP, Dockrell HM. Decreased IFN-gamma and increased IL-4 production by human CD8(+) T cells in response to Mycobacterium tuberculosis in tuberculosis patients. *Tuberculosis* (Edinb). 2002;82:7-13.

[57] Dlugovitzky D, Torres-Morales A, Rateni L, et al. Circulating profile of Th1 and Th2 cytokines in tuberculosis patients with different degrees of pulmonary involvement. FEMS *Immunol Med Microbiol.* 1997;18:203-207.

[58] Jimenez-Martinez MC, Linares M, Baez R, et al. Intracellular expression of interleukin-4 and interferon-gamma by a Mycobacterium tuberculosis antigen-stimulated CD4+ CD57+ T-cell subpopulation with memory phenotype in tuberculosis patients. *Immunology.* 2004;111:100-106.

[59] Montiel M, Rivera S, Hernandez R, et al. [Immune response and anergy. Study in tuberculosis patients from the Universitary Hospital, Maracaibo, Venezuela]. *Acta Cient Venez.* 2002;53:36-43.

[60] Bhattacharyya S, Singla R, Dey AB, Prasad HK. Dichotomy of cytokine profiles in patients and high-risk healthy subjects exposed to tuberculosis. *Infect Immun.* 1999;67:5597-5603.

[61] Sharma SK, Mitra DK, Balamurugan A, Pandey RM, Mehra NK. Cytokine polarization in miliary and pleural tuberculosis. *J Clin Immunol.* 2002;22:345-352.

[62] Wang L, Cai Y, Cheng Q, Hu Y, Xiao H. [Imbalance of Th1/Th2 cytokines in patients with pulmonary tuberculosis]. *Zhonghua Jie He He Hu Xi Za Zhi.* 2002;25:535-537.

[63] Relloso M, Puig-Kroger A, Pello OM, et al. DC-SIGN (CD209) expression is IL-4 dependent and is negatively regulated by IFN, TGF-beta, and anti-inflammatory agents. *J Immunol.* 2002;168:2634-2643.

[64] Tailleux L, Schwartz O, Herrmann JL, et al. DC-SIGN is the major Mycobacterium tuberculosis receptor on human dendritic cells. *J Exp Med.* 2003;197:121-127.

[65] Fischer K, Collins H, Taniguchi M, Kaufmann SH, Schaible UE. IL-4 and T cells are required for the generation of IgG1 isotype antibodies against cardiolipin. *J Immunol.* 2002;168:2689-2694.

[66] Suzuki N, Kudo K, Sano Y, Ito K. Can Mycobacterium tuberculosis infection prevent asthma and other allergic disorders? *Int. Arch. Allergy Immunol.* 2001;124:113-116.

[67] Fenhalls G, Wong A, Bezuidenhout J, van Helden P, Bardin P, Lukey PT. In situ production of gamma interferon, interleukin-4, and tumor necrosis factor alpha mRNA in human lung tuberculous granulomas. *Infect. Immun.* 2000;68:2827-2836.

[68] Martino A, Sacchi A, Sanarico N, et al. Dendritic cells derived from BCG-infected precursors induce Th2-like immune response. *J Leukoc Biol.* 2004.

[69] Chieppa M, Bianchi G, Doni A, et al. Cross-linking of the mannose receptor on monocyte-derived dendritic cells activates an anti-inflammatory immunosuppressive program. *J Immunol.* 2003;171:4552-4560.

[70] Manca C, Reed MB, Freeman S, et al. Differential Monocyte Activation Underlies Strain-Specific Mycobacterium tuberculosis Pathogenesis. *Infect Immun.* 2004;72:5511-5514.

[71] 7Agrewala JN, Wilkinson RJ. Differential regulation of Th1 and Th2 cells by p91-110 and p21-40 peptides of the 16-kD alpha-crystallin antigen of Mycobacterium tuberculosis. *Clin Exp Immunol.* 1998;114:392-397.

[72] Krutzik SR, Ochoa MT, Sieling PA, *et al. Activation and regulation of Toll-like receptors 2 and 1 in human leprosy.* Nat Med. 2003;9:525-532.

[73] Voskuil MI, Schnappinger D, Visconti KC, et al. Inhibition of respiration by nitric oxide induces a Mycobacterium tuberculosis dormancy program. *J Exp Med.* 2003;198:705-713.

[74] Ordway D, Costa D, Martins M, et al. Increased IL-4 production by CD8 and γδ T cells in health care workers is associated with the subsequent development of active tuberculosis. *J Infect Dis.* 2004;190:756-766.

[75] van Crevel R, Karyadi E, Preyers F, et al. Increased production of interleukin 4 by CD4+ and CD8+ T cells from patients with tuberculosis is related to the presence of pulmonary cavities. *J Infect Dis.* 2000;181:1194-1197.

[76] Mazzarella G, Bianco A, Perna F, et al. T lymphocyte phenotypic profile in lung segments affected by cavitary and non-cavitary tuberculosis. Clin Exp Immunol. 2003;132:283-288.

[77] Tramontana JM, Utaipat U, Molloy A, et al. Thalidomide treatment reduces tumor necrosis factor alpha production and enhances weight gain in patients with pulmonary tuberculosis. *Mol. Med.* 1995;1:384-397.

[78] Atamas SP, Choi J, Yurovsky VV, White B. An alternative splice variant of human IL-4, IL-4 delta 2, inhibits IL- 4-stimulated T cell proliferation. *J. Immunol.* 1996;156:435-441.

[79] Gautherot I, Burdin N, Seguin D, Aujame L, Sodoyer R. Cloning of interleukin-4 delta2 splice variant (IL-4delta2) in chimpanzee and cynomolgus macaque: phylogenetic analysis of delta2 splice variant appearance, and implications for the study of IL-4-driven immune processes. *Immunogenetics.* 2002;54:635-644.

[80] Yatsenko OP, Filipenko ML, Voronina EN, Khrapov EA, Sennikov SV, Kozlov VA. Alternative splicing of murine interleukin-4 mRNA. *Bull Exp Biol Med.* 2004;137:179-181.

[81] Vasiliev AM, Vasilenko RN, Kulikova NL, et al. Structural and functional properties of IL-4delta2, an alternative splice variant of human IL-4. *J Proteome Res.* 2003;2:273-281.

[82] Seah GT, Gao PS, Hopkin J, Rook GAW. Interleukin-4 and its alternatively spliced variant (IL-4d2) in atopic asthmatics. *Am. J. Resp. Crit. Care Med.* 2001;164:1016-1018.

[83] Sakkas LI, Tourtellotte C, Berney S, Myers AR, Platsoucas CD. Increased levels of alternatively spliced interleukin 4 (IL-4delta2) transcripts in peripheral blood mononuclear cells from patients with systemic sclerosis. *Clin Diagn Lab Immunol.* 1999;6:660-664.

[84] Demissie A, Abebe M, Aseffa A, et al. Healthy individuals that control latent infection with *M. tuberculosis* express high levels of Th1 cytokines and the IL-4 antagonist IL-4delta2. *J Immunol.* 2004;172:6938-6943.

[85] Fletcher HA, Owiafe P, Jeffries D, et al. Increased expression of mRNA encoding IL-4 and its splice variant IL-4δ2 in cells from contacts of *Mycobacterium tuberculosis* in the absence of in vitro stimulation. *Immunology.* 2004;112:669-673.

[86] Rook G, Dheda K, Zumla A. Do successful tuberculosis vaccines need to be immunoregulatory rather than merely Th1-boosting? *Vaccine*. 2005;In press.

[87] Malhotra I, Mungai P, Wamachi A, et al. Helminth- and Bacillus Calmette-Guerin-induced immunity in children sensitized in utero to filariasis and schistosomiasis. *J Immunol*. 1999;162:6843-6848.

[88] Fine PE, Floyd S, Stanford JL, et al. Environmental mycobacteria in northern Malawi: implications for the epidemiology of tuberculosis and leprosy. *Epidemiol Infect.* 2001;126:379-387.

[89] Harries AD, Hargreaves NJ, Gausi F, Kwanjana JH, Salaniponi FM. High early death rate in tuberculosis patients in Malawi. *Int J Tuberc Lung Dis.* 2001;5:1000-1005.

[90] Barker RD, Millard FJ. High death rates for tuberculosis patients in rural South Africa. *Int J Tuberc Lung Dis.* 1998;2:1049-1050.

[91] Wilkinson D, Moore DA. HIV-related tuberculosis in South Africa--clinical features and outcome. S Afr Med J. 1996;86:64-67.

[92] Riley RL. Airborne pulmonary tuberculosis. *Bacteriol Rev.* 1961;25:243-248.

[93] Fennelly KP, Martyny JW, Fulton KE, Orme IM, Cave DM, Heifets LB. Cough-generated aerosols of Mycobacterium tuberculosis: a new method to study infectiousness. *Am J Respir Crit Care Med.* 2004;169:604-609.

[94] Golub JE, Cronin WA, Obasanjo OO, et al. Transmission of Mycobacterium tuberculosis through casual contact with an infectious case. *Arch Intern Med.* 2001;161:2254-2258.

[95] Lienhardt C, Fielding K, Sillah J, et al. Risk factors for tuberculosis infection in sub-Saharan Africa: a contact study in The Gambia. *Am J Respir Crit Care Med.* 2003;168:448-455.

[96] Lienhardt C, Sillah J, Fielding K, et al. Risk factors for tuberculosis infection in children in contact with infectious tuberculosis cases in the Gambia, West Africa. *Pediatrics.* 2003;111:e608-614.

[97] Wiegeshaus E, Balasubramanian V, Smith DW. Immunity to tuberculosis from the perspective of pathogenesis. *Infect Immun.* 1989;57:3671-3676.

[98] Horwitz MA, Harth G. A new vaccine against tuberculosis affords greater survival after challenge than the current vaccine in the guinea pig model of pulmonary tuberculosis. *Infect Immun.* 2003;71:1672-1679.

[99] Skeiky YA, Alderson MR, Ovendale PJ, et al. Differential immune responses and protective efficacy induced by components of a tuberculosis polyprotein vaccine, Mtb72F, delivered as naked DNA or recombinant protein. *J Immunol.* 2004;172:7618-7628.

[100] Goonetilleke NP, McShane H, Hannan CM, Anderson RJ, Brookes RH, Hill AV. Enhanced immunogenicity and protective efficacy against Mycobacterium tuberculosis of bacille Calmette-Guerin vaccine using mucosal administration and boosting with a recombinant modified vaccinia virus Ankara. *J Immunol.* 2003;171:1602-1609.

[101] Okkels LM, Doherty TM, Andersen P. Selecting the components for a safe and efficient tuberculosis subunit vaccine--recent progress and post-genomic insights. *Curr Pharm Biotechnol.* 2003;4:69-83.

[102] Hess J, Miko D, Catic A, Lehmensiek V, Russell DG, Kaufmann SH. Mycobacterium bovis Bacille Calmette-Guerin strains secreting listeriolysin of Listeria monocytogenes. *Proc Natl Acad Sci U S A.* 1998;95:5299-5304.

[103] Zuany-Amorim C, Sawicka E, Manlius C, et al. Suppression of airway eosinophilia by killed Mycobacterium vaccae-induced allergen-specific regulatory T-cells. *Nat Med.* 2002;8:625-629.

[104] Waddell RD, Chintu C, Lein AD, et al. Safety and immunogenicity of a five-dose series of inactivated Mycobacterium vaccae vaccination for the prevention of HIV-associated tuberculosis. *Clin. Infect. Dis.* 2000S309-315.

[105] Moreira AL, Tsenova L, Aman MH, et al. Mycobacterial antigens exacerbate disease manifestations in Mycobacterium tuberculosis-infected mice. *Infect Immun.* 2002;70:2100-2107.

[106] Turner J, Rhoades ER, Keen M, Belisle JT, Frank AA, Orme IM. Effective preexposure tuberculosis vaccines fail to protect when they are given in an immunotherapeutic mode. *Infect. Immun.* 2000;68:1706-1709.

[107] Hernandez-Pando R, Pavon L, Orozco EH, Rangel J, Rook GAW. Interactions between hormone-mediated and vaccine-mediated immunotherapy for pulmonary tuberculosis in Balb/c mice. *Immunology.* 2000;100:391-398.

[108] Lowrie DB, Tascon RE, Bonato VL, et al. Therapy of tuberculosis in mice by DNA vaccination. *Nature.* 1999;400:269-271.

[109] Turner OC, Roberts AD, Frank AA, et al. Lack of Protection in Mice and Necrotizing Bronchointerstitial Pneumonia with Bronchiolitis in Guinea Pigs Immunized with Vaccines Directed against the hsp60 Molecule of Mycobacterium tuberculosis. *Infect. Immun.* 2000;68:3674-3679.

[110] Johnson JL, Kamya RM, Okwera A, et al. Randomised controlled trial of *Mycobacterium vaccae* immunotherapy in non human immunodeficiency virus infected ugandan adults with newly diagnosed pulmonary tuberculosis. *J. Infect. Dis.* 2000;181:1304-1312.

[111] Mwinga A, Nunn A, Ngwira B, et al. Mycobacterium vaccae (SRL172) immunotherapy as an adjunct to standard antituberculosis treatment in HIV-infected adults with pulmonary tuberculosis: a randomised placebo-controlled trial. *Lancet.* 2002;360:1050-1055.

[112] Luo Y, Lu S, Guo S. [Immunotherapeutic effect of Mycobacterium vaccae on multi-drug resistant pulmonary tuberculosis]. *Zhonghua Jie He He Hu Xi Za Zhi.* 2000;23:85-88.

[113] Luo Y. [The immunotherapeutic effect of Mycobacterium vaccae vaccine on initially treated pulmonary tuberculosis]. *Zhonghua Jie He He Hu Xi Za Zhi.* 2001;24:43-47.

In: Vaccinations: Types, Potential Complications…
Editors: D. B. Steen and H. L. Dyson

ISBN: 978-1-60692-969-8

Chapter II

Vaccinations in Health Care Students from Germany, Iran, Lithuania and Spain*

Joerg Klewer[1,*], Laura Sasnauskaite[2], Alvydas Pavilonis[2], Parvin Tajik[3], Vahid Ziaee[3], Francisco Guillen-Grima[4], Ines Aguinaga-Ontoso[4] and Joachim Kugler[5]

[1]Department of Health and Nursing Sciences, University of Applied Sciences Zwickau, Zwickau, Germany,
[2]Department of Microbiology, Kaunas Medical University, Kaunas, Lithuania,
[3]Forum for Dynamic Thoughts, Tehran University of Medical Sciences, Tehran, Iran,
[4]Department of Health Sciences, Public University of Navarre, Pamplona, Spain.
[5]Public Health, Dresden Medical School, Dresden, Germany

Abstract

Infectious diseases are an increasing global health problem. Comparative studies about vaccination behavior in health care students from different countries are lacking. Due to working close to patients and infected specimens, they are in risk of contracting infectious diseases. The study analyzed vaccinations in health care students against tetanus, diphtheria, poliomyelitis, measles, mumps, rubella and hepatitis A+B. Furthermore, the study tried to investigate assessments on the importance of vaccinations and possible influences on the vaccination behavior. In an international multi-center-study, 182 German medical/dental students, 121 Iranian medical students, 70 Lithuanian medical students and 201 Spanish nursing students participated by working on an

* * A version of this chapter was also published in *Trends in Diptheria Research*, edited by Ben S. Wheeler published by Nova Science Publishers, Inc. It was submitted for appropriate modifications in an effort to encourage wider dissemination of research.

* Correspondence concerning this article should be addressed to Prof. Joerg Klewer, MD PhD, Department of Health and Nursing Sciences, University of Applied Sciences Zwickau, Dr.-Friedrichs-Ring 2a, 08056 Zwickau, Germany – joerg.klewer@fh-zwickau.de

anonymous questionnaire related to demographic data and vaccinations. The response rates were between 76% and 100%.
Altogether, the investigated students were not sufficiently vaccinated, except in the case offull coverage against hepatitis B in Spanish students. In the Lithuanian and Spanish samples, 30-50% of the students did not know if they have been vaccinated, especially against diphtheria and poliomyelitis. Gender differences, with better immunizations in female students, were found in the German and in the Iranian sample. Nearly all investigated students regarded vaccinations as important to prevent infectious diseases.

It becomes obvious that medical training does not affect personal preventive behavior in health care students. Insufficient coverage by vaccinations and lack of professional skills endangers health care students to contract and transmit infectious diseases.

The education of health care students should focus more on infectious diseases and vaccinations to optimize immunization in future health professionals. This will protect them against preventable infections. Additionally, they will be better skilled to prevent infectious diseases by educating and vaccinating the general population.

Keywords: vaccinations, students, infectious diseases, prevention.

Introduction

Infectious diseases are a worldwide health problem (World Health Organization, 2003). The spreading of HIV (human immunodeficiency virus) and tuberculosis in Sub-Saharan Africa, the endemic nature of malaria in tropical regions of the world provide evidence of it. Due to global air traffic, international streams of refugees, and deterioration of East European health systems, medical staff in industrialized countries, like Western Europe and the United States, are faced more and more with infectious diseases, some of which already seemed to be defeated (Armstrong et al., 1999; Reingold, 2000). Further more, it is known that infectious diseases do not follow simple rules: If someone falls ill or not depends on many factors, including environment, nutritional state, immune system, and / or mental health (Abiodun, 1994).

Considering the increase of infectious diseases, one could assume that education of health care students about infectious diseases and the causing agents would have been intensified. Because during their training and after graduating, by working close to patients, they are at risk of contracting infectious diseases (DeVries et al., 1991; Leliopoulou et al., 1999). They are expected to know about the clinical manifestations of infectious diseases and to protect themselves and their patients.

Nevertheless, current studies, focusing on vaccinations against common vaccine-preventable infectious diseases, like tetanus, diphtheria, or hepatitis B, in medical staff have shown that there are gaps in immunizations. Furthermore, their knowledge about infectious diseases often was incomplete or distorted by lack of education on this topic (Kohi & Horrocks, 1994; Thierney, 1995; Leliopoulou et al., 1999; Klewer et al., 2000).

Vaccinations in Medical Staff

The Centers for Disease Control and Prevention (CDC) and the World Health Organization strongly recommend that all health-care workers should be vaccinated (or have documented immunity) against tetanus, diphtheria, hepatitis B, measles, mumps, rubella, influenza and varicella (chicken pox). Despite these international recommendations, vaccination schedules in Germany, Iran, Lithuania and Spain do not include obligatory vaccinations for students in health care sciences, as it is common for example in the United States (Centers for Disease Control, 1997). In Germany, Spain and Lithuania vaccinations are financially covered by the government and/ or the health insurances of the students. In Iran, no national vaccination programs for mumps and rubella do exist. Nationwide vaccination against hepatitis B has been introduced in 1993. Thus, the health care students' risk of contracting vaccine-preventable infectious diseases is higher than in the three other countries. Furthermore, their vaccine uptake during childhood is less than in other countries with national vaccination programs (Ziaee et al., 2004).

Studies investigating vaccinations in medical staff revealed still incomplete coverage with vaccinations against vaccine-preventable diseases. In a German study on 238 medical students in the fifth year between one and nine percent of the medical students reported no vaccinations against hepatitis B (Radon et al., 2001). The relative frequency of medical students not vaccinated against hepatitis A was between 36 and 41%. The prevalence of vaccination especially against German measles among female students was not sufficient. Individual vaccination status of the students depended on their personal attitude towards vaccinations. The authors concluded, that in order to enhance the prevalence of hepatitis B vaccination among medical students, they should be informed more intensively about the free of charge vaccination early during their education, e.g., before the beginning of their medical training.

Another study on vaccinations against hepatitis B in medical staff of a German hospital has shown, that only 74.7% of the medical staff (n = 2204, nurses and doctors) have been vaccinated against hepatitis B (Borchert & Horst-Schaper, 2001). The authors assumed, that further activities are required to enhance the level of vaccinated medical staff.

In a study from the United Kingdom in a sample of 520 junior doctors only 27% reported complete vaccination against hepatitis B (Llewellyn & Harvey, 1994). A proportion of 29% stated that they have not received any vaccination against hepatitis B. The rest of the investigated junior doctors reported incomplete vaccination uptake. The authors demanded a vaccine program for junior doctors to increase the uptake of hepatitis B vaccinations.

Concerning the motivation for hepatitis B vaccine acceptance in 162 medical and physician assistant students, a complete vaccination uptake of 885 was found (Diekema et al., 1995). The most important reason given for vaccination was “recommendation by information from professional sources”. Overall, the vaccine acceptance among the investigated students was excellent and the authors concluded, that recommendations of authority figures are important motivators for hepatitis B vaccine acceptance among students.

Aims of the Study

Comparative studies related to vaccination behavior and vaccine coverage in health care students from different countries are lacking. Caring for adequate personal vaccination coverage reflects the awareness of personal risk for contracting infectious diseases and the infectious diseases itself. These reflections base on subjective perceptions of personal infection risks and of concepts of the etiology of the infectious disease. Due to this, the study analyzed in different samples of health care students from Germany, Iran, Lithuania and Spain

- vaccination coverage against tetanus, diphtheria, poliomyelitis, measles, mumps, rubella, hepatitis A, and hepatitis B;
- assessments on the importance of vaccinations; and
- whether there are gender differences in vaccination behavior.

Methods and Samples

Samples

The study was designed as a descriptive comparative international multi-center-study, consisting of four samples of students in health care sciences (medicine / nursing) from different countries. By using anonymous questionnaires, data from 182 German medical/ dental students, 121 Iranian medical students, 70 Lithuanian medical students and 201 Spanish nursing students have been obtained (Table 1). Participation was voluntary for all students.

Table 1. Demographic data of the investigated student samples.

	German medical/ dental students (n = 182)	*Iranian medical students (n = 121)*	*Lithuanian medical students (n = 70)*	*Spanish nursing students (n = 201)*
Average age and range (years)	*23.4 [20 – 34]*	*24.5 [21 – 32]*	*20.5 [19-40]*	*21.0 [18-39]*
Proportion females (%)	*56.4*	*36.4*	*76.5*	*94.0%*

The German sample included 96 third year medical and 86 fourth year dental students from the Dresden Medical School. Average age over both samples was 23.4 years, and the proportion of females was 56.4%. These medical and dental students underwent similar training in microbiology and infectious diseases. Therefore their knowledge in infection control and vaccinations was comparable. The students have been informed by their lecturers about the purpose of the study and asked for their participation. The anonymous questionnaires have been distributed to all students to be completed at home. Response rate was 76% in medical students and 87% in dental students.

In the Lithuanian sample, 176 medical students in the second and forth years of the Kaunas Medical University were included. Average age of the combined samples was 20.5 years, and the proportion of females was 76.5%. During their courses in microbiology, these medical students have been informed by their lecturers about the aims of the study and asked for their participation. The anonymous questionnaires in Lithuanian language have been distributed to all students to be completed at home. All students participated.

The 201 Spanish students in nursing sciences were recruited through a survey on health behavior and preventive lifestyles at the Public University of Navarre in Pamplona. Due to existing co-operations with Public University of Navarre and the lack of a medical school at this place, students in nursing sciences have been investigated. All students have been informed by the research team about the purpose of the entire study. After being physically examined, the students were asked to work on anonymous questionnaires also including questions going on vaccinations. Average age in this sample was 21.0 years, the proportion of females was 94%, and all students co-operated.

The Iranian sample, all 150 medical students in the 7th year (final year) of the Tehran University of Medical Sciences were invited to participate in the survey. Each student who agreed to participate was informed about the objectives and method of the study. Altogether 121 medical students returned a completed self-administered anonymous questionnaire, resulting in a response rate of 81%. Average age of the Iranian students was 24.5 years, and the proportion of females was 36.4%.

Methods

The study consisted on self-administered, anonymous questionnaires. The questionnaire used in Germany, Lithuania and Spain has been developed and approved in Germany. It was dived in two parts: the first part obtained demographic data (e.g. age, gender, years of study), and the second part was related to vaccination coverage. The questions related to vaccinations included vaccine coverage for infectious diseases like tetanus, diphtheria, poliomyelitis, mumps, measles, rubella (German measles), hepatitis A, and hepatitis B. For each disease vaccine coverage was investigated by using four different categories:

- “not vaccinated”,
- “only basic vaccination”,
- “basic vaccination and booster injections”, and
- “unknown/ I don’t know”.

Serological investigations were not performed.

Table 2. Reported vaccinations against tetanus, diphtheria, poliomyelitis, measles, mumps, rubella, varicella, hepatitis A, and hepatitis B by health science students from Germany, Lithuania, and Spain.

Vaccine-preventable disease	*German medical/ dental students (n = 182)*	*Lithuanian medical students (n = 70)*	*Spanish nursing students (n = 201)*
Tetanus (%)	*not vaccinated = 1.7* *basic vaccination = 12.5* *booster = 82.4* *don't know = 3.4*	*not vaccinated = 18.2* *basic vaccination = 28.8* *booster = 24.2* *don't know = 28.8*	*not vaccinated = 2.5* *basic vaccination = 46.2* *booster = 40.6* *don't know = 10.7*
Diphtheria (%)	*not vaccinated = 3.0* *basic vaccination = 23.1* *booster = 57.4* *don't know = 16.6*	*not vaccinated = 10.8* *basic vaccination = 40.0* *booster = 15.4* *don't know = 33.8*	*not vaccinated = 5.1* *basic vaccination = 38.9* *booster = 21.9* *don't know = 33.2*
Poliomyelitis (%)	*not vaccinated = 2.9* *basic vaccination = 28.6* *booster = 61.1* *don't know = 7.4*	*not vaccinated = 8.1* *basic vaccination = 25.8* *booster = 9.7* *don't know = 56.5*	*not vaccinated = 0.0* *basic vaccination = 44.1* *booster = 28.7* *don't know = 27.2*
Measles (%)	*not vaccinated = 15.1* *basic vaccination = 32.5* *booster = 23.5* *don't know = 28.9*	*not vaccinated = 7.9* *basic vaccination = 42.9* *booster = 3.2* *don't know = 46.0*	*not vaccinated = 13.0* *basic vaccination = 42.7* *booster = 15.1* *don't know = 29.2*
Mumps (%)	*not vaccinated = 28.9* *basic vaccination = 21.1* *booster = 19.3* *don't know = 30.1*	*not vaccinated = 20.0* *basic vaccination = 40.0* *booster = 1.5* *don't know = 38.5*	*not vaccinated = 17.8* *basic vaccination = 27.7* *booster = 6.8* *don't know = 47.6*
Rubella (German measles) (%)	*not vaccinated = 24.9* *basic vaccination = 24.3* *booster = 30.2* *don't know = 20.7*	*not vaccinated = 10.8* *basic vaccination = 44.6* *booster = 4.6* *don't know = 40.0*	*not vaccinated = 3.1* *basic vaccination = 55.0* *booster = 24.6* *don't know = 17.3*
Varicella (chicken pox) (%)	*not vaccinated = 40.9* *basic vaccination = 20.7* *booster = 9.8* *don't know = 28.7*	*not vaccinated = 26.6* *basic vaccination = 32.8* *booster = 1.6* *don't know = 39.1*	*not vaccinated = 50.0* *basic vaccination = 23.2* *booster = 7.9* *don't know = 18.9*
Hepatitis A (%)	*not vaccinated = 47.6* *basic vaccination = 13.9* *booster = 31.3* *don't know = 7.2*	*not vaccinated = 23.8* *basic vaccination = 20.6* *booster = 3.2* *don't know = 52.4*	*not vaccinated = 44.7* *basic vaccination = 8.9* *booster = 10.0* *don't know = 36.3*
Hepatitis B (%)	*not vaccinated = 11.8* *basic vaccination = 33.5* *booster = 52.9* *don't know = 1.8*	*not vaccinated = 22.2* *basic vaccination = 15.9* *booster = 1.3* *don't know = 60.3*	*not vaccinated = 0.0* *basic vaccination = 42.1* *booster = 57.9* *don't know = 0.0*

Basic vaccination = first course completed, no booster injections received.
Booster = basic vaccination completed and booster injections (according to vaccination schedule).

Furthermore, an additional question related to assessments on the importance of vaccinations was added. Four categories have been given to the students to answer on the question, how important to their own opinion vaccinations are (Table 3). The four categories have been:

- "absolutely necessary",
- "sometimes necessary",
- "normally not necessary", and
- "useless and dangerous".

The questionnaires have been translated into Lithuanian and Spanish language respectively, and retranslated to control possible mistakes due to invalid translations.

Table 3. Assessments on the importance of vaccinations in general by health science students from Germany, Lithuania and Spain.

	German medical/ dental students (n = 182)	*Lithuanian medical students (n = 70)*	*Spanish nursing students (n = 201)*
Vaccinations are …			
absolutely necessary	*62.8%*	*42.4%*	*63.6%*
sometimes necessary	*36.6%*	*57.6%*	*34.8%*
normally not necessary	*0.6%*	*0.0%*	*1.5%*
useless and dangerous	*0.0%*	*0.0%*	*0.0%*

The questionnaire used in Iran had a different structure than the questionnaires used in the European samples. This was due to the fact, that the Iranian research group joined the international multi-center-study after completing their survey on medical students in Tehran. In Iran, the survey focused mainly on vaccinations against hepatitis B. Therefore, vaccination coverage was not obtained by detailed questions related to the other infectious diseases. Vaccination coverage against tetanus and diphtheria, and mumps, measles and rubella (MMR) respectively were combined, mainly by investigating the age of the last injection. No questions going on poliomyelitis and hepatitis A were included.

Results

Vaccinations Against Tetanus

Altogether 82.4% of the German medical/ dental students reported a completed vaccination scheme against tetanus, including booster injections during the previous ten years (Table 2). The percentage of students reporting only basic vaccine uptake, without booster injections, was 12.5%. Around 3.4% of the investigated German students admitted, that they do not know, if they are vaccinated against tetanus, and three students declared that they are not vaccinated against tetanus.

In the Lithuanian student sample, 24.2% of the investigated medical students reported full uptake of vaccinations against tetanus and regular booster injections. Additional 28.8% of the Lithuanian medical students stated that they received only basic vaccination against tetanus. The same percentage of students reported, that they do not know their vaccination status for tetanus. Twelve students told that they have not received any tetanus vaccinations.

In total, 40.6% of the Spanish nursing students declared themselves as fully vaccinated against tetanus, including booster injections. A percentage of 46.2% of the nursing students reported that they have received basic vaccination against tetanus, without booster injections. About 10.7% of the students stated, that they are not knowing whether they were vaccinated against tetanus or not, and five students mentioned that they did not get any vaccination against tetanus.

Due to the different questionnaire used in Iran, differing findings have been obtained. Altogether 61.2% of the investigated medical students reported that they have received a vaccination against tetanus during the previous ten years. Average time since the last injection was 4 years, ranging from less than one year up to 18 years.

Vaccinations Against Diphtheria

In the German student sample, 57.4% of the investigated medical/ dental students stated that have received full vaccination against diphtheria, including booster injections (Table 2). Basic vaccination against diphtheria was reported by 23.1% of the German medical/ dental students. The percentage of German students not knowing if they were vaccinated against diphtheria was 16.6%. Other five students stated that they were no immunized against diphtheria.

About 15.4% of the Lithuanian medical students declared that they were fully vaccinated against diphtheria. Forty percent of the Lithuanian students reported only basic vaccination against diphtheria, without booster injections. More than one third (33.8%) of the Lithuanian medical students mentioned that they do not know their vaccination status for diphtheria, and ten students stated that they were not vaccinated against diphtheria at all.

In the sample of Spanish nursing students, the percentage of students reporting full vaccination uptake against diphtheria, including booster injections, was 21.9%. Only basic vaccination, without booster injections, was declared by 39.8% of the Spanish students. Approximately one third of the Spanish nursing students (33.2%) answered that they do not know their vaccination status for diphtheria. Additional ten nursing students mentioned that they did not receive any immunization against diphtheria.

Similar to the findings for tetanus, altogether 61.2% of the investigated Iranian medical students reported that they have received a vaccination against diphtheria during the previous ten years. Average time since the last diphtheria vaccination was 4 years, ranging from less than one year up to 18 years.

Vaccinations Against Poliomyelitis

Nearly two third of the German medical students (61.1%) reported a full vaccination uptake against poliomyelitis, including booster vaccinations (Table 2). Basic vaccination, without booster vaccinations, was reported by 28.6% of the German medical students. About 7.4% of the German students mentioned that they are not knowing if they are vaccinated against poliomyelitis. Additional five students declared not being vaccinated against poliomyelitis.

Less than 10% of the Lithuanian medical students (9.7%) reported complete vaccination against poliomyelitis, including booster vaccinations. Around on quarter of the Lithuanian students (25.8%) stated that they have received basic vaccination against poliomyelitis. Half of the Lithuanian student sample admitted, that they were not aware if they are vaccinated against poliomyelitis or not. Five of the Lithuanian medical students reported that they are not vaccinated against poliomyelitis.

In the Spanish sample, altogether 28.7% of the students had received complete vaccination against poliomyelitis, including booster vaccinations. Nearly half of the student sample (44.1%) reported basic vaccination against poliomyelitis, without booster vaccinations. More than one quarter of the Spanish students (27.2%) mentioned that they do not know their vaccination status for poliomyelitis. None of the students reported no being vaccinated against poliomyelitis.

Due to the different questionnaire used in Iran, no results for the uptake of vaccinations against poliomyelitis in the Iranian medical students were available.

Vaccinations Against Mumps

Complete vaccination against mumps was reported by 19.3% of the German medical/ dental students (Table 2). Only one injection was mentioned by 21.7% of the German students. Nearly one third (30.1%) of the German students stated that they do not know, if they have received immunization against mumps, and forty-eight German students declared that they were not vaccinated against mumps.

Only one Lithuanian medical student reported complete vaccination against mumps. About 40% reported the receipt of one vaccination against mumps, and 20% declared themselves as not being vaccinated against mumps. More than one third of the Lithuanian medical students (38.5%) mentioned that they are not knowing, if they have been vaccinated against mumps.

Around 6.8% of the Spanish nursing students reported complete vaccination against mumps. More than one quarter (27.7%) confirmed the receipt of one injection. Nearly the half of the Spanish nursing students (47.6%) answered that they do not know whether they were vaccinated against mumps or not. Thirty-five of the Spanish students declared that they did not receive any vaccination against mumps.

Due to the different questionnaire used in Iran, differing findings for vaccinations against mumps have been obtained. In the Iranian survey, vaccinations against mumps, measles and rubella (German measles) (MMR) were put together in one question. Reception of at least one MMR vaccination was reported by 34.3% of the Iranian medical students. Fifty percent of the Iranian medical students denied a MMR-vaccine injection, and seventeen medical students did no know if they have ever received a MMR-vaccination. Average age of the Iranian medical students at time of MMR-vaccination was 20.6 years, ranging from one year to twenty-five years.

Vaccinations Against Measles

A complete uptake of measles vaccination was reported by nearly one quarter of the German medical/ dental students (23.5%) (Table 2). Approximately one third (32.5%) of the German students had received at least one vaccine injection against measles. Almost the same percentage (28.9%) of the German students mentioned that they are not knowing if they have ever been vaccinated against measles, and twenty-five of the German medical/ dental students stated that they have never received a vaccination against measles.

Only two Lithuanian medical students reported complete vaccination uptake against measles. More than 40% of the Lithuanian medical students mentioned that they had only received on time vaccination against measles (42.9%) or that they did not know their vaccination status (46%) respectively. Additional five medical students declared that they have not been not vaccinated against measles.

About 15.1% of the Spanish nursing students answered that have been completely vaccinated against measles. Just one vaccination against measles was reported by nearly half of the student sample (42.7%). About 29.2% of the Spanish students mentioned that they do not know whether they have received a vaccination against measles or not, and twenty-five of the Spanish nursing students reported that they have never received a vaccination against measles.

Vaccinations Against Rubella (German Measles)

Nearly one third (30.2%) of the German medical/ dental students reported that they were fully vaccinated against rubella (German measles) (Table 2). More or less one quarter of the German students stated that they had received only one time vaccination against rubella (24.3%) or that they did not receive any vaccination against rubella (24.9%) respectively. Around 20.7% of the German medical/ dental students mentioned, that they do not know if they have been vaccinated against rubella.

In the Lithuanian medical student sample, only three students reported two vaccinations against rubella. Above 40% of the Lithuanian medical students stated that they had only received on time vaccination against rubella (42.9%) or that they did not know their vaccination status (40%) respectively. Additional seven Lithuanian students answered, that they were not vaccinated against rubella.

Approximately one quarter of the Spanish nursing students (24.6%) reported that they are completely vaccinated against rubella. Only one vaccination against rubella was mentioned by 55% of the nursing students. Around 17.3% of the Spanish nursing students stated, that they do not know, if they have received vaccination against rubella, and six students declared, that they have not been vaccinated against rubella.

Vaccinations Against Varicella (Chicken Pox)

Around 9.8% of the German medical/ dental students reported vaccinations against varicella (chicken pox) and booster injections (Table 2). Additional 20.7% of the students mentioned at least basic vaccinations against varicella, and 40.9% of the investigated students denied that they have received vaccinations against chicken pox. The rest of the German students stated, that they do not know if they have been vaccinated against varicella.

Only one Lithuanian medical student reported basic vaccination against varicella and additional booster injections. Around one third of the Lithuanian students (32.8%) declared that they have been vaccinated against varicella. One quarter of the students (26.1%) stated that they did not receive any vaccination against varicella, and twenty-five students mentioned, that they were not knowing, if they have ever received a vaccination against varicella.

In the sample of Spanish nursing students, 7.9% of the students reported, that they have received basic vaccination and booster injections against varicella. Altogether 23.2% of the Spanish students stated to have basic vaccination against varicella. Half of the student sample answered that they have not been vaccinated against varicella, and 18.9% did not know, if they got vaccinations against varicella.

In the Iranian student sample, vaccination against varicella was not investigated. Only one question was going on history of chickenpox. Altogether 72.6% of the medical students reported a history of chicken pox, 17.7% denied it, and 9.7% of the students reported, that they do not know whether they have ever suffered from chicken pox or not.

Vaccinations Against Hepatitis A

Nearly one third of the German medical/ dental students (31.3%) reported that they have received basic vaccinations and boosters injections against hepatitis A (Table 2). Additional 13.9% of the German students reported at least basic vaccinations against hepatitis A. Almost half of the German students (47.6%) answered, that they did never receive any vaccinations against hepatitis A, and twelve German students were not informed about their vaccination status against hepatitis A.

Only two Lithuanian medical students declared, that they got basic vaccination and booster injections against hepatitis A. Around 20.6% of the Lithuanian students reported, that they have received basic vaccination against hepatitis A. Nearly of quarter of the Lithuanian medical students (23.8%) denied any vaccinations against hepatitis A, and more than half of the Lithuanian students (52.4%) mentioned that they do not know, if they have been vaccinated against hepatitis A.

Around 10% of the Spanish nursing students reported, that they have received basic vaccination and booster injections against hepatitis A. Additional 8.9% of the Spanish students mentioned, that they have received at least basic vaccinations against hepatitis A. Nearly half of the student sample (44.7%) denied any vaccinations against hepatitis A, and more than one third of the Spanish students (36.3%) answered, that they were not knowing, if they have been vaccinated against hepatitis A or not.

Vaccinations Against Hepatitis B

More than half of the German medical/ dental students (52.9%) reported, that they have received basic vaccinations and booster injections against hepatitis B (Table 2). Additional 33.5% mentioned, that they have received basic vaccinations against hepatitis B. Around 11.8% of the German students denied any vaccinations against hepatitis B, and three German students did not know whether they have been vaccinated against hepatitis B or not.

Only one Lithuanian medical student reported basic vaccinations against hepatitis B and booster injections. Additional 15.9% of the Lithuanian students mentioned, that they have received basis vaccinations against hepatitis B. Nearly one quarter of the Lithuanian students (22.2%) denied any vaccinations against hepatitis B, and more than half of the Lithuanian medical students (60.3%) stated, that they do not know if they have ever received vaccinations against hepatitis B.

All Spanish nursing students have received vaccinations against hepatitis B. Around 42.1% of them reported basic vaccinations against hepatitis B, the rest also reported about booster injections.

Due to the different questionnaire used in the Iranian sample, the findings differ from the results in the European samples. Altogether 90.9% of the Iranian medical students reported that they have completed basic vaccination against hepatitis B. Around 13.2% of them also reported booster injections against hepatitis B. Hundred-eight of the Iranian medical students have been vaccinated against hepatitis B during their training at medical school.

Gender Differences in Vaccination Status

In the German medical/ dental student sample significant differences in vaccination status (χ^2) between male and female students were found in vaccinations against poliomyelitis ($p = .011$) and rubella (German measles) ($p = .000$). Around 95% of the females students declared, that have been vaccinated against poliomyelitis, 68% of them also reported booster vaccinations. Only two females students were not aware, if they have been vaccinated against poliomyelitis. In the male sample, 82.4% of the students reported at least basic vaccination against poliomyelitis, and 52.7% of them had received booster vaccinations. Nearly 15% of the male students (14.9%) did not know, if they have been vaccinated against poliomyelitis.

Altogether 71.4% of the German female students reported that they have received at least basic vaccination against rubella, around 40.8% of them had received extra booster injections. In the female sample, 18.4% of the students stated, that they are not vaccinated against rubella, and additional 10.2% of the female students did not know their vaccinations status for rubella. Compared with the German female students, only 30% of the male students declared, that they have received at least basic vaccination against rubella, and 14.3% of them reported booster injections. More than one third of the male students denied vaccinations against rubella (34.3%), or did not know, if they have been vaccinated (35.7%) respectively.

In the Spanish nursing student sample, significant differences in vaccination status (χ^2) between male and female students in vaccinations against mumps, measles and rubella (German measles) (MMR) were found. In general, the percentages of female students not knowing, if they have been vaccinated against one of the three diseases, were higher than in the male sample.

Due to the different questionnaire in the Iranian survey, only the uptake of vaccinations against mumps, measles and rubella (German measles) (MMR) was investigated. A significant difference was found between female and male medical students by the way, that in the female sample 48.8% of the students reported MMMR-uptake, compared to 25.4% in the male sample (χ^2, $p = .003$). The percentage of students denying vaccinations against MMR was nearly 50% in both samples, but 23.9% of the male students and 2.4% of the female students declared that they do not know, if they have received vaccinations against mumps, measles and rubella.

Assessments on the Importance of Vaccinations

Nearly two thirds of the German medical/ dental students (62.8%) declared vaccinations as absolutely necessary (Table 3). For more than one third of the German students (36.6%) vaccinations were sometimes necessary. Only one German student declared vaccinations as normally not necessary.

In the Lithuanian medical student sample, around 42.4% of the investigated students declared vaccinations as absolutely necessary, the rest of the Lithuanian students declared them as sometimes necessary.

Nearly two thirds of the Spanish nursing students (63.6%) declared vaccinations as absolutely necessary. For an additional third of the Spanish students (34.8%) vaccinations were sometimes necessary. Only three Spanish students declared vaccinations as normally not necessary.

Due to the focus on vaccinations against hepatitis B in the Iranian survey, the findings are related to assessments on the importance of vaccinations against hepatitis B. Around 85.5% of the Iranian medical students declared, that they strongly agree with the statement "Every medical student has to receive vaccination against hepatitis B!" Additional 13.7% of the Iranian students declared, that they just agree with the mentioned statement. Only one female Iranian medical student answered, that she neither agrees nor disagrees with the statement.

Discussion

Adequate personal vaccination coverage reflects the awareness of personal risk for contracting infectious diseases. Therefore, the study analyzed in different samples of health care students from Germany, Iran, Lithuania and Spain vaccination coverage, assessments on the importance of vaccinations, and whether there are gender differences in vaccination behavior.

Methods of Analyzing Vaccination Coverage

The results of the study base on reported uptake of different vaccinations mentioned in an anonymous questionnaire. No serological parameters have been obtained. On the other hand, one can expect that in medical staff sufficient knowledge about the personal vaccination status should be present. Taking merely the reported vaccination status is a common method to investigate coverage with vaccinations in specific groups, like medical staff, or in the general population (Reiter & Rasch, 2000; Seibt et al., 2000). By using this method, the vaccination status of the investigated medical staff could be obtained in a cheap and easy way. Taking blood and serological testing for adequate antibody levels would have been the most accurate method, but requiring several times higher technical efforts, and maybe causing lower acceptance of the study, due to the procedure of taking blood. Controlling all vaccinations cards would perhaps reveal more precise results, but this requires intensive announcement of the planned investigations already weeks in advance. Despite this, the problem of students forgetting their vaccination remains. In addition, some of the students do not have this card with them at their room in the student hostel, because they keep it at their parents' home. In a conservative setting, all these students being at time of the study without a valid vaccination card would have been counted as not vaccinated. This would have an important influence on the results. Therefore the option to mark the answer "do not know" was added to avoid the problem, that high percentages of students would be classified as "not vaccinated", because of having not their vaccination card with them.

Vaccinations Against Tetanus, Diphtheria and Poliomyelitis

It became obvious, that the vaccination coverage against tetanus, diphtheria and poliomyelitis in the investigated students was not satisfactory. Even by assuming that all students who stated that they are not knowing their vaccination status were well vaccinated, adequate vaccination coverage against the different diseases would not have been achieved. Due to the fact, that in general in Germany booster vaccinations against poliomyelitis are not recommend any more (Robert Koch-Institut, 2001), some of the German students reporting basic vaccinations could be added to the group of students vaccinated adequately. On the other hand, it remains unclear, how the immunity against the three different types of the poliomyelitis virus develops, due to the absence of unintentional booster by contact to viruses deriving from oral vaccinations (Franck et al., 1999). Compared to the student groups from the other countries, the German students presented the highest proportions of students adequately vaccinated against poliomyelitis. Similar to the vaccine coverage for poliomyelitis, the reported vaccine coverage against tetanus and diphtheria was not satisfactory. The proportion of German students reporting adequate vaccination coverage against tetanus and diphtheria was higher than in the student samples from Lithuania and Spain.

A major problem in all investigated student samples were the high proportions of the students not knowing whether they were vaccinated against tetanus, diphtheria or poliomyelitis or not. The reasons for these findings remain unclear. One reason could be the different structures of the health care systems in the different countries. In Lithuania and Spain vaccinations are offered by the public health service, and vaccinations cards of schoolchildren and students are regularly controlled by public health nurses. Therefore it is likely, that the students trusted in official reminders to attend booster injections by the public health service, not caring so much about the vaccination schedule. Conversely, in Germany no public health service checking automatically vaccination cards of students does exist. Everybody is responsible on his own to get appropriate vaccinations and booster, only sometimes assisted by a reminder of the private general practitioner. This was maybe the reason, why a higher proportion of German students were aware if the were vaccinated against tetanus, diphtheria and poliomyelitis or not.

Accordingly, best possible vaccination coverage has not been reached in all investigated student samples. Especially tetanus is a worldwide health problem, without being strictly related to medical procedures, and with high letality, as well in minor injuries. Therefore vaccine coverage of 100% is required, to protect medical staff and the general population.

Vaccinations Against Mumps, Measles, Rubella and Varicella

The proportions of students reporting vaccinations against mumps, measles, rubella and varicella were approximately between 9 and 30%. Additionally, the proportions of students not knowing whether they were vaccinated or not were approximately between 20 and 48%. One problem in interpreting these findings results in different vaccinations schedules and availability of vaccinations against mumps, measles, rubella and varicella in the different countries. In Western Europe, vaccinations against mumps, measles and rubella were available from the middle of the seventies of the last century, in Eastern Europe some years later, especially combinations of different vaccinations within one syringe. Vaccinations against varicella are available since the end of the nineties of the last century, and not generally recommended. Therefore a proportion of students will have experienced natural infection with mumps, measles, rubella or varicella, leading to natural immunity, not requiring vaccinations or booster any more. Due to this, comparing of the findings is difficult. Although it comes clear, that the high proportions of students reporting that are not knowing their vaccination status reflect the problem of unawareness related to the personal medical history, including experienced infections with the mentioned diseases, and their personal vaccinations status. Like for tetanus, diphtheria and poliomyelitis, the lack of knowledge about the personal vaccination status probably derives from the activities of the public health service (see above). The results correspond to findings in German students, showing insufficient vaccination coverage for example against measles (Radon et al., 2001).

It is likely, that in the general population the awareness of experienced infections and the need for vaccinations against mumps, measles, rubella and varicella will be less developed than in medical staff. Therefore increased efforts to increase vaccination coverage against these diseases in the general population are required.

Vaccinations Against Hepatitis A

Vaccinations against hepatitis A are not recommend for the general population, but useful to prevent medical staff from hepatitis A. Due to introduction of vaccinations against hepatitis A at the beginning of the nineties of the 20th century, and a period of at least ten years until a booster is required, students reporting merely basic vaccinations should be classified as adequately vaccinated. On the other hand, especially in Spain and Lithuania high rates of naturally acquired hepatitis A infections can be assumed, causing natural immunity not requiring further vaccinations against hepatitis A. In Germany the rates of natural infections are much lower and still decreasing (Reiter & Rasch, 2000).

Despite this, the proportions of students not knowing their vaccinations status against hepatitis A were very high, especially in the Spanish and Lithuanian samples. The findings in the German sample are comparable to findings from a different German study (Radon et al., 2001). Furthermore, due to the age of the students, the students are likely to travel to countries where hepatitis A is endemic, causing an infection risks apart from the field of medicine. This requires increased efforts to improve the vaccination coverage against hepatitis A in health care students.

Vaccinations Against Hepatitis B

Vaccinations against hepatitis B in medical staff are strongly recommended (Centers for Diseases Control, 1997). The protective effect of vaccinations against hepatitis B last at least ten years. Therefore, all students reporting merely basic vaccinations should be classified as adequately vaccinated. Compared to the vaccination uptake in American medical students, vaccination uptake in the investigated medical students was lower (Diekema et al., 1995), but higher than in British junior doctors (Llewellyn & Harvey, 1994). Merely the Spanish nursing students presented outstanding results by being completely vaccinated against hepatitis B.

Due to the fact, that all medical students participating in the study could get vaccinations against hepatitis B free of charge from their university, the question rises up, why they are not appropriately vaccinated. The Spanish nursing students, and to some extent the Iranian medical students, have proven the effectiveness of increased efforts by the university to reach full vaccine coverage. Therefore different efforts to promote vaccinations in medical students are required, to prevent them from occupational acquired hepatitis B infections. Particularly clinical situations, like taking blood or dealing with infective specimens, include increased infection-risks for hepatitis B, because the freshmen are not well trained to handle complicated situations with higher infection risks. While training the students in procedures with potential risk of infection, intensive education about the need for vaccinations against hepatitis B are essential.

Health care students often do not realize, that becoming a carrier for hepatitis B means suffering from a chronic disease, sometimes shortening their life due to liver cirrhosis, and being a source of infection for the patients. Consequently, hepatitis B carrier are often excluded from direct contacts to patients, especially in the fields of surgery and gynecology. This means, than they are likely to loose their job, without having good chances to find a new one (Tereskerz et al., 1996). Because of the low number of years they have worked, they will often get no reimbursement from pension founds.

Besides, hepatitis B belongs to the sexual transmitted diseases. Due to their age and the increased number of opportunities for sexual intercourses, students are endangered to acquire hepatitis B in private settings. Therefore vaccinating health care students against hepatitis B protects them in a very effective way.

Gender Differences in Vaccination Status

An interesting finding was, that female students reported better vaccination coverage than male students, and that the proportion of females not knowing their vaccination status was lower than in the male sub-samples. This is maybe due to the circumstance, that females becoming health care professionals present a well-developed awareness towards their own health conditions (Schank & Lawrence, 1992); combined with the fact, that in general females are caring more for their physical and mental well-being than males (Hessel et al., 1999).

Due to the proportion of 94% of females in the Spanish sample, the opposite results are limited and difficult to explain.

However, taking these findings into consideration gender-specific education and promotion on vaccination are required. Therefore increased efforts to improve the vaccination status of male students are necessary. Further studies are needed to explain the underlying reasons for such a difference, to develop appropriate training and promotion programs chiefly in male students. In the meantime, authority figures at the universities should bear in mind these findings, and focus on reduction of inadequate vaccination status in male students.

Assessments on the Importance of Vaccinations

It became obvious, that nearly all students appreciated the need for vaccinations. It remains unclear, if these students, seeing vaccinations merely as sometimes necessary, subsumed vaccinations only recommend for use in specific conditions, like against cholera, under vaccinations not always necessary. On the other hand, this does not express disapproval of vaccinations. It is remarkable, that none of the students did see vaccinations as unimportant and dangerous, although the answer did exist. Altogether, the findings symbolize positive intentions towards vaccinations in the investigated samples of health care students, and correspond to results in American health care students (Diekema et al., 1995).

In contrast, these findings do not explain, why not all of the investigated students reported adequate vaccination coverage against the mentioned vaccinations. This points to a discrepancy between acceptance of vaccinations and practical personal protective behavior (Ralston, 1993; Schmid et al., 1993). Similar results have been found in final year medical students not being sufficiently vaccinated. Main reason was lack of motivation to attend the vaccination department at medical school (Schmid et al., 1993).

As a result, education of future health professionals should recognize the positive assessments on the importance of vaccinations and focus more on the importance of completed vaccination coverage, maybe by offering vaccinations at several stages during the studies, to reach all students in a way convenient for them. This would be very important to prevent occupationally acquired infections, like hepatitis B (Baumgarten, 1998).

Improving Vaccination Coverage in Health Care Students

The results point to the problem that improved training in infectious diseases and vaccinations is required for health care students. By this, these future health professionals will achieve broad knowledge in preventive medicine, which is essential to promote vaccinations in students populations and the general population as well. Health care professionals are taken as examples in adequate life-style. Without adequate knowledge in the field of vaccine-preventable diseases, they are not sufficiently prepared to advice their patients about vaccination coverage and booster injections. Taking into account, that in the general population acceptance of vaccinations is still high, misleading or absence of information about vaccinations and prevention of infectious diseases will lead to endangering a considerable proportion of the general population. Then prevention of occupationally and sexually transmitted infections, especially of hepatitis B, will be insufficient.

In addition, it is likely, that in students from other faculties than health sciences, lower vaccination rates against the mentioned infectious diseases will be found. Therefore the results demand increased efforts to improve the vaccination coverage by the general practitioners of the students and the universities as well.

Conclusions

Concluding, universities should think about establishing health promoting programs and institutions on campus where students spend most of their time. Considering the discrepancy between high acceptance of vaccinations and low personal vaccine uptake, by having such an institution promoting and offering vaccinations nearby, students are likely to visit this institution to get their vaccinations. As an additional consequence, these institutions would be useful to inform students about healthy-lifestyle, like non-smoking, low fat diet and sports. By offering a broad spectrum of information, students coming for different reasons could get a check of their vaccination status, and in addition completion of their vaccinations. Finally this would be a partial realization of the World Health Organization concept of the "Health promoting university", starting with improving the health conditions of students and ending up with improved health conditions in the general population (Tsouros et al., 1998).

References

[1] Abiodun OA. The role of psychosocial factors in the causation, course and outcome of physical disorders: a review. *East African Medical Journal*, 1994, 71, 55-59.

[2] Armstrong G, Conn LA & Pinner RW. Trends in infectious diseases mortality in the United States during the 20th century. *Journal of the American Medical Association*, 1999, 281, 61-66.

[3] Baumgarten R. Virushepatitiden: Vermeidbare Erkrankungen. *Zeitschrift für ärztliche Fortbildung und Qualitätssicherung*, 1998; 92, 677-680.

[4] Borchert W & Horst-Schaper G. Hepatitis B: Impfstatus und Prävalenz bei den Mitarbeitern eines großen Krankenhauses in Norddeutschland. *Arbeitsmedizin, Sozialmedizin, Umweltmedizin*, 2001, 36, 230-233.

[5] Centers for Disease Control. Immunization of Health-Care Workers: Recommendations of the Advisory Committee on Immunization Practices (ACIP) and the Hospital Infection Control Practices Advisory Committee (HICPAC). *Morbidity Mortality Weekly Report Recommendations Report*, 1997, 46 (RR-18), 1-42.

[6] Diedrich S, Claus H, Thierfelder W, Bellach BM & Schreier E. Bundesgesundheitssurvey 1997/98: Immunitätslage gegen Poliomyelitis. *Deutsche Medizinische Wochenschrift*, 2000; 125, 584-588.

[7] Diekema DJ, Ferguson KJ & Doebbling BN. Motivation for Hepatitis B Vaccine Acceptance among Medical and Physician Assistant Students. *Journal of General Internal Medicine*, 1995, 10, 1-6.

[8] Franck S, Allwinn R & Doerr HW. Zur aktuellen Poliomyelitis-Immunität. Sero-epidemiologische Untersuchung auf der Basis von Patientenseren im Rhein-Main-Gebiet. *Epidemiologisches Bulletin*, 1999; Nr. 8, 49-51.

[9] Hammer K, Rothkopf-Ischebeck M & Meixner M. Aktuelle Impfstatuserhebung für Tetanus, Diphtherie und Poliomyelitis bei Erwachsenen. *Infektionsepidemiologische Forschung*, 1997; Nr. 1, 35-37.

[10] Hessel, A, Geyer M, Plöttner, Schmidt B & Brähler E. Subjektive Einschätzung der eigenen Gesundheit und subjektive Morbidität in Deutschland. *Psychotherapie, Psychosomatische Medizin und Medizinische Psychologie*, 1999; 49, 264-274.

[11] Klewer J, Tracogna U, Lauschke H & Kugler J. Assessments of German and Namibian nursing staff on occupational HIV transmission risks. In: Monduzzi Editore (Ed.): *XIII. International AIDS Conference*. Litosei – Rastignano, Bologna, 2000, 445-450.

[12] Kohi TW & Horrocks MJ. The knowledge, attitudes and perceived social support of Tanzanian nurses when caring for patients with AIDS. *International Journal of Nursing Studies*, 1994, 31, 77-86.

[13] Leliopoulou C, Waterman H & Chakrabarty S. Nurses failure to appreciate the risks of infection due to needle stick accidents: a hospital based survey. *Journal of Hospital Infection*, 1999, 42, 53-59.

[14] Llewellyn LJ & Harvey I. Hepatitis B vaccination: how many doctors are fully covered ? *Journal of Public Health Medicine*, 1994, 16: 352-356.

[15] Radon K, Frankota H, Klewer J & Nowak D. Impfstatus von Medizinstudierenden in München - Ergebnisse einer Fragebogenerhebung. *Das Gesundheitswesen*, 2001, 63, 573-577.

[16] Ralston DL. Medical Student's Well-Being: A Necessary Component of Reform. *Academic Medicine*, 1993; 68: 272-273.

[17] Rasch G & Schöneberg I. Tetanus in Deutschland - Ergebnisse der Einzelfallerfassung seit 1995. *Bundesgesundheitsblatt*, 1998; 41: 67-69.

[18] Reingold AL. Infectious Disease Epidemiology in the 21st Century: Will It Be Eradicated or Will It Reemerge ?. *Epidemiologic Reviews*, 2000; 22: 57-63.

[19] Reiter S & Rasch G. Schutzimpfungen. *Gesundheitsberichterstattung des Bundes*, 2000; 1, 3-13.

[20] Robert-Koch-Institut. Impfempfehlungen der Ständigen Impfkommission (STIKO) am Robert-Koch-Institut / Stand: Juli 2001. *Epidemiologisches Bulletin*, 2001; Nr. 28, 203-218.

[21] Schank MJ & Lawrence DM. Young adult woman: lifestyle and health locus of control. *Journal of Advanced Nursing*, 1993; 18, 1235-1241.

[22] Schmid K, Schmelz M, Escher S, Raithel HJ & Lehnert G. Akzeptanz von Schutzimpfungen als Mittel der Prävention - Untersuchungen zum Impfstatus bei Medizinstudenten vor Beginn des praktischen Jahres. *Arbeitsmedizin, Sozialmedizin und Umweltmedizin*, 1993; 28, 341-347.

[23] Seibt K, Schulz M & Hensel FJ. Meinungen und Einstellungen zum Thema Impfen bei niedergelassenen Ärzten, und Offizinapothekern und ihrem Personal sowie aktueller Impfstatus dieser Gruppen. *Das Gesundheitswesen*, 2000; 62, 376-382.

[24] Tereskerz P, Pearson RD & Jagger J. Occupational exposure to blood among medical students. *New England Journal of Medicine*, 1996; 335, 1150-1152.

[25] Tierney AJ. HIV / AIDS-knowledge, attitudes and education of nurses: a review of the research. *Journal of Clinical Nursing*, 1995, 4, 13-21.

[26] Tsouros AD, Dowding G, Thompson J & Dooris M (Ed.). *Health Promoting Universities – Concept, experience and framework for action*. World Health Organization, Copenhagen, 1998.

[27] World Health Organization (WHO). *Progress report 2002: Global defense against the infectious disease threat.* WHO, Geneva, 2003, 6-11.

[28] Ziaee V, Tajik P, Tavoosi A, Rostambeigy N &Rahbari H. A Survey of Iranian Final-Year Medical Students: Vaccine Coverage. *Infection Control and Hospital Epidemiology* (under review).

In: Vaccinations: Types, Potential Complications… ISBN: 978-1-60692-969-8
Editors: D. B. Steen and H. L. Dyson

Chapter III

Recent Topics for Hepatitis B Vaccination*

Viroj Wiwanitkit
Department of Laboratory Medicine, Faculty of Medicine, Chulalongkorn University, Bangkok, Thailand

Abstract

Hepatitis B is a highly contagious viral infection. It can lead to chronic carrier state and the hepatocellular carcinoma in the worst case. To prevent is better than to treat athis infection. An effective tool for prevention and control of hepatitis B infection is the vaccination. In this article, topics on the hepatitis B vaccination will be presented. The new concepts on vaccination strategies will be discussed. Also, the new advances on hepatitis B vaccinology will be presented.

Introduction

Hepatitis B virus (HBV) infection is a worldwide viral infection. The main mode of transmission is via blood contact. This infection is highly endemic in many developing countries. The infection is highly prevalent in Asia, Africa, southern Europe and Latin America. In addition, it becomes an important problem for medical personnel. Hospital staff and all other human or veterinary health care workers, including laboratory, research, emergency service, or cleaning personnel are exposed to the risk of occupational infection following accidental exposure to blood or body fluids (BBF) contaminated with this virus [1].

* * A version of this chapter was also published in *Hepatitis B Research Advances*, edited by Alicia P. Willis published by Nova Science Publishers, Inc. It was submitted for appropriate modifications in an effort to encourage wider dissemination of research.

Hepatitis B is a highly contagious viral infection and can lead to chronic carrier state and the hepatocellular carcinoma in the worst case. Around 450 million people worldwide are chronically infected with hepatitis B virus and are therefore at risk of developing chronic liver disease. To prevent is better than to treat this infection. Since 1985, the number of reported cases has declined as a direct result of universal immunization of neonates, vaccination of at-risk populations, lifestyle or behavioral changes in high-risk groups, refinements in the screening of blood donors, and the use of virally inactivated or genetically engineered products in patients with bleeding disorders [2]. At present, vaccination is an effective preventive measure for this disease. HBV vaccination has effectively reduced the acute and chronic infection rates as well as related complications in vaccinated children [3]. The incidence of hepatocellular carcinoma in children has been reduced to approximately 25% of the incidence before the vaccination program, and fulminant hepatitis in children has also been reduced after universal hepatitis B vaccination [3].

In this article, the topics on the hepatitis B vaccination will be presented. The new concepts on vaccination strategies will be discussed. Also, the new advances on hepatitis B vaccinology will be presented.

History of Hepatitis B Vaccine

Although the HBV was discovered about 40 years ago (1967) the hepatitis B vaccine is still new [4-6]. The development of the hepatitis B vaccine started in the late 1970's. At first, progressively sophisticated assays for hepatitis antigens and antibodies have been applied to the study of viral hepatitis epidemiology and biochemical-biophysical characterization of the agents [7]. On early phase, knowledge learned from such studies has been exploited to develop a prototype non-infectious but immunogenic hepatitis B vaccine using hepatitis B surface antigen (HBsAg) purified in large quantities from chronic HBsAg carriers [7]. Briefly, HBsAg was purified from human plasma by gel chromatography, isopyknic centrifugation, and zonal centrifugation [8]. Up to 65 % of the starting antigen was recovered at the end of the purification process. One dose of vaccine (1 ml) has a titre in HBsAg of 1/4 in countercurrent electrophoresis and a protein amount of 2-10 micron/ml [9]. In the early trial, treatment with formaldehyde concentrations up to 0.1% for inactivation of residual infectivity did not significantly reduce antigenicity in vitro and immunogenicity in guinea pigs [8]. The vaccine was also highly potent, inducing antibody in grivet monkeys and chimpanzees [10]. In human trials, the results, 2 years after immunization, suggested that the vaccine was protective against hepatitis B infection in high-risk hemodialysis settings [11]. Preliminary studies with an inactivated hepatitis B vaccine similarly prepared, but with aluminum hydroxide as adjuvant, indicate that such a preparation induces a more rapid and stronger anti-HBs response [11].

In the early 1980's, the first vaccine for hepatitis B was available in the USA [12]. However, there are many limitations for the human-derived hepatitis B vaccine.

The preparation of hepatitis B vaccine from a human source is restricted by the available supply of infected human plasma and by the need to apply stringent processes that purify the antigen and render it free of infectious HBV and other possible living agents that might be present in the plasma [13]. Therefore, the progression of the vaccine to recombinant vaccine started. Human hepatitis B vaccine from recombinant yeast is one of the first launched recombinant hepatitis B vaccines. Such vaccines would be free of the potential safety problems associated with plasma source material and could assure the continued supply of uniform HBsAg for vaccine use [14]. This vaccine was developed from recombinant yeast (*Saccharomyces cerevisiae*) cell culture [13]. With the present advances in biotechnology, recombinant DNA vaccines have been produced in prokaryotic and eukaryotic cells, notably in yeast [15]. The yeast-derived recombinant vaccine has proved safe and effective in extensive clinical trials, eliciting antibodies of equal quantity and quality of specificity to those elicited by plasma-derived vaccine [15].

Besides the attempts in the USA and Europe, there is also much hepatitis B vaccine research and many developments from other countries. For the endemic countries, investigation of HBV vaccine development in China was almost simultaneous with the same kind of work in the international community [16]. It seems that vaccination with the HBV vaccine in China has been successful and has obtained great achievements in the prevention and therapy of HB. Integration of the hepatitis B vaccine into newborn vaccination programmes on a worldwide basis represents a major step in the effort to eliminate this infectious disease and its complications [4]. Knowledge about the virus and the infection it causes led to the development of first, a plasma-derived vaccine and later a recombinant vaccine for the prevention of the infection [4]. However, there are still aspects of the hepatitis B vaccine which could be improved: three doses are needed for a full course of vaccination (which is sometimes difficult to achieve because of poor compliance or difficult logistic situations in some regions), there is a comparably high rate of non-responders to the vaccine (about 5% in adults) and, finally, it is possible that there are strains of HBV showing mutations of HBsAg which could escape the immunity induced by present vaccines [17]. To overcome these problems is the goal of the present hepatitis B vaccine development [17].

Types of Hepatitis B Vaccine

At present, hepatitis B vaccine is produced by a recombinant technique. There are many manufacturers that produce recombinant hepatitis B vaccine. RECOMBIVAX HB (Merck Sharpe & Dohme Ltd) is a good example of recombinant hepatitis B vaccine. It is produced based on *S. cerevisiae* and is indicated for vaccination against infection caused by all known subtypes of HBV [18]. Engerix-B (Smith Kline Biologicals) is another recombinant hepatitis B vaccine and has the same indication as RECOMBIVAX HB [19]. It is produced from genetically engineered yeast (*S. cerevisiae*) [19]. Intramuscular has excellent immunogenicity in healthy neonates and infants, children, adolescents and adults, with seroprotection rates of 85-100% seen approximately, 1 month after the final dose of vaccine [19]. There was a study by Hammond et al. conducted on the immunogenicity of these two yeast recombinant vaccines with different doses [RECOMBIVAX HB vs. Engerix-B] [20]. According to this report, the 95% confidence interval showed an overlap of the means of the GMT for both vaccine groups, and there was no significant difference in immunogenicity of these two vaccines [20]. Rustgi et al. performed another randomized trial to compare the safety and immunogenicity of Engerix-B administered intramuscularly (IM) at 0, 1, 2, and 12 months with RECOMBIVAX HB 10 micrograms administered IM at 0, 1, and 6 months in healthy adults [21]. According to this work, seroprotect rates were similar between the vaccination groups approximately 1 year after administration of the initial dose [21].

Recently, the oral hepatitis B vaccine was proposed. In 2006, oral hepatitis B vaccine formulation was prepared by successful encapsulation of an immunogenic peptide representing residues 127-145 of the immunodominant B-cell epitope of HBsAg in poly(D,L-lactide co-glycolide) (PLG) microparticles [22]. Single oral immunization of mice with BCEM led to the significant induction of specific serum IgG and IgM anti-HB antibodies [22]. After the termination of antibody induction, the orally immunized mice were infected with HBsAg, which resulted in the rapid production of antibodies against HBsAg as a result of secondary immune response [22].

Reported Side Effects of Hepatitis B Vaccination

Safety is a considerable factor for every vaccination. Side effects of vaccine must be closely monitored. Side effects of hepatitis B vaccine are also reported [23-24]. Immune response is believed to be the important factor leading to the side effect. The hypersensitivity type 3 is the possible main cause. Systemic lupus erythematosus (SLE) is an important adverse effect resulting from vaccination against hepatitis B [25-29]. During the past two decades, increasing numbers of reports regarding possible autoimmune side effects of vaccination have been published. However, the existing data does not link the vaccines and the autoimmune phenomena observed in a causal relationship, nevertheless a temporal connection has been described [30]. Hepatitis B vaccine might also be followed by other rheumatic conditions including rheumatoid arthritis and might trigger the onset of underlying inflammatory or autoimmune rheumatic diseases [31]. However, a causal relationship between hepatitis B vaccination and the observed rheumatic manifestations cannot be easily established [31].

Severe acute hepatitis B is another described side effect of hepatitis B vaccination [32-33]. The exact cause of this finding has not yet clarified. Neurological defects are also reported as adverse effects of hepatitis B vaccine. Many cases of multiple sclerosis following hepatitis B vaccination are reported [34-36]. The possibility that hepatitis B vaccine may cause or exacerbate multiple sclerosis stems from several case reports of onset or recurrence of symptoms of central nervous system demyelination shortly following vaccination [34-37]. The question is raised whether infectious agents or vaccines are involved in the pathogenesis or induced worsening of multiple sclerosis [38]. The possibility of activating autoantigen-specific T cells by pathogens or vaccines is raised [38]. According to a recent work, the multivariate relative risk of multiple sclerosis associated with exposure to the hepatitis B vaccine at any time before the onset of the disease was 0.9 and the relative risk associated with hepatitis B vaccination within two years before the onset of the disease was 0.7 [36]. In conclusion, there is only weak, nonspecific evidence to support the biological plausibility of an association between hepatitis B vaccine and multiple sclerosis [34-37]. In addition, epidemiological studies have found that hepatitis B vaccine does not increase the risk of developing multiple sclerosis or cause exacerbations [34-36]. Ascherio et al. conducted a nested case-control study in two large cohorts of nurses in the USA [36].

Expanded Programme for Immunization for Hepatitis B Vaccination

The first three priorities for hepatitis B immunization strategies in order of importance are: a) routine infant vaccination, b) prevention of perinatal HBV transmission and c) catch-up vaccination for older age groups. The infant vaccination is the focused plan for almost all countries. WHO documented that HBV infection is a vaccine preventable infection. Expanded Programme for Immunization (EPI) for hepatitis B vaccination was set. The implementation of the EPI has had a dramatic impact on HBV infection in many endemic countries. Since 1992, hepatitis B vaccine has been an integrated part of Thailand's EPI. According to a recent study of Poovorawan et al. for evaluation of the success of EPI in Thailand, the coverage rate of hepatitis B vaccination after its inclusion into the EPI 71.2-94.3% and only 0.7% of the children born after the implementation of this the novel EPI strategy were HBV carriers [39]. In Malaysia, the implementation of the EPI in 1989 has had a dramatic impact on hepatitis B virus (HBV) infection in school children [40]. The school children vaccinated under EPI had a 0.4% HBsAg carrier rate, which was significantly lower than school children vaccinated on a voluntary basis (HBsAg carrier rate 1.3%) and non-vaccinated school children (HBsAg carrier rate 2.7%), suggesting that HBV vaccination of infants was the most effective measure in preventing vertical transmission of HBV in the hyperendemic region [40]. In the Gambia, high vaccine coverage was achieved with EPI [41].

Table 1. Schedule for Hepatitis B Vaccination

Dose	Schedule
First	at birth
Second	2 months
Third	6 months

* For the general population: first injection - at any given time, second injection - at least 1 month after the first dose, third injection - 6 months after the first dose.

Prevention of Perinatal HBV Transmission

Vertical transmission of HBV is another important mode of infection. The infection by the hepatitis viruses, when appearing during pregnancy, could result in damage to the infant [42]. HBV infection, for which prevalence varies according to areas, is injurious when the mother is a chronic HBsAg carrier [42]. Risk consists of the neonate's contamination during labor, and if contaminated, the neonate becomes a chronic carrier in 80 to 90% of cases [42]. The high prevalence of HBsAg and hepatitis B e antigen (HBeAg) in pregnant women is considered to be the most important factor contributing to the high carrier rate of HBsAg in some populations [43]. The hepatitis B vaccination is a method for control of vertical transmission.

Van Steenbergen et al. said that tracing and immunizing susceptible contacts of women screened as HBsAg-positive, should be an integral component of any country's HBV control program [44]. Briefly, women at high risk for hepatitis B should be screened, including during pregnancy, by testing for hepatitis B core antibody [45]. Those at low risk should be screened by testing for HbsAg [45]. Susceptible high-risk women should be vaccinated;

pregnancy is not a contraindication [45]. Administration of hepatitis B immune globulin and vaccine to newborns is effective in preventing transmission from a hepatitis B-infected mother [45].

HBV Vaccination for the Elderly

For the non - endemic countries, the elderly are a vulnerable group of HBV infection. However, the infection is usually mild. Since the response rate to hepatitis B vaccination decreases with age, developing vaccines with greater immunogenicity is crucial [46]. The role of prophylaxis vaccination in the elderly is limited. The therapeutic vaccination is more frequently used. Since most of hepatitis B infection in the elderly are in the form of chronic carrier. The hepatitis B vaccination decreases serum HBV-DNA levels in the majority of patients with chronic HBV infection and sustained clearance can be achieved in some patients [47]. Combination of interferon-alpha with hepatitis B vaccine is effective for the vaccine failures and may increase sustained response compared to interferon-alpha alone; however, the mechanism of action is yet to be explained [47].

HBV Vaccination in HIV infected Patients

Co-infection between HBV and HIV is common since these two viruses share the common mode of transmission. Pathologically, HIV magnifies HBV viremia and the risk of HBV reactivation, chronic active HBV infection, cirrhosis, and death [48]. Because of these concerns, hepatitis B vaccination is also recommended for all HIV-positive persons lacking prior immunity. However, immune reactivity to hepatitis B vaccines is frequently suboptimal in terms of patients' rate of response, antibody titer, and durability [48]. Relatively high CD4+ T-cell counts (> or =500/mm3) and low levels of HIV viremia (<1,000 RNA genome copies/mL plasma) are necessary to ensure adequate hepatitis B vaccine response [48]. Revaccination should be instituted if post vaccination titers of antibodies to HbsAg are <10 mIU/mL (<10 IU/L) [48].

Winnock et al. performed an interesting study to gain insight into the attitude towards HBV and its vaccination in HIV seropositive patients [49]. According to this work, the main reasons for not prescribing HBV vaccine more often were forgetting, difficulty to identify subjects at risk and being afraid of post-vaccinal complications [49]. Therefore, there is no doubt about the usefulness of hepatitis B vaccination in HIV-infected patients. For HIV-infected with additional immunosuppressive pathology, this recommendation can also be applied. Ahuja et al. found that hepatitis B vaccination should be offered to all HIV-infected end stage renal disease (ESRD) patients because over half of the patients with HIV and ESRD can develop protection. [50].

However, an important problem of hepatitis B vaccination in HIV patient is that the HIV patients are usually vaccine hyporesponsive. CPG 7909, a synthetic oligodeoxynucleotide containing immunostimulatory CpG motifs, is a new adjuvant to hepatitis B vaccine that is reported to enhance the effectiveness of vaccination in HIV-infected cases [51]. Addition of

CPG 7909 achieves rapid, higher, and sustained HBV seroprotection and increases HBV-specific T helper cell response to HBV vaccine in HIV-infected subjects [51].

HBV Vaccination in the Patients Requiring Hemodialysis

Ever since the first outbreaks of hepatitis in hemodialysis units in the late 1960s, a number of hepatotropic viruses transmitted by blood and other body fluids have been identified [52]. HBV was the first significant hepatotropic virus to be identified in hemodialysis centers [52]. HBV infection has been effectively controlled by active vaccination, screening of blood donors, the use of erythropoietin, and segregation of HBV carriers [52]. Hepatitis B vaccination is recommended for the hemodialytic cases [53-54]. Miller et al. suggested that hepatitis B vaccine had a significant protective effect against acquiring HBV infection in chronic hemodialysis patients, and efforts should be expanded to increase the use of hepatitis B vaccine in this patient population [55]. They found that the risk for HBV infection was 70% lower in vaccinated patients [55]. However, the problems of vaccination are reported. The main problem is the low response, which is believed to relate to host-related and immunization-related causes [53]. Various possibilities to improve the vaccine performance through appropriate dosage and schedule, as well as immunopotentiating procedures are reported [53]. Oddone et al. performed an interesting study to assess the cost effectiveness of hepatitis B vaccine in predialysis patients in 1993 [56]. They found that additional HBV infection could be prevented by immunizing predialysis patients, but the cost is high [56]. They concluded that decisions concerning vaccination policy should be influenced by local prevalence of HBV infection [56].

HBV Vaccination for the Traveler

Long distance journeys are more and more frequent [57]. In certain instances, one shall consider vaccination against hepatitis B [57-59]. Routine childhood vaccinations may need to be accelerated for young infants traveling before the standard primary vaccine series can be completed [59]. Since last minute protection of hepatitis B vaccine can be expected, full dosage is required [60-61]. However, many travelers depart within weeks of planning their trip (too late to complete the accelerated 0, 1, 2 month regimen for hepatitis B), and a majority of those traveling depart without being vaccinated [62]. Although extended-stay travelers are at high risk for hepatitis B, short-stay travelers also are at risk [62]. Connor et al. found that most US travelers to hepatitis B endemic regions did not secure pre-travel health advice, and most had not received three doses of hepatitis B vaccine [60]. Substantial shares are candidates for hepatitis B vaccination based on their domestic activities, and/or face hepatitis B risks during travel [60]. A new accelerated, 3-dose regimen on a 0,7 and 21-day schedule suggest that excellent, rapid, and long-term protection might be conferred [62].

HBV Vaccination for Health Care Workers

Health care workers are a population at risk for HBV infection via blood and blood product contact [63]. The outcomes following infection can be significant in terms of both health and employment [64]. It is for these reasons that effective preventative health care is the goal of occupational health practitioners [64]. It therefore is critical for health care workers to encourage the development and assessment of effective preventive and control strategies, including the design and use of safe devices, targeted interventions based on occupation-specific hazards, and surveillance and analysis of exposures in the health care setting [65]. Hepatitis B vaccination is a good preventative for the health care worker. Mihaly et al. said that vaccination was an effective tool in hepatitis B prevention [66]. They noted that every effort had to be made to promote hepatitis B immunity to all health care workers and strictly follow hygienic preventive measures [66]. However, Jefferson et al. performed a metanalysis and found that plasma-derived vaccines appeared to be efficacious and safe for use in high-risk health-care workers, such as the staff of renal dialysis and transplant units [67]. They also found that there was some uncertainty concerning the effectiveness of the vaccine in lower risk health-care workers, although the trend is towards benefit [67]. Chen and Gluud performed another metanalysis to assess the beneficial and harmful effects of hepatitis B vaccination in health-care workers [68]. They found that the intramuscular route with 20 microgram recombinant vaccine was significantly more effective compared with the intradermal route with 2 microgram recombinant vaccine as was the standard schedule compared with a rapid schedule and deltoid intramuscular injection compared with the gluteal intramuscular injection [68]. However, they noted that it was unclear if booster vaccination of non-responders offers higher anti-HBs seroconversion and hepatitis B vaccine prevented the infection of hepatitis B mutants in health-care workers [68]. In addition to the general health care worker, health science students form a high-risk group for infection with blood-borne pathogens, including HBV [69]. Wiwanitkit found that more than 40% of the pre-clinical students did not know their HBV status and fewer than 50% had been vaccinated against the virus [69]. Wiwanitkit proposed that those students entering medical schools for the first time clearly need to be better educated about hepatitis B and to be encouraged to be vaccinated before they begin any clinical practices [69].

Although hepatitis B vaccination is accepted as being useful for health care workers, the cost effectiveness of universal vaccination is still doubtful [67,70]. Pre-selection is considered. Many strategies including interviewing and serological screening are proposed [71]. The decisions must be based on the epidemiological data and the cost effectiveness analysis for each setting.

Vaccine Escape Mutant: a new Problem of Hepatitis B Vaccination

Vaccine escape mutant is a new problem of hepatitis B vaccination. The HBV has evolved a unique life cycle resulting in the production of enormous viral loads during active replication without actually directly killing the infected cell [72]. Because the virus uses reverse transcription to copy its DNA genome, mutant viral genomes are frequently found

[72]. Particular selection pressures, both endogenous (host immune clearance) and exogenous (vaccines and antivirals), readily select out these escape mutants [72]. Cooreman et al. proposed that most escape mutations that influence HBsAg recognition by anti-HBs antibodies were located in the second 'a' determinant loop [73]. Notably, HBsAg with an arginine replacement for glycine at amino acid 145 is considered the quintessential immune escape mutant because it has been isolated consistently in clinical samples of HBIg-treated individuals and vaccinated infants of chronically infected mothers [73]. Cooreman et al. proposed that vaccine- and hepatitis B immune globulin might induce escape mutations of HbsAg [73]. Finding of the new recombinant vaccine to overcome the problem of vaccine escape mutant becomes a new focus on hepatitis B vaccinology. In 1999, Ogata et al. first reported their successful licensed recombinant hepatitis B vaccines that could protect chimpanzees against infection with the prototype surface gene mutant of HBV [74]. Several trials on other new vaccines are presently ongoing.

References

[1] Tarantola A, Abiteboul D, Rachline A. Infection risks following accidental exposure to blood or body fluids in health care workers: a review of pathogens transmitted in published cases. *Am J Infect Control.* 2006 Aug;34(6):367-75.

[2] Hollinger FB, Lau DT. Hepatitis B: the pathway to recovery through treatment. *Gastroenterol Clin North Am.* 2006 Jun;35(2):425-61, x.

[3] Chang MH. Impact of hepatitis B vaccination on hepatitis B disease and nucleic acid testing in high-prevalence populations. *J Clin Virol.* 2006 May;36 Suppl 1:S45-50

[4] Yap SF. Hepatitis B: review of development from the discovery of the "Australia Antigen" to end of the twentieth Century. *Malays J Pathol.* 2004 Jun;26(1):1-12.

[5] Percell RH. Hepatitis B: a scientific success story (almost). *Prog Clin Biol Res.* 1985;182:11-43.

[6] Blumberg BS. The discovery of the hepatitis B virus and the invention of the vaccine: a scientific memoir. *J Gastroenterol Hepatol.* 2002 Dec;17 Suppl:S502-

[7] Katkov WN. Hepatitis vaccines. *Med Clin North Am.* 1996 Sep;80(5):1189-200.

[8] Stamm B, Gerlich W, Thomssen R. Experiments for the development of a hepatitis B vaccine: immunogenicity of HBsAg in guinea pigs (author's transl)]. *Med Microbiol Immunol (Berl).* 1979 May 15;167(2):83-97.

[9] Barin F, Andre M, Goudeau A, Coursaget P, Maupas P. Large scale purification of hepatitis B surface antigen (HBsAg). *Ann Microbiol (Paris).* 1978 Jul;129B(1):87-100.

[10] Buynak EB, Roehm RR, Tytell AA, Bertland AU 2nd, Lampson GP, Hilleman MR. Development and chimpanzee testing of a vaccine against human hepatitis B. *Proc Soc Exp Biol Med.* 1976 Apr;151(4):694-700.

[11] Maupas P, Goudeau A, Coursaget P, Drucker J, Bagros P. Hepatitis B vaccine: efficacy in high-risk settings, a two-year study. I*ntervirology.* 1978;10(3):196-208.

[12] Dienstag JL, Purcell RH. Recent advances in the identification of hepatitis viruses. *Postgrad Med J.* 1977 Jul;53(621):364-73.

[13] McAleer WJ, Buynak EB, Maigetter RZ, Wampler DE, Miller WJ, Hilleman MR. Human hepatitis B vaccine from recombinant yeast. *Nature*. 1984 Jan 12-18;307(5947):178-80.
[14] Gerin JL, Purcell RH. New approaches to hepatitis B vaccines. *Prog Clin Biol Res*. 1983;143:369-77.
[15] Zuckerman AJ. Novel hepatitis B vaccines. *J Infect*. 1986 Jul;13 Suppl A:61-71.
[16] Tao Q, Feng B. Prevention and therapy of hepatitis B. *Chin Med J (Engl)*. 1999 Oct;112(10):942-6.
[17] Jilg W. Novel hepatitis B vaccines. *Vaccine*. 1998 Nov;16 Suppl:S65-8.
[18] Venters C, Graham W, Cassidy W. Recombivax-HB: perspectives past, present and future. *Expert Rev Vaccines*. 2004 Apr;3(2):119-29.
[19] Keating GM, Noble S. Recombinant hepatitis B vaccine (Engerix-B): a review of its immunogenicity and protective efficacy against hepatitis B. *Drugs*. 2003;63(10):1021-51.
[20] Hammond GW, Parker J, Mimms L, Tate R, Sekla L, Minuk G. Comparison of immunogenicity of two yeast-derived recombinant hepatitis B vaccines. *Vaccine*. 1991 Feb;9(2):97-100.
[21] Rustgi VK, Schleupner CJ, Krause DS. Comparative study of the immunogenicity and safety of Engerix-B administered at 0, 1, 2 and 12 months and Recombivax HB administered at 0, 1, and 6 months in healthy adults. *Vaccine*. 1995 Dec;13(17):1665-8.
[22] Rajkannan R, Dhanaraju MD, Gopinath D, Selvaraj D, Jayakumar R. Development of hepatitis B oral vaccine using B-cell epitope loaded PLG microparticles. *Vaccine*. 2006 Jun 12;24(24):5149-57.
[23] Carmeli Y, Oren R. Hepatitis B vaccine side-effect. *Lancet*. 1993 Jan 23;341(8839):250-1.
[24] Fields HA, Mahoney FJ, Margolis HS. Safety of hepatitis B vaccine. *Science*. 1996 May 3;272(5262):633-4.
[25] Tudela P, Marti S, Bonal J. Systemic lupus erythematosus and vaccination against hepatitis B. *Nephron*. 1992;62(2):236.
[26] Guiserix J. Systemic lupus erythematosus following hepatitis B vaccine. *Nephron*. 1996;74(2):441.
[27] Maillefert JF, Tavernier C, Sibilia J, Vignon E. Exacerbation of systemic lupus erythematosus after hepatitis B vaccination: comment on the article by Battafarano et al and the letter by Senecal et al. *Arthritis Rheum*. 2000 Feb;43(2):468-9.
[28] Senecal JL, Bertrand C, Coutlee F. Severe exacerbation of systemic lupus erythematosus after hepatitis B vaccination and importance of pneumococcal vaccination in patients with autosplenectomy: comment on the article by Battafarano et al. *Arthritis Rheum*. 1999 Jun;42(6):1307-8.
[29] Fineschi S. Can recombinant anti-hepatitis B vaccine be a cause of systemic lupus erythematosus? *Lupus*. 2001;10(11):830.
[30] Aron-Maor A, Shoenfeld Y. Vaccination and systemic lupus erythematosus: the bidirectional dilemmas. *Lupus*. 2001;10(3):237-40.
[31] Maillefert JF, Sibilia J, Toussirot E, Vignon E, Eschard JP, Lorcerie B, Juvin R, Parchin-Geneste N, Piroth C, Wendling D, Kuntz JL, Tavernier C, Gaudin P. Rheumatic disorders developed after hepatitis B vaccination. *Rheumatology (Oxford)*. 1999 Oct;38(10):978-83.

[32] Ballinger AB, Clark ML. Severe acute hepatitis B infection after vaccination. *Lancet.* 1994 Nov 5;344(8932):1292.

[33] Lilic D, Ghosh SK. Liver dysfunction and DNA antibodies after hepatitis B vaccination. *Lancet.* 1994 Nov 5;344(8932):1292-3

[34] Salleras L, Bruguera M, Prat A. Hepatitis B vaccine and multiple sclerosis: an unproved association. *Med Clin (Barc).* 2006 Apr 22;126(15):581-8.

[35] DeStefano F, Verstraeten T, Chen RT. Hepatitis B vaccine and risk of multiple sclerosis. *Expert Rev Vaccines.* 2002 Dec;1(4):461-6.

[36] Ascherio A, Zhang SM, Hernan MA, Olek MJ, Coplan PM, Brodovicz K, Walker AM. Hepatitis B vaccination and the risk of multiple sclerosis. *N Engl J Med.* 2001 Feb 1;344(5):327-32.

[37] Demicheli V, Rivetti A, Di Pietrantonj C, Clements CJ, Jefferson T. Hepatitis B vaccination and multiple sclerosis: evidence from a systematic review. *J Viral Hepat.* 2003 Sep;10(5):343-4.

[38] Zipp F, Wandinger KP. Current concepts on vaccinations in multiple sclerosis. *Nervenarzt.* 2001 Oct;72(10):802-6.

[39] Poovorawan Y, Theamboonlers A, Vimolket T, Sinlaparatsamee S, Chaiear K, Siraprapasiri T, Khwanjaipanich S, Owatanapanich S, Hirsch P, Chunsuttiwat S. Impact of hepatitis B immunisation as part of the EPI. *Vaccine.* 2000 Nov 22;19(7-8):943-9.

[40] Ng KP, Saw TL, Baki A, Rozainah K, Pang KW, Ramanathan M. Impact of the Expanded Program of Immunization against hepatitis B infection in school children in Malaysia. *Med Microbiol Immunol (Berl).* 2005 May;194(3):163-8.

[41] Viviani S, Mendy M, Jack AD, Hall AJ, Montesano R, Whittle HC. EPI vaccines-induced antibody prevalence in 8-9 year-olds in The Gambia. *Trop Med Int Health.* 2004 Oct;9(10):1044-9.

[42] Ranger-Rogez S, Alain S, Denis F. Hepatitis viruses: mother to child transmission. *Pathol Biol (Paris).* 2002 Nov;50(9):568-75.

[43] Vranckx R, Alisjahbana A, Meheus A. Hepatitis B virus vaccination and antenatal transmission of HBV markers to neonates. *J Viral Hepat.* 1999 Mar;6(2):135-9.

[44] van Steenbergen JE, Baayen D, Peerbooms PG, Coutinho RA, Van Den Hoek A. Much gained by integrating contact tracing and vaccination in the hepatitis B antenatal screening program in Amsterdam, 1992-1999. *J Hepatol.* 2004 Jun;40(6):979-85.

[45] Culpepper L. Preventing hepatitis B: focus on women and their families. *J Am Board Fam Pract.* 1993 Sep-Oct;6(5):483-91.

[46] Marcus EL, Tur-Kaspa R. Viral hepatitis in older adults. *J Am Geriatr Soc.* 1997 Jun;45(6):755-63.

[47] Senturk H, Tabak F, Akdogan M, Erdem L, Mert A, Ozaras R, Sander E, Ozbay G, Badur S. Therapeutic vaccination in chronic hepatitis B. *J Gastroenterol Hepatol.* 2002 Jan;17(1):72-6.

[48] Laurence JC. Hepatitis A and B immunizations of individuals infected with human immunodeficiency virus. *Am J Med.* 2005 Oct;118 Suppl 10A:75S-83S.

[49] Winnock M, Neau D, Castera L, Viot J, Lacoste D, Pellegrin JL, Dupon M, Jutand MA, Colombani F, Dabis F; Groupe d'Epidemiologie Clinique du SIDA en Aquitaine. Hepatitis B vaccination in HIV-infected patients: a survey of physicians and patients participating in the Aquitaine cohort. *Gastroenterol Clin Biol.* 2006 Feb;30(2):189-95.

[50] Ahuja TS, Kumar S, Mansoury H, Rodriguez H, Kuo YF. Hepatitis B vaccination in human immunodeficiency virus-infected adults receiving hemodialysis. *Kidney Int.* 2005 Mar;67(3):1136-41.

[51] Cooper CL, Davis HL, Angel JB, Morris ML, Elfer SM, Seguin I, Krieg AM, Cameron DW. CPG 7909 adjuvant improves hepatitis B virus vaccine seroprotection in antiretroviral-treated HIV-infected adults. *AIDS.* 2005 Sep 23;19(14):1473-9.

[52] Tang S, Lai KN. Chronic viral hepatitis in hemodialysis patients. *Hemodial Int.* 2005 Apr;9(2):169-79.

[53] Rapicetta M. Hepatitis B vaccination in dialysis centres: advantages and limits. *Nephron.* 1992;61(3):284-6.

[54] Davis JP. Experience with hepatitis A and B vaccines. *Am J Med.* 2005 Oct;118 Suppl 10A:7S-15S.

[55] Miller ER, Alter MJ, Tokars JI. Protective effect of hepatitis B vaccine in chronic hemodialysis patients. *Am J Kidney Dis.* 1999 Feb;33(2):356-60.

[56] Oddone EZ, Cowper PA, Hamilton JD, Feussner JR. A cost-effectiveness analysis of hepatitis B vaccine in predialysis patients. *Health Serv Res.* 1993 Apr;28(1):97-121.

[57] Van Laethem Y. Vaccinations for the traveler. J Pharm Belg. 2002 Nov-Dec;57(6):130-4.

[58] Marchou B, Picot N, Massip P. Vaccinations of the traveller. *Ann Med Interne (Paris).* 1998 Oct;149(6):332-9.

[59] Mackell SM. Vaccinations for the pediatric traveler. *Clin Infect Dis.* 2003 Dec 1;37(11):1508-16.

[60] Connor BA, Jacobs RJ, Meyerhoff AS. Hepatitis B risks and immunization coverage among American travelers. *J Travel Med.* 2006 Sep-Oct;13(5):273-80.

[61] Birkenfeld G. Last minute vaccinations. MMW Fortschr Med. 2006 Jun 29;148(26):24-6.

[62] Keystone JS. Travel-related hepatitis B: risk factors and prevention using an accelerated vaccination schedule. *Am J Med.* 2005 Oct;118 Suppl 10A:63S-68S.

[63] Occupational transmission of hepatitis B. *Plast Surg Nurs.* 2003 Winter;23(4):160-3.

[64] Murphy E. Hepatitis B, vaccination and healthcare workers. *Occup Med (Lond).* 2000 Aug;50(6):383-6.

[65] Lanphear BP. Transmission and control of bloodborne viral hepatitis in health care workers. *Occup Med.* 1997 Oct-Dec;12(4):717-30.

[66] Mihaly I, Nagy E, Ibranyi E, Majoros I, Lukacs A. Effect of vaccination on the risk of hepatitis B infection in hospital personnel. *Orv Hetil.* 1996 Mar 31;137(13):681-5.

[67] Jefferson T, Demicheli V, Deeks J, MacMillan A, Sassi F, Pratt M. Vaccines for preventing hepatitis B in health-care workers. *Cochrane Database Syst Rev.* 2000;(2):CD000100.

[68] Chen W, Gluud C. Vaccines for preventing hepatitis B in health-care workers. *Cochrane Database Syst Rev.* 2005 Oct 19;(4):CD000100.

[69] Wiwanitkit V. How medical students in their pre-clinical year perceive their own hepatitis-B-virus status: the results of a study in a Thai medical school. *Ann Trop Med Parasitol.* 2002 Sep;96(6):627-30.

[70] Lohiya G, Lohiya S, Caires S, Reesal MR. Occupational exposure to hepatitis B virus. Analysis of indications for hepatitis B vaccine. *J Occup Med.* 1984 Mar;26(3):189-96.

[71] Perrillo RP. Screening of health care workers before hepatitis B vaccination: more questions than answers. *Ann Intern Med.* 1985 Nov;103(5):793-5.

[72] Locarnini S, McMillan J, Bartholomeusz A. The hepatitis B virus and common mutants. *Semin Liver Dis.* 2003 Feb;23(1):5-20.

[73] Cooreman MP, Leroux-Roels G, Paulij WP. Vaccine- and hepatitis B immune globulin-induced escape mutations of hepatitis B virus surface antigen. *J Biomed Sci.* 2001 May-Jun;8(3):237-47.

[74] Ogata N, Cote PJ, Zanetti AR, Miller RH, Shapiro M, Gerin J, Purcell RH. Licensed recombinant hepatitis B vaccines protect chimpanzees against infection with the prototype surface gene mutant of hepatitis B virus. *Hepatology.* 1999 Sep;30(3):779-86.

In: Vaccinations: Types, Potential Complications...
Editors: D. B. Steen and H. L. Dyson
ISBN: 978-1-60692-969-8

Chapter IV

Smallpox Vaccine Stockpile and Vaccination Policy*

Judith A. Johnson
Specialist in Life Sciences, Domestic Social Policy Division,
United States of American

Abstract

On June 20, 2002, an advisory panel to the U.S. Centers for Disease Control and Prevention (CDC) voted against mass smallpox vaccination and instead recommended that 10-20 thousand first responders receive the vaccine. The recommendations are currently under review by CDC and the Department of Health and Human Services (HHS). Congress addresses control of the vaccine stockpile in the Homeland Security legislation (H.R. 5005, S. 2452). Although there is little uneasiness over the safety of the only known samples of variola virus, held by the CDC in Atlanta and a laboratory near Novosibirsk in Russia, there is some concern that samples of the virus may have been acquired by terrorists or rogue governments, particularly because of the unrest that occurred during the break up of the Soviet Union. The Public Health Security and Bioterrorism Preparedness and Response Act of 2002 (P.L. 107-188), signed by the President on June 12, 2002, directs the Secretary of HHS to ensure that there is enough smallpox vaccine in the Strategic National Stockpile to meet health security needs and authorizes $509 million for FY2002 and such sums as may be necessary through FY2006 for this purpose. H.R. 5005, the Homeland Security Act of 2002 as passed by the House, would amend P.L. 107-188 by moving authority for the stockpile to the Department of Homeland Security (DHS); HHS would continue to manage the stockpile and determine its contents. S. 2452, the National Homeland Security and Combating Terrorism Act of 2002, as reported by the Governmental Affairs Committee on July 25, 2002, directs DHS to consult with CDC in the administration of the stockpile by CDC. An emergency

* * A version of this chapter was also published in *Focus on Bioterrorism*, edited by George T. Foster published by Nova Science Publishers, Inc. It was submitted for appropriate modifications in an effort to encourage wider dissemination of research.

supplemental appropriation (P.L. 107-117), signed by the President on January 10, 2002, provided $512 million for the purchase of smallpox vaccine by HHS.

On June 20, 2002, an advisory panel to the U.S. Centers for Disease Control and Prevention (CDC) voted against mass smallpox vaccination and instead recommended that 10-20 thousand first responders receive the vaccine. The recommendations are currently under review by CDC and the Department of Health and Human Services (HHS). Congress addresses control of the vaccine stockpile in the Homeland Security legislation (H.R. 5005, S. 2452).

The terrorist attacks of the fall of 2001 resulted in increased attention to preparedness for other such possible events, one being the deliberate release of variola virus, the virus which causes smallpox. Although there is little uneasiness over the safety of the only known samples of variola virus, held by the CDC in Atlanta and a laboratory near Novosibirsk in Russia, there is some concern that samples of the virus may have been acquired by terrorists or rogue governments, particularly because of the unrest that occurred during the break up of the Soviet Union.

Smallpox is transmitted via person-to-person contact or inhalation of saliva droplets in the breath of an infected person. The incubation period of 12-14 days (range 7-17 days) is followed by the sudden onset of flu-like symptoms. After 2-3 days the distinctive rash begins to appear, and it is this stage, which lasts for 7-10 days, that is most infectious. As scabs begin to form infectivity rapidly declines. About 65% to 80% of survivors have deep scars or pockmarks that tend to occur on the face. After a worldwide effort of organized vaccination, smallpox was declared eradicated by the World Health Assembly in May 1980.[1] Smallpox vaccination is achieved via inoculation using live vaccinia virus, a virus linked with cowpox. Vaccination is highly effective and can prevent smallpox even when given 2 to 3 days after exposure to variola. The last recorded natural case of smallpox occurred in Somalia in 1977; a fatal laboratory-acquired case occurred in the United Kingdom in 1978. The last U.S. case was in 1949. The U.S. Public Health Service recommended in 1971 that routine smallpox vaccination be discontinued and the U.S. program stopped in 1972.

An unfortunate side effect of the eradication of smallpox, widely acclaimed as a major public health triumph, is that the U.S. population and the rest of the world are vulnerable to biologic weapon attack using variola virus. In past natural outbreaks, smallpox killed 30% of those who had no immunity. Approximately 119 million U.S. residents born after 1972 lack immunity. The immunity of the 157 million U.S. residents born before 1972 has declined and their level of disease protection is uncertain.

Because of these facts, CDC and HHS asked the Advisory Committee on Immunization Practices (ACIP) to consider if changes were needed in the June 2001 recommendations on smallpox vaccination.[2] Under the June 2001 recommendations, only laboratory workers who directly handle smallpox-related virus are vaccinated. After several public meetings, draft recommendations on smallpox vaccination were approved by ACIP on June 20, 2002. ACIP did not recommend smallpox vaccination of the general public because "the risk of an attack

---

[1] The World Health Assembly determines policy and budget for the World Health Organization.

[2] ACIP is a 15 member group of medical and public health experts that provides advice to HHS and CDC on vaccine use and policy for effective disease control in the civilian population.

was assessed to be low"...[and] "the potential benefits of vaccination do not outweigh the risks of vaccine complications." Instead ACIP recommended that 10 to 20 thousand first responders receive the vaccine. These individuals would act in teams investigating initial smallpox cases and vaccinating the patient's contacts. Under the ACIP plan, healthcare personnel at a limited number of hospitals involved in caring for smallpox patients would also be vaccinated.

The ACIP draft recommendations are now being considered by CDC and HHS.[3] Media reports of July 7, 2002, indicate that the federal government will possibly expand the number of individuals vaccinated to 500,000 first responders and emergency room personnel.[4] However, other media sources indicate that reports of such an expansion in the numbers of those vaccinated are inaccurate; HHS will release its implementation plan by the end of July.[5] States could begin receiving vaccine as early as September.

Increasing the number of healthcare personnel vaccinated may be in response to criticism of the ACIP proposal. The Executive Director of the American Public Health Association, Mohammad Akhter, stated that in the event of a smallpox outbreak, victims would head to the nearest hospital rather than a ACIP designated hospital. He was also concerned that the small number of designated hospitals would become overwhelmed by such patients, and therefore advocated that all emergency room personnel should be vaccinated. The Federation of American Hospitals expressed similar concerns, and supports vaccinating more health care workers than under the ACIP plan.[6]

Federal officials are hesitant to recommend vaccination of the general public because smallpox vaccine has a higher complication rate than any other vaccine in current use. An estimated 28 million people with eczema and 10 million people with a compromised immune system (organ transplant recipients, HIV/AIDS or cancer patients), or 15% of the population, are at high risk for developing serious complications.[7] Such complications will also occur in the rest of the population, but at a lower rate. Liability problems associated with smallpox vaccine could be enormous. The serious complications include:

- postvaccinial encephalitis may be fatal or leave survivors with paralysis or other central nervous system symptoms;
- progressive vaccinia, or growth of the vaccination lesion without healing, occurs in immunocompromised individuals and is often fatal;
- fetal vaccinia, passage of vaccinia to a fetus, may lead to stillbirth;
- eczema vaccinatum, or development of vaccinial lesions over sites where there is or has been eczema, may be fatal.

---

[3] The draft recommendations can be found at: [www.cdc.gov/nip/smallpox/supp_recs.htm].

[4] Broad, W. U.S. to Vaccinate 500,000 Workers Against Smallpox. *The New York Times*, July 7,2002. p. A1, A16.

[5] Hawana, J.S. Advance Smallpox Vaccination Recommended in PNAS Report; HHS plan due by end of July. *Washington Fax*, July 9, 2002.

[6] Young, J. Proposal to Designate Smallpox Response Center Hospitals Evokes Concerns. *Washington Fax*, June 26, 2002.

[7] Kemper, A.M., et al. Expected Adverse Events in a Mass Smallpox Vaccination Campaign. *Effective Clinical Practice*, v. 5, March/April 2002. p. 84-90.

Complications may occur in individuals who don't even receive the vaccine, but are only exposed to someone who has recently been vaccinated. In fact, eczema vaccinatum is more severe among unvaccinated persons exposed to a vaccine recipient than among recent vaccine recipients. One recent study found that even if high risk individuals and their household contacts (25% of the U.S. population) were excluded from vaccination, an estimated 1600 serious adverse events and 190 deaths would occur if people aged 1 to 29 years were vaccinated, and 4600 serious adverse events and 285 deaths would occur if people aged 1 to 65 years were vaccinated.[8] Less serious complications of vaccination include rash, fever, and accidental inoculation, in which the rash occurs elsewhere on the body (from the vaccination site) due to direct contact with vaccinia. Blindness may result if the rash develops near the eye.

Federal vaccination policy must balance the certainty of the adverse effects of smallpox vaccine against the uncertainty of a biowarfare attack using variola virus. In the past, naturally occurring outbreaks of smallpox have been controlled using ring vaccination: all the patient's contacts are tracked down, vaccinated and quarantined until the disease spread is stopped. Such a strategy is logical if there is limited vaccine, or a significant level of smallpox immunity in the population, or if a society wishes to limit the number of adverse events and fatalities caused by mass smallpox vaccination. However, in a modern society with low levels of smallpox immunity, mass transit and rapid forms of long distance travel, ring vaccination may not be feasible especially if the attack occurs in many sites and is relatively large. Moreover, our social and economic system may be greatly stressed by the necessary implementation of quarantine.

Researchers are using mathematical models of disease transmission to determine the outcome of a smallpox attack under a range of different conditions, such as the number of initial infections, the transmission rate (number of secondary cases caused by each initial case), the number of vaccinators, and whether ring or mass vaccination is used to control the outbreak. The models are still under development and provide contradictory results. For example, a model developed by researchers at Emory University found that "ring vaccination, even when it's started only after the 25th case of smallpox, can contain an epidemic almost as well as mass vaccination, provided that at least 80% of those exposed can be found and vaccinated."[9] In contrast, a model developed at Yale University found that "mass vaccination results in far fewer deaths and much faster epidemic eradication."[10] The Yale model predicts that in a smallpox attack on a large city causing 1000 initial cases, ring vaccination results in 367,000 cases and 110,000 deaths over 350 days, but mass vaccination following an attack results in 1,830 cases and 560 deaths over 115 days. However, if 40% of the population is vaccinated prior to attack, the number of deaths under ring vaccination and mass vaccination are 40,000 and 440 respectively. The Yale group concludes "that unless pre-attack vaccination is used ..., serious consideration should be given to replacing the existing CDC policy [with] mass vaccination in the event of a smallpox attack in a large urban center."

---

8 Ibid.

9 Enserink, M. How Devastating Would a Smallpox Attack Really Be? *Science*, May 31, 2002. p. 1592-1595.

10 Kaplan, E.H. et al. Emergency Response to a Smallpox Attack: the Case for Mass Vaccination. *Proceedings of the National Academy of Sciences, Early Edition*, July 8, 2002. [www.pnas.org]

Traditional methods, like ring vaccination, are based on the fact that smallpox spreads through person-to-person contact. A controversial report, presented at a June 2002 meeting on smallpox vaccination policy, indicates that aerosolized smallpox virus from a Soviet bioweapon test may have accidently caused 10 cases of smallpox and three deaths in 1971 in what is now Aralsk, Kazakhstan.[11] Previously, scientists believed that aerosolized smallpox virus would be inactivated by environmental factors, such as UV radiation from the sun. However, the authors believe the best explanation for the outbreak is that the initial case acquired smallpox when her boat entered waters downwind from a Soviet bioweapons test site located on an Aral sea island. Because an aerosol of smallpox virus would have the potential to infect a larger number of people than person to person contact, this chapter is of concern to public health experts.

Although the 119 million unvaccinated people in the U.S. would face a mortality rate of about 30% in a smallpox attack, there is some question over the level of protection remaining in the 157 million individuals who were vaccinated more than 30 years ago. Complete protection from smallpox disease begins to taper off 3 to 5 years after vaccination. However, some historical data indicate that vaccinated individuals may experience milder disease symptoms and a lower mortality rate (5%) even up to 50 years post-vaccination.[12] Additional studies would be needed to confirm this point, but if correct, a smallpox attack might not be as deadly or spread as rapidly as some experts had thought. It might also influence decisions on who in the U.S. population should be the first to receive vaccines if a smallpox attack does take place.

Within the last year, HHS has been successful in greatly increasing the U.S. stockpile of smallpox vaccine via agreements with three separate sources: Wyeth Laboratories, a pharmaceutical company located in Marietta, PA; Acambis, a British drug firm with offices in Cambridge, MA; and Aventis Pasteur, a French vaccine company with a plant in Swiftwater, PA. The policy debate by ACIP and others on how many U.S. residents should be vaccinated has been made possible by HHS efforts to increase the U.S. stockpile of smallpox vaccine.

In the fall of 2001, the National Institute of Health (NIH) funded a study on whether the 15.4 million doses of smallpox vaccine in the U.S. stockpile could be diluted without losing its potency. The vaccine, called Dryvax, was manufactured by Wyeth in 1982. Results of the study, released in April 2002, indicate that the Dryvax can be safely diluted by a factor of 5 or 10. In 97% to 99% of study participants the diluted vaccine produced a "take" or skin lesion, a positive indicator of a protective immune response.[13] Although none of the 680 study subjects, aged 18 to 32, had a serious adverse reaction, there was a high frequency of pain, swelling and redness at the inoculation site as well as fever headache, rash, muscle aches, fatigue and chills. More than a third of the subjects missed work, school, sleep, or other activities because of an adverse reaction.

In November 2001, HHS placed a rush order for an additional 155 million doses of smallpox vaccine (beyond an initial order of 54 million doses) with Acambis. Clinical trials

---

[11] Enserink, M. Did Bioweapons Test Cause a Deadly Smallpox Outbreak? *Science*, June 21, 2002. p. 2116-2117.

[12] Cohen, J. Smallpox Vaccinations: How Much Protection Remains? *Science*, v. 294. November 2, 2001. p. 985.

[13] Frey, S.E. et al. Clinical Responses to Undiluted and Diluted Smallpox Vaccine. *The New England Journal of Medicine*, v. 346, April 25, 2002. p. 1265-1273.

of the vaccine began in March 2002.[14] The vaccine is a single strain of vaccinia, in contrast to the mixture in Dryvax, and is produced in a cell culture rather than the traditional method which used cows or calves. Although animal studies indicate that the Acambis version may have a lower risk of causing encephalitis, the other side effects are expected to be about the same as the traditional vaccine. Acambis expects to deliver the vaccine order by the end of 2002. At the end of March 2002, Aventis announced that it would donate to the U.S. government about 85 million doses of smallpox vaccine that were manufactured in 1958 for the U.S. Department of Defense. Preliminary tests of the vaccine indicate that it is probably as potent as Dryvax.[15] Clinical trials of the Aventis vaccine began in the spring of 2002. Dilution tests of the vaccine will also be conducted.

CDC is negotiating a contract to increase the U.S. stockpile of a product used to treat serious adverse reactions to smallpox vaccine.[16] The product, vaccinia immune globulin intravenous treatment (VIGIV) is expected to be available in 2003. Currently CDC has access to a similar product that could be used to treat adverse reactions in about 675 adults, the number expected when vaccinating 4 to 6 million people. CDC is seeking to increase the stockpile by 30,000 doses, the amount needed if a mass U.S. smallpox vaccination did not include pregnant women. If pregnant women were included, an additional 40,600 doses would be needed.

If the smallpox vaccine could be used without the high rate of serious complications, the threat of a bioterrorism weapon using smallpox virus would be eliminated. The federal government is encouraging both academic scientists and companies to develop a safer vaccine. Aventis Pasteur plans to begin testing a smallpox vaccine using a greatly weakened strain of vaccinia called NYVAC.[17] A combination of the traditional vaccine Dryvax with a primer vaccine called modified vaccinia Ankara (MVA) is also being studied. MVA is given several months before Dryvax and was used in German studies in the 1970s and recent studies by Bavarian Nordic of Copenhagen to eliminate serious side effects in healthy and high risk individuals. However, because MVA was never tested where smallpox virus was endemic and MVA with Dryvax does not produce a typical smallpox vaccine scar, there are concerns that it may not provide adequate disease protection. A monkey model of smallpox, developed by CDC and the U.S. Army Medical Research Institute of Infectious Diseases (USAMRIID), will be used to test the efficacy of MVA. The Food and Drug Administration (FDA) amended its new drug and biological product regulations so that products intended to prevent serious or fatal conditions may be approved for use based on effectiveness data from animal studies when human efficacy studies are not ethical or feasible. The new regulations took effect on June 30, 2002.[18]

---

[14] Enserink, M. Smallpox Vaccines: New Cache Eases Shortage Worries. *Science*, v. 296, April 5, 2002. p. 25, 27.

[15] Ibid., p. 25.

[16] Smallpox Vaccine Adverse Event Treatment Will Be Made Under CDC Contract. *The Pink Sheet*, July 1, 2002. p. 17-18.

[17] Enserink, M. In Search of a Kinder, Gentler Vaccine. *Science*, v. 296, May 31, 2002. p. 1594.

[18] *FDA News*, May 30, 2002, available at: [www.fda.gov/bbs/topics/news/2002/new00811.html]

Scientists at CDC and USAMRIID are working on antiviral treatments for smallpox. One drug, cidofovir, has demonstrated activity against variola virus in preliminary tests. In 2001, an Investigational New Drug (IND) application was filed with FDA for the "use of cidofovir in both the treatment of acute smallpox infection and the management of adverse events associated with vaccinia immunization."[19] Other compounds 25 to 150 times more active than cidofovir have been identified and are under investigation.

Legislation

The Public Health Security and Bioterrorism Preparedness and Response Act of 2002 (P.L. 107-188), signed by the President on June 12, 2002, directs the Secretary of HHS to ensure that there is enough smallpox vaccine in the Strategic National Stockpile to meet health security needs and authorizes $509 million for FY2002 and such sums as may be necessary through FY2006 for this purpose. H.R. 5005, the Homeland Security Act of 2002 as passed by the House, would amend P.L. 107-188 by moving authority for the stockpile to the Department of Homeland Security (DHS); HHS would continue to manage the stockpile and determine its contents. S. 2452, the National Homeland Security and Combating Terrorism Act of 2002, as reported by the Governmental Affairs Committee on July 25, 2002, directs DHS to consult with CDC in the administration of the stockpile by CDC. An emergency supplemental appropriation (P.L. 107-117), signed by the President on January 10, 2002, provided $512 million for the purchase of smallpox vaccine by HHS.

[19] LeDuc, J.W. et al. Smallpox Research Activities: U.S. Interagency Collaboration, 2001. *Emerging Infectious Diseases*, v. 8, July 2002. p. 743-745.

In: Vaccinations: Types, Potential Complications... ISBN: 978-1-60692-969-8
Editors: D. B. Steen and H. L. Dyson

Chapter V

T Cell Vaccination for Multiple Sclerosis*

Sheri M. Skinner, Ying C. Q. Zang, Jian Hong and Jingwu Z. Zhang
Department of Neurology
Baylor College of Medicine
Houston, Texas 77030, USA

Abstract

Autoreactive T cells appear both in healthy individuals and in people suffering from a variety of autoimmune diseases. In Multiple Sclerosis (MS) these cells have been extensively studied and regulatory mechanisms that keep them in check in the healthy individual are the subjects of much current and past research. The dysregulation that brings on the symptoms of multiple sclerosis appears to include aspects of genetic, environmental, and other unknown factors. Much early work aimed toward understanding these mechanisms was done using the experimental allergic encephalomyelitis model (EAE) in rodents. Indeed, a great deal of work on molecular aspects of regulatory function utilizes this model today. The early animal work led to an explosion of research aimed at using immunoreactive T cells as a suppression device to achieve the depletion of autoreactive T cells in human MS. To this end, for over ten years, a number of investigators have been developing and perfecting the use of these cells in a T Cell Vaccination (TCV) paradigm. Not only has this research path shown extensive promise, giving rise to several sets of clinical trials now in progress, but investigation into the array of regulatory mechanisms at work in TCV has opened up several areas of exciting research. Anti-idiotypic and anti-ergotypic T cell responses were identified as being of paramount importance in achieving a favorable TCV response in vaccine recipients. Anti-idiotypic antibody

* * A version of this chapter was also published in *Neuroimmunology Research Focus* , edited by Paulo V. Broglio published by Nova Science Publishers, Inc. It was submitted for appropriate modifications in an effort to encourage wider dissemination of research.

activity was noted and studied. Recently, a great upsurge in research on a newly recognized population of "T-Regulatory" cells has brought to light a major force in TCV success and has opened doors to a further understanding of immune system regulation on a molecular level. Unraveling the mechanisms by which the inflammatory and demyelinating processes take place continues to give rise to additional measures by which these processes may be slowed or stopped, allowing a new lease on life for those looking forward formerly to nothing but increased levels of debilitation. Meanwhile, work continues to increase efficiency of vaccine elaboration, decrease cost to the patient, and provide ever more promising approaches to mastering the regulation of autoimmune attacks on the nervous system of the MS patient. This chapter will detail the ongoing research into the regulatory mechanisms operating in T cell vaccine function within the immune system and will discuss the technical challenges in development of such a vaccine.

1. Introduction

Autoreactive T cells appear both in healthy individuals and in people suffering from a variety of autoimmune diseases. These cells have been extensively studied in an effort to characterize them and to determine their role in disease development. These studies have taken place, most notably, with respect to Multiple Sclerosis (MS). It is accepted that an array of physiological regulatory mechanisms successfully keep such cells in check in a normal homeostatic setting and that dysregulation, allowing demyelination and inflammatory symptoms of MS to develop, take the form of a combination of genetic, environmental and other unknown factors. Work continues apace to delineate the ways in which these factors come together to result in such autoimmune pathologies.

Early development of animal models allowed the study of induction and suppression of MS-like symptoms. Induction of experimental allergic encephalomyelitis (EAE) in susceptible rodent species was central to this approach. Studies using this model gave rise to a greater understanding of the T cell populations active in disease induction and allowed detailed studies of antigens that may be involved. T cell lines grown and used in these studies helped delineate the peptides within these antigenic proteins that were responsible for T cell based interactions resulting in disease production.

The importance of immunoreactive T cells in this animal model led ultimately to the concept that suppression and depletion of their numbers might lead to relief of symptoms in human MS and this conviction led to the development of T Cell Vaccination (TCV), over ten years of studies and ultimately clinical trials that proved these investigators correct in their basic assumptions.

Concurrent with the attempts at perfecting TCV procedures, laboratory investigations continued to determine the molecular bases of MS development and of regulatory suppression of autoimmune mechanisms. Wide ranging studies elucidated the nature and role of CD4+ and CD8+ T cells in these functions. Careful investigation of antigenic proteins pinpointed the peptide sequences active in development of an array of EAE and MS symptoms. TCV became understood as the use of inactivated autoreactive T cells as an immunogen that set into motion a network of regulatory mechanisms to ultimately deplete circulating autoreactive T cells. These regulatory mechanisms became the focus of intense research directed at both cellular and antibody contributions and which resulted in an increasing understanding of the manner in which the human immune system maintains homeostasis.

2. Development of TCV

2.1. Early TCV

Cohen and colleagues pioneered the use of autoreactive T cells specific to myelin antigens to manipulate the mammalian immune system. They determined that these cells were capable, not only of inducing an MS-like disease in rodents, but also of preventing it. The disease induced was known as experimental allergic encephalomyelitis (EAE). Establishment of this disease model was quickly followed by a determination that symptoms could also be ameliorated by judicious use of the autoimmune T cells in a vaccine protocol (Ben-Nun et al., 1981a and b, Ben-Nun and Cohen, 1982, Holoshitz et al., 1983). Indeed, this model was critical for the success of early work identifying anti-idiotypic T cell responses aimed at a target T cell receptor as central to the effectiveness of TCV (Lider et al., 1988; Elias et al., 1999). Animal studies allowed further probing into TCV mechanisms with work by Lohse and Cohen (1989) revealing a newly identified population of autoreactive T cells dubbed "anti-ergotypic" which responded to cell surface activation markers. Details of these mechanisms and more will be discussed in the next section.

The last ten years has seen a rapid progression of TCV trials in human subjects. Beginning in 1991 with the use of autologous CD4+ T cells derived from cerebrospinal fluid (CSF) of MS patients (Hafler et al., 1992), work proceeded toward a vaccine protocol that would be safe, effective, and workable for a larger and larger patient population. A number of hurdles had to be overcome, and numerous small human studies were designed in order to address each of them. T cell choice, expansion and attenuation procedures had to be worked out and protocols were developed to overcome the early lack of information on specific immunodominant regions of the myelin target. Non-specific cloning procedures utilized phytohemagglutinin (PHA) as immunogen. Further, T cell clones were grown and chosen on the basis simply of their CD4+ nature, their ease of expansion in vitro, and the presence of common T cell receptor gene rearrangements to allow choice of a dominant T cell clonotype. Despite the small subject numbers of these studies much was learned about effective vaccine elaboration and continued evidence of protocol safety was accumulated over the ensuing several years, providing continued assurance of the wisdom of this research direction. Some indication of vaccine effectiveness was hinted at with partial and short term alleviation of some symptoms in some patients. However, investigators were a long way from proving safety and effectiveness for TCV in MS.

As increasing information was forthcoming from basic research studies concerning the immunodominant epitopes of MBP and indeed of other likely candidate myelin autoantigens (Zhang et al., 1990, 1994; Chou et al., 1992; Pette et al., 1990; Saruhan-Direskeneli, G., 1993; Martin et al., 1991-1994; and Ota et al., 1990), it became increasingly important to couch human studies to investigate the parameters of successful downregulation of circulating pathological autoreactive T cells, to document a clonotypic response in humans and to finally show long term clinical immunosuppressive response in the MS patient post TCV. More extensive human trials must be undertaken.

2.2. Clinical Trials

A limited phase I trial was entered into by Zhang and colleagues in which an initial 8 patients with several types of MS were followed over 2-3 years with detailed analytical studies (Zhang et al., 1994). This trial determined the parameters and the protocol that was effective in depleting autoreactive T cells in the MS patient. After many years of TCV investigation, the guidelines established here remain the ones universally recognized as fundamental to the practice of TCV in MS and have led to effective depletion or suppression of myelin-reactive T cells in MS patients in a succession of human TCV trials (Achiron et al., 2004, Correale et al., 2000). In this initial trial, selected MBP-reactive T cell clones were derived from the blood of each patient to be vaccinated, providing an essentially inexhaustible cell source and minimal risk to the patient. The clones themselves were selected based upon their reactivity in vitro to two immunodominant regions of MBP (peptides 84-102 and 143-168). Selected vaccine clones were activated with autologous MBP-pulsed APC's in vitro and irradiated to render them incapable of proliferation, all elements of vaccine elaboration that continue to the present time. For all patients, this protocol resulted in T cell responses that corresponded reciprocally with a progressive decrease in the frequency of circulating MBP-reactive T cells. With each vaccination a boosting effect was seen in the decline of circulating MBP-reactive cells. In most patients this decline dropped the number to below the detectable limit (Zhang et al., 1993; Zhang et al., 1995).

Clinical results from the pilot studies were gathered in more detail and outcomes remained promising and free of adverse events, allowing swift follow up with a phase I/II trial incorporating 54 patients for extended study. Here, TCV remained a consistent and powerful procedure for the depletion of circulating MBP-reactive T cells, which effect still correlated favorably with improved clinical variables. With increased numbers of subjects, however, a trend for a lost clinical stability appeared 12 months after the last injection. A number of causes were suspected ranging from clonal shift to epitope spreading (Tuohy et al., 1999) and these are being investigated. In addition, no clinical conclusions could be drawn from this uncontrolled clinical trial and planning ensued for a placebo controlled trial with 150 subjects to evaluate efficacy, safety, and tolerability of a new multi-antigen TCV formulation and will also evaluate biomarkers of effects on epitope spreading.

Concurrent with the studies ongoing in the Zhang laboratory, a number of investigators took a variety of independent approaches to TCV in MS. These included work by Hermans and colleagues showing that TCR- $\alpha\beta$+CD8+ T cells incorporate the most important direct anti-idiotypic effects while CD4+ T cells become the predominant cytokine producers after TCV (Hermans et al., 1999). Meanwhile, Correale's group took an alternative approach, using autologous T cell lines directed against a broad array of epitopes present in their whole bovine myelin antigen, aiming to affect the maximum number of myelin antigens possible with a single vaccine (Correale et al., 2000). Once again, no serious adverse effects were noted, and human myelin peptide-specific lysis activity was seen while secretion of IFN-γ and TNFα/β predominated. In a different approach, Van der Aa and colleagues recognized the difficulty of generating a sufficient variety of specific T cell clones from circulating T cells.

Noting the higher frequency of activated myelin-reactive T cells present in MS CSF, they initiated a pilot clinical trial in which this condition could give rise to a specialized vaccine elaboration (Van der Aa et al., 2003). They utilized earlier optimized expansion T cell techniques to produce a vaccine containing CSF-derived CD4+ activated T cells characterized as being predominantly of the Thl/Th0 TCRαβ+CD4+ phenotype and a restricted clonality. Indeed, they found a significant reduction in circulating MBP-MOG-PLP-reactive T cells after vaccination in two of the five patients studied. Meanwhile, Achiron and colleagues placed their emphasis upon individuals, defined as "non-responders" to earlier vaccine protocols, attempting to rescue this patient group with a cells aimed at particular peptide targets (Achiron et al., 2004). In a 20-patient study, blood samples were stimulated with immunodominant peptide sequences of MBP and MOG and cell lines which were greater than 60% in CD4+ content were used in the vaccine. While MRI analysis demonstrated significant reduction in active brain lesions and a reduction in relapse rate was seen, there were no correlations found between clinical responses and any of the specific epitopes tested.

Ongoing studies (see Table 1 for details) include those investigating control of lesion development (Medaer and colleagues, Karussis and colleagues), studies aimed at influencing the progression of the disease from the earliest possible point in its diagnosis (Achiron and colleagues, Loftus and colleagues), and attempts at treating nonresponding patients with both RR and PP modes of MS (Achiron and colleagues).

3. T Cell Vaccine-Induced Regulatory Mechanisms

3.1. Anti-Idiotypic Responses

T cell vaccination was determined early on in the EAE animal model to induce anti-idiotypic regulators (Lider et al, 1988). That is, T cells could be shown to target TCR peptides (Elias et al, 1999). The discovery of TCR commonality in human brain lesions (Oksenberg et all, 1993) was extended to human myelin-reactive T cells (Hong et al, 1999) in which recognition of an immunodominant MBP peptide was noted in a sampling of MS patients. T cells appearing in vaccinated MS patients have long been recognized as being predominantlyCD8+ cytotoxic T cells (Tejada-Simon et al., 2000; Zhang et al., 1993; Zhang et al., 1995; Correale et al., 2000; Cohen, 1989; Zang et al., 2000). In MS, the targets of vaccination have been identified in the TCR sequences within the CDR3 region (Zang et al, 2000, 2003).

An explanation for the selective activation of this CD8+ response to TCR may reside in the choices made in vaccine preparation such as route of administration and cell surface properties of the final inoculum (Zhang, J., 2004). At any rate, there does appear to be a close correlation between the vaccine-induced depletion of myelin-reactive T cells and the ensuing positive clinical response of the vaccine recipient.

Table 1. TCV Human Trials for MS.

Study Sites	Phase/Yrs	# Pat /MS type	T cell source	Antigen	Dosage Scheme	Immunologic Results	Clinical Results	Status / Reference
Harvard Medical School, Boston, MA, USA	Phase I pilot / 1 year	4 / PP	CSF	None; T cell clones chosen for CD4+, ease of expansion in vitro, presence of common T cell receptor gene rearrangements inicating a dominant T cell clonotype.	1, 2, or 3 inoculations SQ; $4x10^7$ clones per injection.	Partial short-term Immunosuppression	No side effects; No benefit from multiple injections.	Hafler et al., 1992, Clin Immunol Immunopathol, 62 (3), 307-313.
Dr. L. Willems Instituut, Diepenbeek, Belgium.	Limited Phase I / 2-3 years.	5/RR 1/PP 2/SP	PBMC clones	MBP-human brain	2 months; 3 vaccinations, SC; $1.5X10^7$ cells/clone; 4 clones/vaccination	Depletion of MBP autoreactive T cells,	Reduced relapse rate, Reduced MRI lesion load as compared to matched controls	Zhang et al., 1993, Science. 261: 1451-1454. Zhang et al, 1995, J. Immunol. 155: 5868-5877. Hermans et al., 2000, J. Neuroimmunol. 102: 79-84..
Dr. L. Willems Instituut, Diepenbeek, Belgium.	Phase I / 2 years.	49/NG	PBMC clones	MBP	Three SQ immunizations at 2-month intervals;	TCR-αβ+CD8+ T cells showe the most important direct anti-idiotypic effects; CD4+ T cells were predominant cytokine producers (Th1).	No side effects.	Hermans et al., 1999, J. Autoimmun. 13: 233-246..

USC School of Medicine, Los Angeles, CA., USA	Pilot / 3 years.	4/ SP	PBMC; Lines	Whole bovine myelin	3 months; 5-7 injections SC; 40 X 10^6 T cell lines	Circulating T cells reacting against bovine myelin, immunodominant regions of human MBP, MOG and PLP declining over time; IL-10 immunosuppressive response.	EDSS, 2-stable; I-worse; I-better	Correale et al, 2000, J. Neuroimmunol., 107, 130-139.
Baylor College of Medicine, Houston, TX, USA.	Phase I/II ; 2 years	28/RR 26/SP	PBMC clones	MBP protein and MBP immunodominant synthetic peptides 83-99; 151-170	2 months; 3 vaccinations, SC; 3-6 X10^7 cells/vaccination; 2-4 clones/vaccination	Anti-idiotypic T cell and antibody responses; common TCR motif; Th2 cytokine shift.	Prolonged time to progression in both RR- and SP-MS; trend for accelerated progression 12 months after the last injection; slight reduction in MRI lesion activities in the first year and only a 3.3% increase in the second year.	Zhang et al, 2002, J. Neurol., 249, 212-218. Hong et al, 2000, J. Immunol. 165, 6858-6864. Zang et al, 2000, Eur. J. Immunol., 30, 908-913. Tejada-Simon et al, 2000, Int. Immunol. 12, 1641-1650.

Table 1 – (Continued)

Study Sites	Phase/Yrs	# Pat /MS type	T cell source	Antigen	Dosage Scheme	Immunologic Results	Clinical Results	Status / Reference
Limburgs Universitair Centrum, Diepenbeek, Belgium	Pilot trial / 1 year	4/ RR 1/SP	CSF	No antigen; used earlier optimized expansion techniques to produce a vaccine containing CSF-derived CD4+ activated T cells predominantly of Th1/0TCRαβ+CD4+ phenotype and restricted clonality	3 sc; Activated 10^6CD4$^+$ T cells	Significant reduction in circulating MBP-MOG-PLP-reactive T cells; anticlonotypic and antiergotypic responses.	No relapses during or after treatment; clinically stable or reduced EDSS	Van der Aa et al., 2003, Clin. Exp. Immunol, 131, 155-168.
Sheba Medical Center, Tel-Hashomer, Israel	Phase I / 1 year.	20/RR Non-responders.	PBMC	MBP and MOG synthetic peptides	2 months;3 vaccinations, SC; 1.5X 10^7cells/line; up to 5 lines / vaccination	Responses seen to five immunodominant myelin peptides.	Reduction in relapse rate, decreased rate of progression to disability, stabilization MRI	Achiron et al., 2004, Autoimmun. Rev., 3, 25-32.
Opexa Therapeutics, The Woodlands, TX, USA.	Dose escalation study / 3 yr	9 RRMS and SPMS previously receiving monovalent vaccine	PBMC Clones	MRTC lines against MBP, MOG, PLP	subcutaneous injections of either 6-9 million cells (Dose 1) or 30-45 million cells (Dose 2) at weeks 0, 4, 12 and 20.	Vaccine depletes MRTC's in both previously vaccinated and previously unvaccinated subjects	Reduction in relapse rate, alleviations of symptoms, no significant side effects	2002-2005 [http://www.opexatherapeutics.com/toxavintrials.php]

Limburgs Universitair Centrum, Diepenbeek, Belgium	Phase I,/II/ 18 mos Double-blind, placebo controlled / Ongoing	60 RR	CSF	Myelin-specific;CD4+ isolation, expansion and PHA activation	three SQ inoculations of 50 x 106 myelin-specific, attenuated T cells.	Ongoing	Ongoing [change in # active lesions by MRI]	Van der Aa et al., 2003, Clin. Exp. Immunol, 131, 155-168.
Hadassah Hospital, Jerusalem, Israel	Double-blind / 1 year.	30 RR	Ongoing	Ongoing	Ongoing	Ongloing	Ongoing	Ongoing, [karus@cc.huji.ac.il]
Sheba Medical Center, Tel-Hashomer, Israel	Phase I,II, interventional, open label, randomized/ 6 mos	20 RR or PP, non-responders	PBMC T cell lines or clones	Encephalitogenic myelin peptides	NG	Ongloing	Ongoing	Ongoing, [http://www.clinicaltrials.gov/]
Sheba Medical Center, Tel-Hashomer, Israel	Phase III, double-blind, placebo controlled / 1 year.	76 First demyelinating event	PBMC	immunodominant MBP, PLP and MOG peptides	three SQ injections of attentuated T cell lines	Ongoing	Ongoing	Ongoing, [http://www.clinicaltrials.gov/]
Opexa Therapeutics, The Woodlands, TX, USA.	Phase IIb, placebo controlled safety and efficacy / 2 yr	150 CIS or early RRMS	PBMC Clones s	MRTC lines against MBP, MOG, PLP	5 SQ injections at 0,4,8,12,24 wks	Ongoing	Ongoing	Ongoing, [http://www.clinicaltrials.gov/]

While early studies were unable to detect a significant anti-idiotypic antibody response to TCR, more recent studies using samples from a large human trial (Zhang et al, 2002) utilized a more sensitive approach to this task. Hong and colleagues (2000) were able to isolate and clone circulatory B cells producing such antibodies and to test these directly as they were produced in culture. Their reaction against the CDR3 sequence against which they had been made, along with their inhibitory effect upon vaccine T cells expressing this sequence strongly suggests their active participation in myelin-reactive T cell suppression and their involvement in the post-TCV anti-idiotypic network.

3.2. Anti-Ergotypic T Cell Responses

Cohen and Lohse (Lohse et al, 1989) originallly dubbed cell surface activation markers "ergotopes" and over time, a number of these markers were identified. These include a chain of the IL-2 receptor (CD25) (Mimran et al, 2004), HSP60 epitopes and once again, TCR (Cohen, 2004). It is important to note that while TCR is expressed upon resting cells, the ergotypic peptides are present only on activated T cells. It was shown by Cohen and colleagues, among others, that, in animal models, only activated (as opposed to resting) T cells when used in a vaccine could provide full protective effect (Lohse et al., 1989; Cohen et al., 2002). Indeed, TCV was seen to initiate anti-ergotypic responses associated with the suppression of activated T cells in human studies by Van der Aa and colleagues (2003).

Upon depletion of autoreactive T cells by TCV, repair processes must ensue for maintenance of homeostatic functioning. It is thought that such maintenance may be offered by a normally functioning CD4+CD25+ T cell population.

The concept of "suppressor" T cells faded from consideration for a time, but has returned under the designation of regulatory T cells or "Tregs". Generally, this term refers to CD4+ Tcells that constitutively express a variety of markers such as CD25 (alpha chain IL-2 receptor), GITR (Glucocorticoid Induced TNF Receptor), and the transcription factor, FoxP3. More specifically, in the CD4+ compartment, at least three different types of Treg subsets are known: the best known one mentioned above possessing the CD25 marker (most especially that possessing a CD25high phenotype (Sakaguchi, 2004; Baecher-Allan et al, 2004)), Tr1 cells which can be activated in the presence of IL-10 and become anergic upon activation (Roncarolo et al, 2001), and finally, Th3 cells which are seen to be involved in oral tolerance phenomena (Weiner, 2001; Levings et al, 2002). These Treg subsets differ in their suppression mechanisms which range from cell-cell contact, to IL-10 or TGF-beta secretory activity.The first of these, $CD4^+$ $CD25^+$ T cells, are some of the best-characterized of the immunoregulatory subsets and are known to prevent both activation and effector function of activated responder T cells (Shevach, 2000). It is thought that while CD4+CD25+ T cells are antigen-activated via their TCR to become suppressive, their resulting suppressor effector function is completely nonspecific (Thornton and Shevach, 2000). Indeed, this lack of specificity in suppressive response has led to the assumption that this population of Tregs operates like the Th1, Th2 and Th3 classes of cells in controlling the magnitude and class specificity of the immune response (Cohn, 2004; von Herrath and Harrison, 2003).

Although much work has been done on CD4+CD25+ T cells in general, it is wise to remember that not all $CD4^+CD25^+$ T cells are functionally regulatory cells and not all $FoxP3^+$ T cells are regulatory T cells (Fontenot et al, 2005). It would perhaps simplify matters to pay particular attention to a subset of T cells noted by Sakaguchi and colleagues (Sakaguchi, 2004) and identified by particularly high expression of surface CD25. These CD25^{Hi} cells have several characteristics recently determined to recommend them as particularly useful in studies of MS and the effects of TCR in ameliorating its symptoms. It is reassuring that much of the extensive work on this subset of T cells has been clarified and reinforced in a particularly cleanly executed study by Haas and colleagues (2005) which was limited to samples obtained from MS patients who suffered from early, clinically active and untreated RRMS. These treatment-naïve patients offered a glimpse into the behavior of a regulatory T cell population as yet unaffected by the many immunoreactive treatments that render many other such patient studies inconclusive in their attempts at data interpretation. Further, the study is exemplary in limiting its sampling to the CD25^{Hi} subset of T cells on the basis of questionable regulatory properties offered by CD25^{Low} or CD25^{Int} populations (Baecher-Allan et al, 2001; Wing et al., 2002) and the observation that the CD25^{Int} population contains cells that are recently activated and proliferating and only transiently upregulate CD25 (Kohm et al., 2002). Therefore, whereas these other populations may indeed be active in the regulatory phenomenon as a whole, it is helpful to obtain data unconfounded by cell populations whose behavior has yet to be clearly defined. In this carefully regulated setting, Haas and colleagues were able to confirm that the CD4+CD25^{Hi} T cell subset possessed the following characteristics: a) their frequency is no different in MS patients than in healthy controls, b) in an acute relapse they do not seem to be sequestered in the CNS as their proportions in the peripheral circulatory CD4+ population did not differ from that in the CSF, c) these cells show reduced suppressive properties in in vitro studies that appear related to functional impairment, a condition appearing whether the patient is in or out of remission. They do present a cautionary statement, however, to the effect that these findings cannot be applied to studies of other autoimmune diseases given that current data in, for example, RA, suggest that CD4+CD25^{Hi} cellular dynamics may differ greatly from those operative in MS.

It should be noted that a considerable overlap has been identified between the anti-ergotypic and the regulatory T cell compartments of the immune response. Early work by Vandenbark and colleagues first suggested such a regulatory possibility (Buenafe et al 2004). However, it is not clear that the anti-ergotypic T cell population identified in animal models is truly representative of CD4+ regulatory T cells under study in humans. Indeed, CD4+ regulatory T cells evident in human populations continue to be the subject of intensive study. Recent work by Hong et al (2006) shows that almost all of the CD4+ activity mounted against the T cell clone vaccinogen is indeed anti-ergotypic. Moreover, these cells constituted two subsets of regulatory T cells, CD25+ cells that were mechanistically classifiable according to their FoxP3 expression. The FoxP3+ population utilized an IL10 secretion mechanism while the FoxP3- group, while secreting both IL10 and IFN gamma, did not appear to rely on IL10 for its effect. It is noteworthy that these anti-ergotypic regulatory T cells were not detectable in the same MS patients before TCV. These two populations are suspected to provide a slowly responding yet longer lasting support of overall immune balance. It appears that effective replacement of the regulatory balance lost in the disease state is key to TCV success against autoimmune dysfunction.

4. Technical Improvements

As more is being learned about the regulatory networks impacted by MS and the ways in which TCV re-invigorates these networks such that disease processes are slowed or halted and repair mechanisms are allowed to proceed, protocols for TCV become more complete and better suited to a larger population of MS patients. TCV is, of necessity, a highly individual and therefore highly labor intensive undertaking. However, research is intensifying around a number of regulatory pathways that allow continued improvements and additions to be made to the protocols. Along with the breakthroughs at the research bench, a good deal of dogged testing and tweaking of procedural mechanisms is needed to optimize the steps in the TCV process. It is the wish of investigators and physicians in the field to eventually arrive at a close approximation to a one-size-fits-all procedure that minimizes cost to the patient and time spent in the laboratory and the clinic. Among the considerations in this vein are those discussed below.

4.1. T Cell Acquisition

The T cell populations that give rise to the lines and clones that will seek out the autoimmune targets are the most critical aspect of TCV. Targeting has recently widened to include multi-antigen T cell populations that should cover a wider number of MS patients (Zhang 2002). In many cases the aim is to clone vaccinogen cells from circulatory PBMC. In some cases, investigators are testing the possibility of accessing T cells from the CSF; in effect, allowing the patient's own body to do the sorting with the expectation that the truly optimal selection of activated and appropriately antigen-sensitive populations will be acquired in this manner. Technical problems remain in both camps and attempts to balance efficiency with specificity continue.

4.2. Activation and Expansion

Cohen's group has determined that only activated T cells, not resting ones, can effectively induce protective immune response, as activation markers are necessary for induction of anti-ergotypic T cell responses. Hence, all TCV procedures must include pre-activation of vaccinating cells. In addition to specificity, one must acquire sufficient numbers of activated cells for the vaccination needs of the patient. Because of the technical difficulties in developing antigen-specific clones, it is usually necessary to rely largely upon patient T cell lines for the bulk of the vaccinogen. Specificity choices do dictate, to some extent, the means used for expansion and activation of these cells. Expansion exclusively by antigen stimulation will safeguard the specificity of the cell population, but with repetition will lead eventually to cellular anergy and loss of that specificity. Mitogen stimulation (as with PHA or IL-2) can relieve this problem, but does not achieve specificity. Hence, mitogen stimulation is best used with clones. However, a compromise may be achieved by alternating antigen stimulation with mitogen stimulation until sufficient vaccinogen cell numbers are reached.

On the other hand, a population of cells that is likely to include antigenically non-specific groups, such as one might isolate from the CSF, may require an extra selection step before expansion. After the in vivo expansion of relevant cells that is thought to take place in the CNS during the disease process (Zhang 2004), further selection of appropriate populations is possible using TCR CDR3 DNA sequence analysis or immunoscope technology (Sun et al, 2005). Final expansion can then be done with in vitro PHA or anti-CD3 antibody treatment.

4.3. Timing of Inoculations

Experience with TCV trials has determined a few guideposts in choosing cell dosage levels and inoculation frequency. It is necessary, for example, to allow a period of 1-2 months between active immunizations in order that the immune processes active in TCV have a chance to establish themselves. After that point, the process becomes one of testing for the presence of effector cells and further inoculation as needed. It has been noted that, for most MS patients, more than one active immunization will be needed for sufficient response. Trials are in progress to determine long term needs for continued inoculations over time. It may be that old clones may renew themselves over time (Hermans et al, 2000) or that new clones with other antigen specificities (a clonal shift) may grow up in the place of depleted ones (Tuohy et al, 1999), necessitating isolation and preparation of fresh antigenically specific populations for vaccination. With continued clinical trials, injection schedules are honed to suit the immunogen(s) and the patient, and newer approaches continue to be developed. One such is Cohen's approach of building numbers of T regulatory members of the cellular population by addition of ergotopic peptide vaccines to the current TCV protocol (Cohen 2002). The process remains a highly individualized one with many questions left to answer concerning the nature of the TCV response, the immunologic environment it sets in motion, and the long-term responses of the patients.

Conclusion

In the near future, development in three critical areas will be central to the evaluation and improvement of T cell vaccination for the treatment of MS. Firstly, the focus of clinical research should be to address whether T cell vaccination is indeed efficacious for the treatment of MS and other autoimmune diseases such as rheumatoid arthritis. Within the next five years, at least two Phase I/II clinical trials should have been completed to provide some clinical data and at least one pivotal trial should have started in 2006. Therefore, in no more than 10 years we should be able to see clear indications of the treatment efficacy of T cell vaccination in MS. Moreover, there is likelihood that T cell vaccination may be used in combination with other therapeutic agents, such as beta-interferons and Copolymer-I, to show synergistic treatment efficacy. Further, it is anticipated that at least one clinical trial using substantially different technology to isolate pathogenic T cells and to prepare T cell vaccine will begin in the area of rheumatoid arthritis.

Secondly, it is our belief that within the next few years, significant technical improvements will be made, concurrently with the clinical studies, in the selection and preparation of more reliable and specific T cell vaccines. Such improvements will owe their development to the advancement of new procedures such as tetramer technology coupled with cell sorting. These technical improvements are likely to make the preparation of T cell vaccines remarkably simple and easily standardized, all of which would also significantly reduce the manufacturing cost. In addition, research discoveries centering upon new autoantigen(s) and new T cell subsets closely associated with MS pathology may further improve the quality and specificity of T cell vaccine and make the treatment more powerful. If T cell vaccination is proven efficacious in pivotal clinical trials for relapsing-remitting or secondary progressive MS patients, it may provide a treatment option for selected MS patients who are refractory to and unable to take beta-interferon and/or Copoxane. However, considering the rigors of vaccine preparation and shipment, the problem remains as to how such a cell-based therapy might be used to treat a large population of MS patients living in different geographical locations. Our experience in two clinical trials involving over 100 patients indicates that it is technically feasible to treat a large population of patients at different geographic locations. In preparing such trials, at least two possibilities have been discussed. One approach involves the preparation of T cell vaccine in a central GMP facility where blood specimens are received. The vaccine is subsequently distributed to satellite GMP facilities within the continents. Success of this approach would rely upon a reasonably long shelf-life for the vaccine and a reliable distribution system. A second plan requires that T cell vaccine be manufactured uniformly in multiple GMP facilities that are geographically distributed and then administered locally. Both possibilities would involve significant regulatory considerations.

The third area of focus moves beyond cell-based therapies. As discussed above, it is realistic to predict that a peptide-based vaccine or a DNA vaccine, corresponding to a T cell receptor sequence commonly expressed on and characteristic of myelin autoreactive T cells associated with MS, may be developed into preliminary clinical trials within the next five years. Such a TCR peptide vaccine would be as convenient as conventional therapeutics for the treatment of MS. However, the major hurdle in this regard is related to the discovery of a common T cell receptor sequence(s) that must fulfill certain criteria. These include (1) its specificity for a dominant myelin autoreactive T cell population(s) and (2) its presence/coverage in a significant portion of MS patients. It is our belief that, although peptide-based or DNA-based vaccination is appealing in its concept, its immunologic and clinical effectiveness may be limited. This limitation arises from the possibility that specific depletion of a dominant subset of the myelin-reactive T cell population may not be sufficient to suppress autoreactive T cell responses to the candidate myelin antigen(s) in many individuals with MS. It has been noted that there is significant heterogeneity within the T cell repertoire utilized by myelin autoreactive T cells among different MS individuals, a circumstance which is further complicated by epitope spreading issues. In this regard, T cell vaccine tailor-made to contain all dominant autoreactive T cell clones recognizing multiple myelin antigens/peptides found in a given patient is likely to be the more effective option. It is our expectation that these issues will develop more clarity in the near future and that greater and greater numbers of autoimmune disease patients will benefit.

References

[1] Achiron, A., Lavie, G., Kishner, I., Stern, Y., Sarova-Pinhas, I., Ben-Aharon, T., Barak, Y., Raz, H., Lavie, M., Barliya, T., Faibel, M., Cohen, I.R., and Mandel, M. (2004). T cell vaccination in multiple sclerosis relapsing-remitting nonresponders patients. *Clin. Immunol.* 113: 155-160.

[2] Baecher-Allan, C., Brown, J. A., Freeman, G. J. and Hafler, D. A. (2001).$CD4^{+}CD25^{high}$ regulatory cells in human peripheral blood. *J. Immunol.* 167: 1245-1253.

[3] Baecher-Allan, C., Viglietta, V. and Hafler, D.A. (2004). Human $CD4^{+}CD25^{+}$ regulatory T cells, *Semin. Immunol.* 16: 89-98.

[4] Ben-Nun, A., Wekerle, H., and Cohen, I.R. (1981a). The rapid isolation of clonable antigen –specific T –lymphocte lines capable of mediating autoimme ecephalomyelitis. *Eur. J. Immunol.* 11: 195-199.

[5] Ben-Nun, A., Wekerle, H., and Cohen, IR. (1981b). Vaccination against autoimmune encepahlomyelitis with T-lymphocte line cells reactive against myelin basic proteins. *Nature.* 292: 60-61.

[6] Ben-Nun, A. and Cohen, I.R. (1982). Spontaneous remission and acquired resistance to autoimmune encephalomyelitis (EAE) are associated with suppression of T cell reactivity: suppressed EAE Effector T cells recovered as T cell lines. *J. Immunol.* 128 (3): 1450-1457.

[7] Buenafe, A.C., Tsaknaridis, L., Spencer, L., Hicks, K.S., McMahan, R.H., Watson, L., Culbertson, N.E., Latocha, D., Wegmann, K., Finn, T., Bartholomew, R., Burrows, G.G., Whitham, R., Bourdette, D.N., Jones, R.E., Offner, H., Chou, Y.K., Vandenbark, A.A. (2004). Specificity of regulatory CD4+CD25+ T cells for self-T cell receptor determinants. *J. Neurosci. Res.* 76: 129-140.

[8] Chou YK, Bourdette DN, Offner H, Whitham R, Wang RY, Hashim GA, Vandenbark AA. (1992). Frequency of T cells specific for myelin basic protein and myelin proteolipid protein in blood and cerebrospinal fluid in multiple sclerosis. *J. Neuroimmunol.* 38(1-2):105-13.

[9] Cohen, I.R. (1989). Natural id-anti-id networks and the immunological homunculus. In: Atlan, H., Cohen, I.R. (eds), *Theories of Immune Networks*, Springer-Verlag, Berlin, pp.6-12.

[10] Cohen, I.R. (2002). T-cell vaccination for autoimmune disease: a panorama. *Vac.* 20: 706-710.

[11] Cohen, I.R., Quintana, F.J., and Mimran, A. (2004). Tregs in T cell vaccination: exploring the regulation of regulation. *J. Clin. Invest.* 114(9): 1227-1232.

[12] Cohn, M. (2004). Whither T-suppressors: if they didn't exist would we have to invent them? *Cell Immunol.* 227:81-92.

[13] Correale, J., Lund, B., McMillan, M., Ko, D.Y., McCarthy, K., and Weiner, L.P. (2000). T cell vaccination in secondary progressive multiple sclerosis. *J. Neuroimmunol.* 107: 130-139.

[14] Elias, D., Tikochinsky, Y., Frankel, G., and Cohen, I.R. (1999). Regulation of NOD mouse autoimmune diabetes by T cells that recognize a T-cell receptor CDR3 peptide. *Int. Immunol.* 11: 957-966.

[15] Fontenot, J.D., Rasmussen, J.P., Williams, L.M., Dooley, J.L., Farr, A.G., Rudensky, A.Y. (2005). Regulatory T cell lineage specification by the forkhead transcription factor foxp3. *Immunity*. 22: 329-341.

[16] Haas, J., Hug, A., Viehöver, A., Fritzsching, B., Falk, C.S., Filser, A., Vetter, T., Milkova, L., Korporal, M., Fritz, B., Storch-Hagenlocher, B., Krammer, P.H., Suri-Payer, E. and Wildemann, B. (2005). Reduced suppressive effect of CD4+CD25^{high} regulatory T cells on the T cell immune response against myelin oligodendrocyte glycoprotein in patients with multiple sclerosis. *Eur.J.Immunol.* 35:3343-3352.

[17] Hafler, D., Cohen, I.R., Benjamin, D., and Weiner, H.L. (1992). T-cell vaccination in multiple sclerosis: a preliminary report. *Clin. Immunol. Immunopath.* 62: 307-312.

[18] Hermans, G., Denzer, U., Lohse, A., Raus, J. and Stinissen, P. (1999) Cellular and humoral immune responses against autoreactive T cells in multiple sclerosis patients after T cell vaccination. *J. Autoimmun.* 13: 233-246.

[19] Hermans, G., Medaer, R., Raus, J., and Stinissen, P. (2000). Myelin reactive T cells after T cell vaccination in multiple scelerosis: cytokine profile and depletion by additional immunizations. *J. Neuroimmunol.* 102: 79-84.

[20] Holoshitz, J., Naparstek, Y., Ben-Nun, A., and Cohen, I.R. (1983). Lines of T lymphocytes induce or vaccinate against autoimmune arthritis. *Science.* 129: 56-58.

[21] Hong, J., Zang, Y.C., Tejada-Simon, M.V., Kozovska, M., Li, S., Singh, R.A., Yang, D., Rivera, V.M., Killian, J.K., and Zhang, J.Z. (1999). A common TCR V-D-J-sequence in V beta 13.1 T cells recognizing an immunodominant peptide of myelin basic protein in multiple sclerosis. *J. Immunol.* 163: 3530-3538.

[22] Hong, J., Zang, Y.C.Q., Tejada-Simon, M.V., Li, S., Rivera, V.M., Killian, J., and Zhang, J.Z. (2000). Reactivity and regulatory properties of human anti-idiotypic antibodies induced by T cell vaccination. *J. Immunol.* 165: 6858-6864.

[23] Hong, J., Zang, Y.C.Q., Nie, H., and Zhang, J.Z. (2006). CD4+ regulatory T cell responses induced by T cell vaccination in patients with multiple sclerosis. *Proc. Nat. Acad. Sci.* 103:5024-5029.

[24] Kohm, A. P., Carpentier, P. A., Anger, H. A. and Miller, S. M. (2002).Cutting edge: $CD4^{+}CD25^{+}$ regulatory T cells suppress antigen-specific autoreactive immune responses and central nervous system inflammation during active experimental autoimmune encephalomyelitis. *J. Immunol.* 169: 4712-4716.

[25] Levings, M.K., Sangregorio, R., Sartirana, C., Moschin, A.L., Battaglia, M., Orban, P.C. and Roncarolo, M.G. (2002). Human $CD25^{+}CD4^{+}$ T suppressor cell clones produce transforming growth factor β, but not interleukin 10, and are distinct from type 1 T regulatory cells. *J. Exp. Med.* 196: 1335-1346.

[26] Lider, O., Reshef, T., Beraud, E., Ben-Nun, A., and Cohen, I.R. (1988). Anti-idiotypic network induced by T cell vaccination against experimental autoimmune encephalomyelitis. *Science*. 239: 181-184.

[27] Lohse, A.W., Mor, F., Karin, N. and Cohen, I.R. (1989). Control of experimental autoimmune encephalomyelitis by T cells responding to activated T cells. *Science.* 244: 820-822.

[28] Martin R, Howell MD, Jaraquemada D, Flerlage M, Richert J, Brostoff S, Long EO, McFarlin DE, McFarland HF. 1991 A myelin basic protein peptide is recognized by cytotoxic T cells in the context of four HLA-DR types associated with multiple sclerosis. *J. Exp. Med.* Jan 1;173(1):19-24.

[29] Martin R, Utz U, Coligan JE, Richert JR, Flerlage M, Robinson E, Stone R, Biddison WE, McFarlin DE, McFarland HF. 1992 Diversity in fine specificity and T cell receptor usage of the human CD4+ cytotoxic T cell response specific for the immunodominant myelin basic protein peptide 87-106. *J. Immunol.* Mar 1;148(5):1359-66.

[30] Martin R, Whitaker JN, Rhame L, Goodin RR, McFarland HF. 1994 Citrulline-containing myelin basic protein is recognized by T-cell lines derived from multiple sclerosis patients and healthy individuals. *Neurology.* Jan;44(1):123-9.

[31] Mimran, A., Mor, F., Carmi, P., Quintana, F.J., Rotter, V., and Cohen, I.R. (2004). DNA vaccination with CD25 protects rats from adjuvant arthritis and induces an antiergotypic response. *J. Clin. Invest.* 113: 924-932.

[32] Oksenberg, J.R., Panzara, M.A., Begovich, A., Mitchell, D., Erlich, H.A., Murray, R.S., Shimonkevitz, R., Sherritt, M., Rothbard, J., and Bernard, C.C. (1993). Selection for T–cell receptor V beta-D beta-J beta gene rearrangements with specificty for a myelin basic protein peptide in brain lesions of multiple sclerosis. *Nature*. 362: 68-70.

[33] Ota K, Matsui M, Milford EL, Mackin GA, Weiner HL, Hafler DA.1990 T-cell recognition of an immunodominant myelin basic protein epitope in multiple sclerosis. *Nature.* Jul. 12;346(6280):183-7.

[34] Pette M, Fujita K, Wilkinson D, Altmann DM, Trowsdale J, Giegerich G, Hinkkanen A, Epplen JT, Kappos L, Wekerle H. (1990). Myelin autoreactivity in multiple sclerosis: recognition of myelin basic protein in the context of HLA-DR2 products by T lymphocytes of multiple-sclerosis patients and healthy donors. *Proc. Natl. Acad. Sci. U S A.* 87(20):7968-72.

[35] Roncarolo, MG, Bacchetta, R., Bordignon, C. Narula, S. and Levings, M.K. (2001). Type 1 T regulatory cells, *Immunol. Rev* 182: 68-79.

[36] Sakaguchi, S. (2004). Naturally arising $CD4^+$ regulatory T cells for immunologic self-tolerance and negative control of immune responses, *Annu. Rev. Immunol.* 22: 531-562.

[37] Saruhan-Direskeneli, G., Weber, F., Meinl,E., Pette, M., Giegerich, G., Hinkkanen, A., Epplen, J.T., Hohlfeld, R., and Wekerle, H. (1993). Human T cell autoimmunity against myelin basic protein: CD4+ cells recognizing epitopes of the T cell receptor β chain from a myelin basic protein-specific T cell clone. *Eur. J. Immunol.* 23: 530-540.

[38] Shevach E. (2000). Regulatory T cells in autoimmunity. *Ann. Rev. Immunol.* 18: 423-449.

[39] Sun, W., Nie, H., Li, N., Zang, Y.C.Q., Zhang, D., Feng, G., Ni, L., Xu, R., Prasad, S., Robinson, R.R., Ho, W., Sercarz, E., and Zhang, J.Z. (2005). Skewed T-cell receptor BV14 and BV16 expression and shared CDR3 sequence and common sequence motifs in synovial T cells of rheumatoid arthritis. *Genes Immun.* 6: 248-261.

[40] Tejada-Simon, M.V., Yang, D., Zang, Y., Rivera, V., and Zhang, J. (2000). T-cell reactivity to myelin antigens and their structural and functional properties at different clinical stages of multiple sclerosis. *Int. Immunol.* 12: 1641-1650.

[41] Thornton, A.M. and Shevach, E.M. (2000). Suppressor effector function of CD4+CD25+ immunoregulatory T cells is antigen nonspecific. *J. Immunol.* 164:183-90.

[42] Tuohy, V.K., Yu, M., Yin, L., Kawczak, J.A., and Kinkel, R.P. (1999). Spontaneous regression of primary autoreactivity during chronic progression of experimental autitoimmune encephalomyelitis and multiple sclerosis. *J. Exp. Med.* 189: 1033-1042.

[43] Van der Aa, A., Hellings, N., Medaer, R., Gelin, G., Palmers, Y., Raus, J., and Stinissen, P. (2003). T cell vaccination in multiple sclerosis patients with autologous CSF-derived activated T cells: results from a pilot study. *Clin. Exp. Immunol.* 131: 155-168.

[44] von Herrath, M.G., Harrison, L.C. (2003). Antigen-induced regulatory T cells in autoimmunity. *Nat. Rev. Immunol.* 3:223-32.

[45] Weiner, H.L. (2001). Induction and mechanism of action of transforming growth factor-β-secreting Th3 regulatory cells, *Immunol. Rev* 182: 207-214.

[46] Wing, K., Ekmark, A., Karlsson, H., Rudin, A. and Suri-Payer, E. (2002). Characterization of human $CD25^+CD4^+$ T cells in thymus, cord and adult blood. *Immunology.* 106: 190-199.

[47] Zang, Y.C.Q., Hong, J., Tejada-Simon, M., Li, S., Rivera, V.M., Killian, J., and Zhang, J.Z. (2000). Th2 immune regulation induced by T cell vaccination in patients with multiple sclerosis. *Eur. J. Immunol.* 30: 908-913.

[48] Zang, Y.C.Q., Hong, J., Rivera, V.M., Killian, J., and Zhang, J.Z. (2003). Human anti-idiotypic T cells induced by TCR peptides corresponding to a common CDR3 sequence motif in myelin basic protein-reactive T cells. *Int. Immunol.* 15(9): 1073-1080.

[49] Zhang, J. (2002). T-cell vaccination for autoimmune diseases: immunologic lessons and clinical experience in multiple sclerosis. *Exp. Rev. Vac.* 1(3): 285-292.

[50] Zhang, J. (2004). T cell vaccination as an immunotherapy for autoimmune diseases. *Cell. Molec. Immunol.* 1(5): 321-327.

[51] Zhang, J.W., Chou, S.J., Hashim, G.A., Medaer, R. and Raus, J.C.M. (1990). Preferential peptide and HLA restriction of MBP specific T cell clones derived from MS patients. *Cell. Immunol.* 129; 189-198.

[52] Zhang, J., Medaer, R., Stinissen, P., Hafler, D., and Raus, J. (1993). MHC-restricted depletion of human myelin basic protein-reactive T cells by T cell vaccination. *Science.* 261: 1451-1454.

[53] Zhang, J., Markovic, S., Lacet, B., Raus, J., Weiner, H.L., and Hafler, D.A. (1994). Increased frequency of inerleukin-2-responsive T-cells specific for myelin basic protein and proteolipid protein in peripheral blood and cerebrospinal fluid of patients with multiple sclerosis. *J. Exp. Med.* 179: 973-984.

[54] Zhang, J., Vandevyver, C., Stinissen, P., and Raus, J. (1995). In vivo clonotypic regulation of human myelin basic protein-reactive T cells by T cell vaccination. *J. Immunol.* 155: 5868-5877.

[55] Zhang, J.Z., Rivera, V.M., Tejada-Simon, M.V., Yang, D., Hong, J., Li, S., Haykal, H., Killian, J. and Zang, Y.C.Q. (2002). T cell vaccination in multiple sclerosis: results of a preliminary study. *J. Neurol.* 249: 212-218.

In: Vaccinations: Types, Potential Complications…
Editors: D. B. Steen and H. L. Dyson

ISBN: 978-1-60692-969-8

Chapter VI

Binding Properties of Antibodies to Bacterial Capsular Polysialic Acids: Implications to Vaccination Against Meningitis*

Jukka Häyrinen*

Department of Biochemistry, University of Kuopio, Finland

Abstract

Bacterial meningitis is a serious health risk to the newborn. No effective vaccines against the important causative agents *E. coli* K1 and *N. meningitidis* group B exist, apparently due to tolerance induced by host tissue glycans structurally similar to the bacterial capsular polysaccharides. Insufficient data on these cross-reactivities and poor understanding of the antibody interaction with the immunologically evasive capsular polysialic acid have hindered the development of polysaccharide vaccines against meningitis. Recent advance in analytical techniques and novel immonotherapeutic approaches have however, improved the situation significantly. The nature of polysialic acid–antibody interaction is now established and new promising therapeutical strategies have emerged. In this article, studies of immunological properties of polysialic acid and vaccine development spanning more than quarter of century are reviewed.

Key words: meningitis, bacterial; Escherichia coli; Neisseria meningitidis; bacterial capsules; polysaccharides, bacterial; binding sites, antibody; antigen-antibody reactions; cross-reactions; glycoproteins; sialic acids; vaccines.

---

* * A version of this chapter was also published in *Monoclonal Antibodies: New Research,* edited by Marie A. Simmons published by Nova Science Publishers, Inc. It was submitted for appropriate modifications in an effort to encourage wider dissemination of research.

* Correspondence concerning this article should be addressed to Department of Biochemistry, University of Kuopio, P.O.Box 1627, FIN-70211 KUOPIO; FINLAND. Tel. +358-17-16-3640; Fax +358-17-281-1510; E-mail: jukka.hayrinen@uku.fi.

Introduction

Bacterial meningitis is one of the most persisting serious world wide health problems (Eickhoff et al. 1964, Baker et al. 1973, Peltola 1983, Harrison 1995). Even today, in the beginning of the third millenium, we are faced with reports relating to separated incidents (Warren et al. 2003) and to wider outbreaks of the infection (WHO 2003). Despite new diagnostic tools (Mölling et al. 2002, Bennet & Cafferkey 2003) and progress in therapeutic treatment (de Gans et al. 2002), the disease still has a high mortality with death resulting within hours after onset, and it frequently causes serious sequelae to the survivors.

The most common meningitis-causing bacteria are encapsulated strains of *Streptococcus agalactiae* group B (GBS), *Escherichia coli* K1, *Neisseria meningitidis* serogroups A, B and C (MenA, B and C, respectively), *S. pneumoniae* and *Hemophilus influenzae* type b (Robbins 1978, Baker & Kasper 1985). Also *S. suis*, a common porcine pathogen, causes meningitis in humans (Arends & Zanen 1988, Kay et al. 1995). Although the number of infections due to some bacteria is expected to diminish (Saukkonen et al. 1989), *N. meningitidis* causes frequently epidemics (Harrison 1995, Defilippis et al. 1995, Edmond et al. 1995, Marwick 1991, Poolman 1995) and is currently spreading to new areas in developing countries (Suri et al. 1994, Djibo et al. 2003, Lepow & Hughes 2003).

Although the prognosis of patients suffering from bacterial meningitis has improved with the use of anti-inflammatory drugs in combination with antibiotics, vaccination is generally thought to be the best way to control the disease (Kornelisse et al. 1995). Bacterial surface polysaccharides are widely used and they are considered to be among the safest vaccine preparations, with low rates of side-effects (Jennings 1983, Frasch 1990).

Unfortunately some of the bacterial capsules, especially those rich in α2–8 linked sialic acids, are weak immunogens (Gotschlich et al. 1969, Jennings & Lugowski 1981). This has prevented the development of polysaccharide vaccines against *E. coli* K1 and MenB, two of the most the common meningitis causing bacteria. The poor immunogenicity of the α2–8 linked polysialic acid (PSA or polySia) capsules has been suggested to result from host tolerance due to structural similarity of the capsules to tissue glycans (Finne 1982). This conclusion was supported by the observed cross-reactivity of anti-MenB antibodies with purified tissue components (Finne et al. 1983), formation of tissue cross-reactive auto-antibodies in patients recovering from MenB meningitis (Nedelec et al. 1990), the disruption of functional recovery in injured nerves by antibodies to the polysialylated neural cell adhesion molecule, NCAM (Remsen et al. 1990) and the amnesic action of anti-NCAM antibodies during learning processes (Regan 1993). These findings suggested that capsule-based immunogens should be carefully evaluated prior to actual vaccination trials, and that a thorough understanding of the underlying mechanisms of the polysaccharide-antibody interaction is essential (Finne 1982, Jennings 1988).

Different approaches have been utilized in circumventing the autoimmune dilemma. Today, rational drug design is based on established structure-function relationships and characterized interactions. Several studies have shown antibodies against polysialic acids to require an unusual epitope for ligand binding (Finne & Mäkelä 1985, Jennings et al. 1985, Häyrinen et al. 1989a, 1995). These findings were recently confirmed by the resolving of the mechanism and kinetics of the PSA–antibody interaction (Evans et al 1995, Brisson & Jennings 2001, Häyrinen et al. 2002). The structural basis of immunological response to chemically modified MenB polysaccharide was also recently elucidated (MacKenzie & Jennings 2003). These and other new results give new insight in vaccine development and prevention of autoimmune side-effects. This review tries to summarize our current knowledge of the polysialic acid–antibody interaction and its implications to immunotherapeutic applications such as vaccines against meningitis.

Capsular Polysaccharides of Bacteria Causing Meningitis

The polysaccharide capsule material forms an acidic and hydrophilic layer covering the entire bacterium (Gottschlich et al. 1981). The thick, viscous capsule effectively protects bacteria from dehydration, chemical agents and host cell defense mechanisms including opsonization, phagocytosis and enzymatic lysis (Kasper 1986). The polysaccharides have an effect on bacterial invasion and may act as receptors for recognition by specific bacteriophages (Troy 1992). The encapsulated bacterial strains are generally more virulent than their non-encapsulated counterparts. This is thought to reflect the capsule's role in target cell recognition, serum resistance, antigenicity and protection against the host complement system (Jennings 1983, Kasper 1986, Leying et al. 1990). As the outermost membrane components of bacteria, they have a strong impact on the immunological properties of bacteria and thus have a marked role in the onset, prevention and treatment of the infection (Kasper 1986). Interestingly, all bacteria (such as the Group B Streptococci and *S. Suis*) with capsular polysaccharides having terminal sialic acid are effective human pathogens, and the sialic acid residues have been shown to be important virulence factors (Jennings et al. 1984).

Table 1. Repeating units of serogroup determining capsular polysaccharides of *N. meningitidis*.

Structure	Source
–6ManNAc1–P–	MenA (Liu et al. 1971)
–8Neu5Ac2–	MenB, *E. coli* K1 (Bhattacharjee et al. 1975)
–9Neu5Ac2–	MenC (Bhattacharjee et al. 1975)

The capsular polysaccharides are high-molecular-weight polymers of smaller oligosaccharide "building blocks", referred to as repeating units. The structures of GBS repeating units show striking resemblance to the sialylated terminal carbohydrate sequences of tissue glycoproteins and glycolipids (Rauvala & Finne 1979, Ando et al. 1973, Li et al. 1973, Krusius et al. 1978, Watanabe et al. 1979, Liukkonen et al. 1992). The chemically identical capsular polysaccharides of *E. coli* K1 and MenB are homopolymers of α2–8-linked *N*-acetylneuraminic acid, an ubiquitous nine carbon sugar, that are loosely attached to the bacterial outer membrane via phospholipid anchors (Table 1). The individual polysaccharide chains can be hundreds of monosaccharides long (Pelkonen et al. 1988) and the polymers are extremely flexible due to participation of the Neu5Ac 8- and 9-OH- groups on the formation of the □2–8/9 glycosidic bond. These groups are located in the extended side chain of the monosaccharide, which introduces several relatively freely rotating single bonds between the more rigid ring structures.

Polysaccharide Immunogenicity

Immunochemically, polysaccharides have several distinct features different from those of the protein antigens (Feizi & Childs 1987). First, in the primary immune response the antibodies generated against polysaccharides are usually of IgM type. Although the IgM antibodies are capable of activating complement, IgG antibodies can also utilize the alternative pathway and act directly on the pathogen. Bacterial capsular polysaccharides are also known to inhibit the alternative complement pathway by binding to inactivating proteins (Kasper 1986). Second, when IgG antibodies against polysaccharides are generated, they are invariably of IgG2 subtype, which have generally lower avidities and lower complement activating capabilities than IgG1 antibodies obtained after immunization with protein immunogens. Third, the polysaccharides are T cell independent (TI) antigens, i.e. incapable of utilizing helper T cells in the activation of antibody-producing B cells. The inability of the TI antigens to induce maturation of the immune response results in the lack of switching the response from IgM to IgG. Thus, only a transient and delayed response is achieved without any booster-effect by successive immunizations (Käyhty et al. 1984). This results in short term protection and the lack of development of the immunological memory, requiring repetitive inoculation times to maintain protective levels of circulating antibodies. Also, protection does not occur in immunocompromised individuals (Lesinski & Westerink 2001).

Meningococcal A and C polysaccharides have been shown to be immunogenic in animals but the response to MenB is markedly weaker (Gotschlich et al. 1969, Jennings & Lugowski 1981). Polyclonal MenB antibodies have been previously obtained by immunization of animals with heat-killed whole bacteria (Lifely et al. 1989). An important advance was the development of the autoimmune NZB-mouse system, which was successfully used in producing a monoclonal antibody specific to the MenB/ K1 capsule (Frosch et al. 1985). Protective MenB antibodies have been obtained in a rat model (Saukkonen et al. 1989) and also in humans after passive exposure or MenB infection (Zollinger et al. 1984). Immunization with purified MenA and C polysaccharides has earlier resulted in an induced response only in adults, whereas MenB has failed to elicit antibodies in any age group (Gotschlich et al. 1969). Immunization with group B polysaccharide complexed with meningococcal outer membrane proteins has, however, produced MenB-reactive antibodies (mainly IgM) both in animals (Lifely et al. 1987, Lifely & Esdaile 1991) and in man (Lifely et al. 1991), that were protective in *in vitro* bactericidal assays and in an *in vivo* murine passive protection model.

Capsular Polysaccharides as Vaccines

Vaccination is established as the most cost-effective strategy to control infectious diseases (Kornelisse et al. 1995). The observed worldwide increase in the number of bacterial strains resistant to antibiotics also favors prevention rather than treatment of the disease (Robbins 1978). Although bacterial surface polysaccharides are preferred as vaccine preparations, (Frasch 1990), they are usually weaker immunogens than e.g. proteins. Thus their use in vaccination or in the production of therapeutic antibodies requires additional considerations.

1. Multivalency, Conjugation, Chemical Modification and Choice of Adjuvant

The basic production methodology (isolation, purification and formulation) and administration principles of polysaccharide-based vaccines are well established (Frasch 1990). Additional methods introduced to improve their properties in actual use have included conjugation of the polysaccharide to a protein (Avery & Goebel 1931), chemical modification of the polysaccharide (Jennings 1988), and use of selective adjuvants (Moreno et al. 1985).

If a single-antigen vaccine, based on some epitope common to all relevant serotypes of the pathogen, is not available, serotype-specific antigens must be individually administered. Multivalency (inclusion of several serotypes in a single preparation) has been used to minimize the number of immunization times (Frasch 1990). This approach, however, could create problems. The response to weak immunogens is easily masked by the stronger immunogens in the preparation. Also, the different antigens could simultaneously recruit too many cells of the immune system, resulting in exclusion of some of the clones via apoptosis. Thus, both mechanisms could lead to weakened protective efficacy of the vaccine. Additionally, the vaccine must be continuously re-formulated to allow the inclusion of new emerging serotypes.

The objectives for conjugation of weak immunogens to proteins, such as diphteria toxoid, tetanus toxoid (TT) and outer membrane proteins (OMPs), are to induce stronger response and to convert it to T-cell dependent (Avery & Goebel 1931). T-cell response is essential for the desired long-term protection in young children. Because of the lack of TI-activated B cells, only short-term protection is achieved in infants under 6 months of age, due to lack of development of the immunological memory (Käyhty et al. 1984). Conjugation, however, could be disadvantageous to antigen presentation and it may even generate artificial epitopes. The latter was demonstrated in a study, where MenB polysaccharide was coupled to tetanus toxoid protein via adipic acid dihydrazide (ADH) spacer (Bartoloni et al. 1995): Although specific IgM and IgG MenB antibodies were detected, most of the response was directed towards the ADH-TT-junction not present in the native polysaccharide on the bacterial surface.

The adjuvant used in the immunization can also have a significant effect on the antibody titer and specificity of the response (Frasch 1990). Aluminium ions have been reported to selectively increase the titers against MenB (Moreno et al. 1985). They are postulated to act by binding to the polysaccharide and stabilizing the structure against intra-molecular esterification and cleavage by host sialidases (Jennings 1994, Moreno et al. 1985). This is supported also by a recent study, where metal cations were shown to promote the PSA–antibody interaction (Häyrinen et al. 2002).

Another strategy in production of polysaccharide-based vaccines and immunoprophylactic antibodies employs chemical modification of naturally poor immunogens (Jennings 1988). *N*-alkylation of the de-*N*-acetylated polysaccharide is known to increase the immunogenicity of polysaccharides, resulting in higher antibody titers in the antisera. *N*-propionylation and subsequent conjugation of the derivatized MenB polysaccharide to tetanus toxoid were found to promote the formation of IgM and IgG antibodies to weakly immunogenic MenB (Jennings et al. 1986, Jennings et al. 1987). Periodate oxidation, which is used in the tetanus toxoid conjugation neither introduced any new epitopes nor modified the existing ones (Häyrinen et al. 1995). The antibodies, which also recognized unmodified PSA, were bactericidal *in vitro* and could readily enter the fetal circulation through the placenta (Granoff et al. 1998). Although low levels of native polysaccharide-reactive antibodies are also detected, they are not protective and recognize a different terminal epitope (Mackenzie & Jennings 2003). *N*-Propionylation of the MenB polysaccharide was originally suggested to mimic a unique epitope present on bacterial, but not on host cell surface (Jennings 1989). Later another compound, presumably a lipid, was also suggested to be present (Pon et al. 1997). This hypothesis was recently confirmed by SPR: The authors were able to show that the binding of a protective antibody to MenB glycan occurs only when the polysaccharide is cell-associated, or when it is an attached to a lipid (MacKenzie & Jennings 2003). This concludes, that the recognized epitope is present on both *N*-Pr-MenB and cell-associated polysaccharide. Interestingly, aliphatic propionyl chains are also major structural components of spermine – a compound shown to promote the observed antibody binding of PSA. Whether these phenomena are related to those observed with lipid conjugated polysialic acids, is still unclear (Sato et al. 1995). With proper choice of adjuvant *N*-Pr-MenB could well become a usable therapeutic (Jennings 1989, Poolman 1995). Recently, promising advance was reported in treatment of small cell Lung cancer by vaccination with both N-Propionylated and unmodified PSA conjugated to keyhole limpet hemocyanin (Krug et al. 2004).

2. Prevention of Bacterial Meningitis with Polysaccharide Vaccines

Polysaccharides have been successfully employed in the prevention of meningitis caused by streptococci: Capsular based conjugate vaccines have been developed for most GBS serotypes: Ia (Wessels et al. 1993), II (Paoletti et al. 1992), III (Lagergard et al. 1990). Vaccine components are already available against serotypes IV and VII (Paoletti & Kasper 2002) and VI and VIII (Paoletti & Madoff 2002), although they are not currently included in the multivalent formulations in clinical use. The IgG (mainly IgG1) antibodies elicited in response have sufficiently high titers and are protective without any observed side-effects (Lagergard et al. 1990, Paoletti et al. 1994) and their potential reactivities with tissue antigens have also been studied (Häyrinen et al. 1989b, Tikkanen et al. 1995). Preparation of type-specific polysaccharides to be used as vaccine-components against GBS is well documented (Carlo et al. 1983, Jennings & Kasper 1992, Paoletti & Madoff 2002). The non-capsular streptococcal group B polysaccharide was also shown to promote the formation of protective IgM antibodies (Raff et al. 1991). However, in another experiment the TT-conjugated group B polysaccharide antibodies bound to fewer sites on the bacterial surface and failed to activate the complement (i.e. deposit complement protein C3), which resulted in a lower degree of protection as compared with the antibodies against TT-conjugated type-specific GBS type III polysaccharide (Marques et al. 1994).

Polysaccharide vaccines were also tried in the prevention of meningitis caused by *H. inluenzae* (Peltola et al. 1984). Although the preparation was proven safe and efficient (Shapiro et al. 1989), no protection was achieved in the infants younger than 18 months of age, who are the main age group susceptible to *H. inluenzae* infections. Better protection was obtained through conjugation of the polysaccharide to a protein (Eskola et al. 1985). The conjugate was immunogenic also in infants and it was highly (94%) protective. Protein complex–conjugate polysaccharide vaccines have also been experimentally applied in the prevention of pneumococcal diseases (Käyhty et al. 1995, Bethell & Pollard 2002).

Considerable effort has been put to development of new immunotherapeuticals against *N. meningitidis*. Although the capsular polysaccharides of Men A and C have been successfully employed as vaccines for more than 20 years (Peltola et al. 1977), they induce only a relatively short-lasting T-cell independent immune response, are not effective in young children under two years of age (Broker 2003), although some progress has also recently been made (Segal & Pollard 2003). In the development and phase I clinical trials of a licensed Men A/C conjugate vaccine (Centers for Disease Control 1978), increased antibody titers without any marked side-effects were achieved (Constantino et al. 1992). A tetravalent polysaccharide vaccine against serotypes A, C, Y and W135 (Menomune®) was licensed in 1981 and is successfully administered (Centers for Disease Control 1985).

Although news on the development of a MenC/B conjugate preparation have been published (Marwick 1991), licensed preparations are yet to become commercially available. Thus currently no vaccines exist, capsular or other, for *E. coli* K1 or MenB, which is the culprit in 10% (Tsang et al. 2001) to over 50% of the cases (Kyaw et al. 2002) and therefore a leading cause for meningitis in Europe and North America. Trials with MenB-polysaccharide complexed with outer membrane proteins, using aluminium hydroxide as adsorbing adjuvant (Moreno et al. 1985) have resulted in only transient IgM-responses. In addition, similar vaccine preparations are sometimes found not even to be immunogenic (Frasch et al. 1988). However, in one experiment, protective antibodies were detected in adult male volunteers 12 months after vaccination (Lifely et al. 1991). The antibodies (mainly IgM) were also effective in *in vitro* bactericidical assays and in an *in vivo* murine passive protection model.

3. Alternatives to Capsular Vaccines

Immunizations with antigens other than the capsular polysaccharides alone, such as outer membrane proteins (OMP) and lipopolysaccharides (LPS), have produced protective antibodies but only against individual strains (Saukkonen et al. 1989). This has limited their use in mass scale vaccination programs. Recently, some advance was made using attenuated strains of live bacteria in a rodent model and human volunteers (Li et al. 2004).

Outer membrane vesicles (OMV's) from MenB have been shown to elicit a strong immune response (Aase et al. 1995, Haneberg et al. 1998). Also, in a recent follow-up study no adverse effects were detected in using MonoMen® OMV-booster injection previously vaccinated with a hexavalent MenB vaccine (Lafeber et al. 2000). The high-throughput isolation of OMV-generated high affinity antibodies directly from human single chain Fv antibody (scFv) expression libraries was recently demonstrated (Stacy et al. 2003). Promising results were also obtained in testing of an experimental liposome vaccine, composed of meningococcal OMP P1-protein complexed with LPS, in mice (Idänpään-Heikkilä et al. 1995).

Protein-based vaccines are an alternative to the poorly immunogenic polysaccharide in the vaccination against MenB. Iron-inducible OMPs have been suggested as potential vaccine candidates (Frasch 1990). In a study with an experimental MenB(15:P1.3)OMP conjugate vaccine, 70% protection was achieved in the age group of 5–21 years, but again no protection could be achieved in children under 5 years of age (Boslego et al. 1995). The membrane proteins are highly conserved and they are shown to induce the formation of bactericidal antibodies (Jodar et al. 2002). The genomic sequencing of *N. meningitidis* is helping us to understand the mechanisms of meningococcal invasion (Nassif 2002) and its analysis by DNA arrays has already revealed many new promising vaccine candidates (Grifantini et al. 2002). Most recent product of the *N. meningitidis* group B strain MC58 genome-sequencing project is the genome-derived neisserial antigen 2132 (GNA2132) (Welsch et al. 2003). Although the antibodies had little detectable bactericidal activity with human or infant-rat complement, anti-GNA2132 antiserum protected infant rats against meningococcal bacteremia. The suitability of the recently actualized concept of DNA vaccines against meningococcal infections is also presently under investigation (Lesinski & Westerink 2001).

A novel strategy in circumventing the possible generation of autoantibodies is the use of peptidomimetics. In a recent study (Moe & Granoff 2001), murine monoclonal antibodies (mAbs) prepared against the *N*-propionyl derivative (*N*-Pr) of the MenB polysaccharide were found reacting with capsular polysaccharide epitopes, distinct from host polysialic acid. The antibodies were protective and they were used to fish out several cross-reactive peptides and peptoids from phage display and combinatorial libraries. Another experiment with *Escherichia coli* K1 produced hybridomas secreting monoclonal IgM antibodies that bound also to MenB. Approximately 50% of the antibodies were classified as autoantibodies as defined by binding to a neuroblastoma cell line expressing PSA (Shin et al. 2001). Several mimotopes were again detected, ranging from linear sequences of seven amino acids to circular peptides.

Cross-reactivity of the Capsular Polysialic Acids with Tissue Antigens

The MenB and K1 capsules are structurally similar to polysialic acids present in human tissue (Table 2) (Finne 1982, Finne et al. 1983). This "molecular mimicry" well represents the evolution of bacterial defense mechanism against host immune system (Finne et al. 1983, Bitter-Suermann 1993). Although PSA is also present in the Na^+-channels of the neural cells (Zuber et al. 1993) and developing muscle (Lackie et al. 1993), capsules of some pathogenic bacteria, other than *E. coli* K1 and MenB (*Pasteurella haemolytica* A2, *Moraxella nonliquefaciens*), salmonoid fish eggs and several human tumors (e.g. Wilms tumor, leukemia, breast cancer, various neuroblastomas) (Troy 1992), the major PSA-carrying glycoprotein in human tissues is the neural cell adhesion molecule, NCAM (Edelman 1983). NCAM plays a crucial role in axonal guidance during embryonal development and has marked effects on organogenesis, repair of nerve injury and formation of neural connections during learning processes (Lackie et al. 1993, Remsen et al. 1990). PSA is postulated to induce plasticity by negatively modulating the homophilic binding of N-CAM through electrostatic repulsion (Hoffman & Edelman 1983). NCAM-PSA expression is strictly temporally regulated, peaking in humans at the time of birth (Troy 1992), when the newborn are also most susceptible to acute bacterial meningitis and are challenged by the pathogens in the birth channel.

Table 2. Polysialic acids present in tissue glycoconjugates.

Structure	Source
–8Neu5Ac2–	Glycoproteins (NCAM, Na^+-channel) (Finne et al. 1982, Zuber et al. 1993)
–9Neu5Ac2–	Glycoproteins (rare) (Fukuda et al. 1985)

Since the onset of neonatal meningitis usually occurs during the first weeks or months after birth, it would be feasible to vaccinate young women of fertile age in order to get placentally transferred maternal IgG antibodies into the fetal circulation (Baker & Kasper 1985). This approach, however, presents potential problems: The placentally transferred antibodies could cross-react with structurally similar fetal tissue components (Finne 1982, Finne et al. 1983, Häyrinen et al. 1995, 2002). This view has been criticized (Zollinger et al. 1984, Lifely & Moreno 1986), based on lack of observed ill-effects after trial vaccination of adult volunteers with MenB polysaccharide, presence of endogenous antibodies after exposure to MenB, and the apparent lower avidity of the IgM at body temperature (Lifely & Moreno 1986). Also, the circulating cross-reactive auto-antibodies associated both in patients with MenB meningitis (Nedelec et al. 1990) and serum M-component gammopathies (Azmi et al. 1995) could not be shown to cause any clinical symptoms[1].

Ganglioside GD2 antibodies have been reported to bind specifically to the polysialylated form of NCAM (Cheung et al. 1985, Patel et al. 1989). This was demonstrated to result from cross-reaction between the disialosyl-galactose-glucose sequence of the ganglioside and a similar sequence containing *N*-acetylglucosamine in the polysialyl glycopeptides (Finne 1982) rather than a polysialic acid epitope (Häyrinen et al. 1995). This is in accordance with previous experiments, in which the IgM^{NOV} polysialic acid antibody did not bind to gangliosides (Kabat et al. 1988). The reported cross-reactivities might also result from occasional co-purification of gangliosides observed in the isolation of NCAM from neuronal tissue. Some reactivities with NCAM were likely directed towards another part of the molecule, for example the phosphatidylinositol anchor present in the NCAM 120 kD isoform (He et al. 1987). In another study the epitope recognized by the antibody included the ligand-coupled dipalmitoyl phosphatidylethanolamine used as a linking agent in ELISA (Sato et al.

[1] It is suggested, that even though epitopes of various length are expressed on the bacterial surface, only the shorter epitopes, similar to the tissue antigens, are rendered tolerant in the host. Also, the cross-reactive antibodies could bind to the tissue antigens already *in vivo* in the human volunteers, thus being cleared from the sera studied. Thus, only cross-reactivities to antigens not tolerized or not able to absorb the antibodies (for example inaccessible due to blood-brain barrier), could have been detected.

1995). The lipidated trisialyl conjugate bears a marked structural resemblance to trisialogangliosides, having a similar phosphatidylethanolamine-containing ceramide backbone.

Polysialic acid–Antibody Interaction

1. Analytical Advances in Study of Polysaccharide Antibody Binding

Traditional immunological methods used to analyze the polysaccharide–antibody interactions have included ligand binding assay (Farr 1958, Finne et al. 1983), equilibrium dialysis (Munson 1983), ELISA (Wessels et al 1991), immunodiffusion (Jennings et al. 1980b) and dot blot assays (Rodríguez-Aparicio et al. 1993). An immunoblotting method is now available and it has been applied in the screening of reactions of bacterial capsular polysaccharides with serotype-specific antibodies (Tikkanen et al. 1995). Most recent addition in the analytical arsenal is surface plasmon resonance (SPR), which has been used in charcterization of binding properties of antibodies against native and modified PSA (Häyrinen et al. 2002, MacKenzie & Jennings 2003). The technique allows simultaneous determination of both the kinetic and steady state reaction constants from the binding data[2].

2. Epitope Chain Length Requirement

Antibodies against polysialic acids have earlier been shown to require an unusually long epitope for binding (Finne & Mäkelä 1985, Jennings et al. 1985, Finne et al. 1987, Kabat et al. 1988). A similar requirement for long chains was observed also with antibodies generated against the *N*-propionylated derivative of MenB polysaccharide (Granoff et al. 1998, Mackenzie & Jennings 2003). The minimum chain length for binding is now estimated to be approximately 8 to 10 sialic acid residues (Häyrinen et al.1989, 1995, 2002). Although the degree of binding increases with each additional monosaccharide unit and the first ten residues contribute to more than 90% of the maximum calculated free energy change ($\Delta G = -7782$ cal/ mol) in the binding reaction of MAb 735 (Häyrinen et al. 1989a). However, a single antibody combining site is traditionally considered to encompass maximally only 6 to 7 monosaccharide units (Kabat 1960)[3]. This discrepancy was originally suggested to result from

---

[2] Independent of the method of choice, one should be careful in carrying out the binding experiments: The bacteria have also other surface components, such as peptidoglycan, teichoic acids and lipopolysaccharides and outer membrane proteins in gram-negative and M-proteins and serogroup-specific polysaccharides in gram-positive bacteria, which may co-purify with the desired compounds and interfere with their analysis (Frasch 1990). The risk of contamination is even larger with eukaryotic antigens as the starting material is more complex, with gangliosides, glycosaminoglycans etc. present, often in much larger concentrations as the polysialylated molecules targeted. Thus, it is advisable to characterize the ligands prior to their use in immunobinding studies (Häyrinen et al. 2002).

[3] Different results previously reported for polysialic acid minimum chain length binding requirement were likely to result from experimental paradigms and settings: An estimate of 25-mer in immunoblot is high due to steric hindrance of the membrane typical for solid phase assays (Tikkanen et al. 1995). A low minimum size of a pentamer was reported in a dot blot assay (Rodríguez-Aparicio et al. 1993), but a more stringent analysis of the data suggests an epitope of at least 6 to 7 residues. ELISA results suggesting minimum sizes of tri- and pentamers were expressed as maximum lengths of non-reactive oligosaccharides, yielding minimum chain lengths of tetra- and hexamers needed for binding, respectively (Sato et al. 1995). In theses studies, sialyl chains

a conformational epitope present on the antigen (Michon et al. 1987). Studies by NMR, potential energy calculations and X-ray diffraction predicted the binding of the combining site to a polysaccharide of 8 or more residues in length. Based on these results the PSA-antibodies were postulated to recognize an extended helical epitope with a pitch of six Neu5Ac residues per turn (Michon et al. 1987, Brisson et al. 1992, Evans et al. 1995). This model is now widely accepted and a refinement was recently published, where the inherent flexibility of the polysaccharide was better taken into account (Brisson & Jennings 2001).

3. Number of Antibody Binding Sites in Polysialic Acid–Antibody Interaction

The observed requirement for an unusually long epitope could have resulted from bivalent binding of the two antibody binding sites to one polysaccharide molecule, or from a conformational epitope of the polysialic acid molecule. According to the bivalency model, binding of a single binding site would exhibit a weak interaction not detectable by common immunochemical methods (such as RIA and ELISA) requiring the separation of bound and free molecules (Kabat 1960). This hypothesis has been later tested in a ligand binding assay with an intact mouse monoclonal IgG2a antibody mAb735 (Frosch et al. 1985) and its Fab-fragment (Häyrinen et al. 1989a): One binding site was found sufficient for binding and no co-operative effects were observed in solution. The biphasic Scatchard plots obtained in surface plasmon resonance analysis (Häyrinen et al. 2002) show however, that concentration-dependent bivalent binding could be achieved with closely spaced immobilized antibodies using ligand excess, as also previously observed (Evans et al. 1995, Lookene et al. 1996).

4. Affinity and Reaction Kinetics

Affinity is the key factor determining antibody avidity and its opsonophagocytic efficacy. Several studies made have, however produced unambiguous and sometimes controversial results (Kabat et al. 1988, Wessels et al. 1987, Mandrell & Zollinger 1987, Häyrinen et al. 1989a, Diaz-Romero & Outschoorn 1993). The methods employed in these earlier studies, such as ELISA, equilibrium dialysis and microcalorimetry, could not assess the contributions of the association and dissociation phases to the observed net affinities. Micromolar K_D-values have been determined for binding of MAb735 antibody and its Fab-fragment to short PSA's (16-mer) (Häyrinen et al. 1989a). Although the value obtained for the affinity constant of antibody 735 by SPR was slightly higher (2×10^6 M^{-1}) than that obtained by recently by calorimetry (3×10^5 M^{-1}), the differences could merely reflect the large entropy loss associated with binding to long fragments or the large standard deviations observed in the measurement of $-T\Delta S°$, as indicated by the authors (Evans et al. 1995). In a more recent study a chain-length dependent increase in the affinity of PSA–antibody interaction was

were covalently linked to lipid and lipopolysaccharide antibodies have been shown to readily react with short-chain LPS components (Nelson et al. 1990). The control equine antibody H.46 studied by Sato et al. also required a long epitope of eight residues or more for binding (Sato et al. 1995), as also previously shown (Finne & Mäkelä 1985).

observed: The difference between the K_D-values for d.p. 16 and 200 was more than 10,000-fold (Häyrinen et al. 2002), possibly due to co-operative binding of both binding sites to the long glycan. This could also have significance *in vivo* enabling medium affinity antibodies to bind bacterial capsules with a higher avidity: The antibodies could simultaneously recognize more than one closely spaced overlapping epitopes, as observed on binding of low affinity antibodies to clustered CD147 molecules on activated T cells (Koch et al 1999). In the central nervous system PSA is less abundant on cell surface, so it is possible, that no high-affinity multivalent interaction (and hence no marked cross-reaction) can take place, as also previously suggested (Jennings et al. 1987).

5. Antibody Isotype and Host Species

A significant difference in opsonic activity and protective efficacy *in vivo* between the different GBS antibody isotypes (IgM and IgG) has been demonstrated (Raff et al. 1991). The observed 1000-fold activity of IgM over that of IgG was suggested to result from differences in the regions other than the actual binding sites responsible for fixation and complement activation (the so-called Fc-region). However, all PSA-antibodies studied so far, including IgG and IgM from various species (human, mouse, rat, rabbit, horse), have showed a similar requirement for a long oligosaccharide segment for binding, as was also concluded in a study using human IgG/IgM switch variant antibodies (Häyrinen et al. 1995). The dissimilarities in bactericidal activity could derive from differences in the complement activation, as recently shown (Mandrell et al. 1995) — the IgM isotype of the antibody 5E1 was protective and dependent on the source of complement whereas the IgG isotype was not. The bactericidal activity of rabbit complement was also more than 1000-fold, when compared with human complement (Mandrell et al. 1995). The enhancement of the activity was observed with IgM but not with IgG isotypes of *H. influenzae* type b antibodies, indicating differences in the complement activation or greater ability of the IgM to cross-link epitopes on different polysaccharides, as suggested by the authors. Also, IgM is better conserved during evolution, so the observed difference may be due to the action of the more potent rabbit complement on human IgM, which is phylogenetically closer to the rabbit than human IgG.

6. Temperature

Several explanations for observed temperature dependencies of the corresponding antibody binding activities have been suggested: An increased dissociation of the MenB polysaccharide from antibody at elevated temperatures (Mandrell & Zollinger 1987), temperature dependency of the affinity constants (Diaz-Romero & Outschoorn 1993) and loss of three-dimensional structure or defined conformation of the polysaccharide in the elevated temperatures (Lifely et al. 1987). However, in another study no temperature dependency was observed (Häyrinen et al. 1995). Later using more sophisticated techniques, this discrepancy was resolved: Although, changes in temperature have no apparent effect on the on-rate of the reaction, the complex dissociates slightly slower at +4 °C (Häyrinen et al. 2002) as also previously suggested (Mandrell & Zollinger 1987). Although this has propably marginal significance *in vivo*, it should be considered when evaluating *in vitro* data.

7. Effects of pH, Ionic Strength

The PSA–Ab binding reaction is thought to involve an electrostatic component (Häyrinen et al. 1989a, 1996 Evans 1995). Opposing ionic charges create potential differences, which are the main element in the reaction energetics of electrostatic interactions. Both components of the interaction exhibit marked charge structures: The pKa-values of carboxyl groups in PSA are higher when compared to Neu5Ac-mono- and oligomers (Aubin & Prestegard 1993). Also the combining sites of the mAb735 are exceptionally basic (pI ~ 9.0) (Häyrinen et al. 1989a) due to several lysine residues present. This reflects the observed generation of positively charged antibodies to anionic antigens (Sela & Mozes 1966). Interestingly, α2–8-polysialyltransferase from embryonic chick brain also has a high pI of ~ 10.5 (Troy 1992). The experimental evidence supports the above conclusions: Electrostatic component are strongly dependent on ionic strength and high concentrations of sodium ions were shown to facilitate the dissociation of the PSA–Ab-complex (Häyrinen et al. 2002, Kiss 1998). Fast association rates observed for PSA–Ab binding (Häyrinen et al. 2002) are also typical for electrostatic interactions (Lookene et al. 1996).

8. Di- and Polyvalent Cations

In addition to its well established second messenger functions and its prominent role in mineralization, calcium is involved in several adhesion related events in the central nervous system. Many of these functions have now been linked to (poly)sialic acids: The regulation of polysialylation (Brusés & Rutishauser 1998), modulation of aggregation properties of NCAM (Rouiller et al. 1990, Kiss et al. 1994), and regulation of NCAM iso-form expression and polysialylation in the developing muscle (Rafuse & Landmesser 1996).

Although Ca^{2+} is shown to bind Neu5Ac and PSA with millimolar affinity constants (Jacques et al. 1976, Shimoda et al. 1994, Bystricky et al. 1997, Häyrinen et al. 2002), the rationale behind Ca^{2+}–PSA interaction is still not completely established. Although calcium ions could as act as "counter ions" and regulate the effective hydration volume of PSA – which is considered as the main role of PSA in NCAM function (Troy 1992) – Ca^{2+} does not seem to have marked effects on the conformation of PSA (Aubin & Prestegard 1993). The results from ligand binding and CD-spectroscopy show, that Neu5Ac and colominic acid are chelating Ca^{2+} in different sites (Shimoda et al.1994, Bystricky et al. 1997). However, Ca^{2+} is shown to increase the affinity of PSA–Ab interaction and it may have a role in PSA aggregation (Toikka et al. 1998).

The observed interactions of spermine with PSA suggest that polyamines could have effects on PSA analogous to inorganic cations (Häyrinen et al. 2002). Polyamines and PSA have some intriguing similarities: They are both expressed excessively during the growth and metastasis of brain tumors. Both are also charged molecules which are suggested to involve helical motifs in their interactions: Spermine, the biologically "active" polyamine, is known to bind to major groove of dsDNA stabilizing the helical structure (Tabor & Tabor 1984).

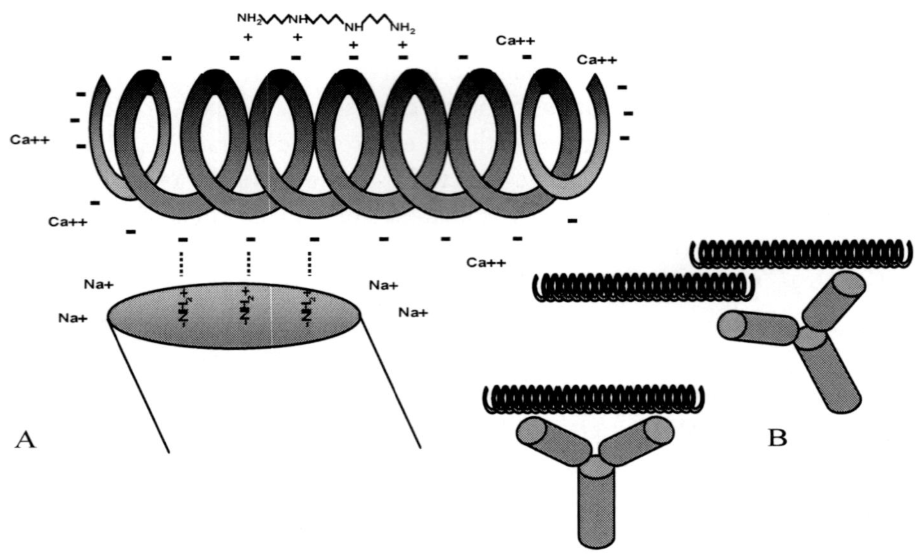

Figure 1. Schematic model of polysialic acid–antibody epitope recognition (see text for details). (A) A long segment of the helical polysaccharide is recognized by the antibody combining site. Three salt bridges between the surface lysine residues of the binding site and the carboxylate groups in the polysaccharide are indicated (dashed line). At least six additional hydrogen bonds are presumed to stabilize the complex. The terminal trisaccharides are in different shorter conformation which prevents them from binding. Polyamines and divalent cations (Ca^{2+}) may modulate the interaction by stabilizing the epitope. High salt concentrations (Na^{+}) disrupt the binding by dissociating the complex (B) High affinity binding is observed when both antibody combining sites of an IgG bind to one or more long polysaccharide chains. In binding of antibodies against *N*-alkylated antigens to bacterial cell surface, the presence of a lipid molecule is also required in the formation of the epitope.

9. The Molecular Mechanism of Polysialic Acid–Interaction

Based on the results with the antibody 735 and other polysialic acid antibodies, the following mechanism for the interaction of polysialic acid antibodies has been established (Fig. 1). Eight to ten Neu5Ac-residues are needed to form the polysaccharide epitope recognized. The epitope is presumably part of an extended helix with six residues per turn (Brisson et al. 1992), and with the carboxylate groups responsible for the negative charge pointing outwards. The terminal segments of three sialic acids are in different, less extended conformation than the inner residues (Michon et al. 1987). *N*-propionylation does not seem to interfere with the formation of the epitope on MenB polysaccharide, which is conceivable since the substituted NAc-groups are most likely located on the outer surface of the helix. The epitope is possibly stabilized *in vivo* by di- and/ or polyvalent cations.

Only one antibody binding site is required for the reaction, although both sites of an IgG can be saturated using ligand excess (Häyrinen et al. 2002). The binding site, accommodating a polysaccharide chain of eight to ten residues, is of a "groove" type rather than a "pocket" type (Kabat et al. 1988), as suggested by ligand binding, thermodynamic and X-ray data (Häyrinen et al. 1989a, Evans et al. 1995). Interaction is largely electrostatic, although the complex is also stabilized by several hydrogen bonds. The main amino acid residues responsible for the interaction are the lysine side chains, and notably their ε-NH_2-groups, which largely contribute to the basic characteristics of the combining sites. Binding of oligosaccharides is rapid but exhibits only moderate affinity, whereas longer polysaccharides (up to more than hundred units) bind slower but with higher affinity. In SPR experiments co-operative binding of long polysialic acids is observed (Häyrinen et al. 2002). Whether this is possible *in vivo* on bacterial – and even more importantly on neuronal – cell surface, remains to be evaluated.

Implications of PSA–Ab Interaction to Vaccine Design

The development of immunotherapeuticals against meningitis causing bacteria is still in progress, but the extensive literature clearly indicates that caution must be exercised in the use of native capsular polysaccharides as vaccines. The data obtained supports the suggested selection of long epitopes by immune system in the production of protective antibodies against MenB (Evans et al. 1995). Unfortunately the interaction of the PSA-antibodies with both bacterial capsular polysaccharides and tissue-derived polysialic acid undisputedly shows, that the conformational epitope critical for the recognition is present in polysialic acids of both bacteria and man: The nM binding affinity of MAb 735 to meningococcal polysaccharide is only roughly 5-fold when compared to binding of human embryonal brain PSA (Häyrinen et al. 2002, Del Rio et al. 1998).

The lack of observed ill-effects *in vivo* could result from the inaccessibility of the cross-reactive epitope: If the invading bacterial population is reduced by antibiotics, the blood-brain-barrier has time to close before the primary immune response and starts the production of antibodies (within few days). However, tolerance can develop if similar antigens are expressed in other tissues more accessible to the immune system. Breaking this tolerance by vaccination with preparations structurally similar to tissue components could endanger the health of the fetus by autoimmune reactivity of the antibodies generated (Finne 1982). It is clear, that for vaccine development, more data is needed on the *in vivo* effects of the cross-reactive antibodies.

The recent progress in vaccine development has been considerable and there are now several strategies to follow: Carbohydrate based vaccine development could simultaneously include *N*-propionylation of the capsular polysaccharide, conjugation with tetanus toxoid and use of aluminium hydroxide as adjuvant as suggested. Promising results have been obtained in immunization with other components, such as membrane proteins, vesicles and mimetic peptides, that do not posess the problems inherent with polysaccharides. The possiblities of DNA vaccines are also only just emerging. The findings reviewed here have already opened new prospects for rational vaccine development, and give hope for effective prevention of the group B meningococcal meningitis in the future.

References

[1] Aase A, Bjune B, Hoiby EA, Rosenqvist E, Pedersen AK & Michaelsen TE (1995) Comparison among opsonic activity, antimeningococcal immunoglobulin G response and serum bactericidical activity against meningococci in sera from vaccinees after immunization with a serogroup B outer membrane vesicle vaccine. *Infect Immun 63*, 3531.

[2] Ando S, Kon K, Isobe M &Yamakawa T (1973) Structural study on tetraglycosyl ceramide and gangliosides isolated from human red blood cells. *J Biochem 73*, 893.

[3] Arends JP & Zanen HC (1988) Meningitis caused by *Streptococcus suis* in humans. *Rev Infect Dis 10*, 131.

[4] Aubin Y & Prestegard JH (1993) Structure and dynamics of sialic acid at the surface of a magnetically oriented membrane system. *Biochemistry 32*, 3422.

[5] Avery OT & Goebel WF (1931) Chemo-immunological studies on conjugated carbohydrate-proteins. V. The immunological specificity of an antigen prepared by combining the capsular polysaccharide of type III *Pneumococcus* with foreign protein. *J Exp Med 54*, 437.

[6] Azmi FH, Lucas AH, Spiegelberg HL & Granoff DM (1995) Human immunoglobulin M paraproteins cross-reactive with *Neisseria meningitidis* group B polysaccharide and fetal brain. *Infect Immun 63*, 1906.

[7] Baker CJ, Barnett FF, Gordon RC & Yow MD (1973) Suppurative meningitis due to streptococci of Lancefeld group B: A study of 33 infants. *J Pediatr 82*, 724.

[8] Baker CJ & Kasper DL (1985) Group B streptococcal vaccines. *Rev Infect Dis 7*, 458.

[9] Bartoloni A, Norelli F, Ceccarini C, Rappuoli R & Constantino P (1995) Immunogenicity of meningococcal B polysaccharide conjugated to tetanus toxoid or CRM197 via adipic acid dihydrazide. *Vaccine 135*, 463.

[10] Bennett DE & Cafferkey MT (2003) Multilocus restriction typing: A tool for Neisseria meningitidis strain discrimination. *J Med Microbiol 52*, 781.

[11] Bethell D & Pollard AJ (2002) Meningococcal vaccines. *Expert Rev Vaccines 1*, 75.

[12] Bhattacharjee AK, Jennings HJ, Kenny CP, Martin A & Smith ICP (1975) Structure determination of the sialic acid polysaccharide antigens of *Neisseria meningitidis* serogroups B and C with carbon-13 nuclear magnetic resonance. *J Biol Chem 250*, 1926.

[13] Bitter-Suermann (1993) Influence of bacterial polysialic capsules on host defense: Masquerade and mimicry. *In: Roth J, Rutishauser U & Troy II FA (eds.) Polysialic acid: From microbes to man. Birkhäuser Verlag, Basel, Switzerland*, 11.

[14] Boslego J, Garcia J, Cruz C, Zollinger W, Brandt B, Ruiz S, Martinez M, Arthur J, Underwood P, Silva W, Moran E, Hankins W, Gilly J & Mays J (1995) Efficacy, safety and immunogenicity of a meningococcal group B (15:P1.3) outer membrane protein vaccine in Iquique, Chile. *Vaccine 13*, 821.

[15] Brisson JR, Baumann H, Imberty A, Perez S & Jennings HJ (1992) Helical epitope of the group B meningococcal α(2–8)-linked sialic acid polysaccharide. *Biochemistry 31*, 4996.

[16] Brisson JR & Jennings HJ (2001) NMR and molecular modeling of complex carbohydrates and carbohydrate-protein interactions. Applications to anti-bacteria vaccines. *Adv Exp Med Biol 491*, 543.

[17] Broker M (2003) Development of new vaccines against meningococcal disease. *Arzeneimittelforschung 53*, 805.

[18] Brusés JL & Rutishauser U (1998). Regulation of neural cell adhesion molecule polysialylation: Evidence for nontranscriptional control and sensitivity to an intracellular pool of calcium. *J Cell Biol 140*, 1177.

[19] Bystricky S, Pavliak V & Szu SC (1997) Characterization of colominic acid by circular dichroism and viscosity analysis. *Biophys Chem 63*, 147.

[20] Carlo DJ, Nollstadt KH, Stoudt TH & Maigetter RZ (1983) Group B streptococcal capsular polysaccharides. *US Patent* no 4,413,057.

[21] Centers for Disease Control (1978) Recommendations of the Immunization Practices Advisory Committee on Immunization Practices—Meningococcal polysaccharide vaccines. *Morb Mortal Weekly Rep 27*, 327.

[22] Centers for Disease Control (1985) Recommendations of the Immunization Practices Advisory Committee (ACIP)—Meningococcal vaccines. *Morb Mortal Weekly Rep 34*, 255.

[23] Cheung NKV, Saarinen VM, Neely JE, Landmeier B, Donovan D & Coccia PF (1985) Monoclonal antibodies to a glycolipid antigen on human neuroblastoma cells. *Cancer Res 45*, 2642.

[24] Constantino P, Viti S, Podda A, Velmonte MA, Nencioni L & Rappuoli R (1992) Development and phase 1 clinical testing of a conjugate vaccine against meningococcus A and C. *Vaccine 10*, 691.

[25] Defilippis I, Soares BEC, Valentim JC & Dealmeida AECC (1995) Development of a collection of bacteria causing meningitis in Rio de Janeiro from 1990 to 1991. *Memor Inst Oswaldo Cruz 90*, 21.

[26] Del Rio M, Demoly P, Koros AMC, Laurent JC, Mani JC, Pau B & Pujol J-L (1998) Characterization and assessment in detection and immunotargeting of PSA-NCAM in lung cancer. Polysialic acid: Biochemistry, Cell biology Diseases, October 2–6, Ile des Embiez, France.

[27] Diaz-Romero J & Outschoorn IM (1993) Detection of antibodies to *Neisseria meningitidis* group B capsular polysaccharide by a liquid-phase ELISA. *In: Roth J, Rutishauser U & Troy II FA (eds.) Polysialic acid: From microbes to man. Birkhäuser Verlag, Basel, Switzerland*, 39.

[28] Djibo S, Nicolas P, Alonso JM, Djibo A, Couret D, Riou JY & Chippaux JP (2003) Outbreaks of serogroup X meningococcal meningitis in Niger 1995-2000. *Trop Med Int Health 8*, 1118.

[29] Edelman GM (1983) Cell adhesion molecules. *Science 219*, 450.

[30] Edmond MB, Hollis RJ, Houston AK & Wenzel RP (1995) Molecular epidemiology of meningococcal disease in a university community. *J Clin Microbiol 33*, 2209.

[31] Eickhoff TC, Klein JO, Daly AK, Ingall D & Finland M (1964) Neonatal sepsis and other infections due to Group B beta-hemolytic streptococci. *New Engl J Med 271*, 1221.

[32] Eskola J, Käyhty H, Peltola H, Karanko V, Samuelsson J & Gordon LK (1985) Antibody levels achieved in infants by course of polysaccharide/diphteria toxoid conjugate vaccine. *Lancet 1*, 1184.

[33] Evans SV, Sigurskjold BW, Jennings HJ, Brisson J-R, To R, Tse WC, Altman E, Frosch M, Weisgerber C, Kratzin HD, Klebert S, Vaesen M, Bitter-Suermann D, Rose DR, Young NM & Bundle DR (1995) Evidence for the extended helical nature of polysaccharide epitopes. The 2.8 Å resolution structure and thermodynamics of ligand binding of an antigen binding fragment specific for α-(2→8)-polysialic acid. *Biochemistry 34*, 6737.

[34] Farr RS (1958) A quantitative immunochemical measure of the primary interaction between I*BSA and antibody. *J Infect Dis 103*, 239.

[35] Feizi T & Childs RA (1987) Carbohydrates as antigenic determinants of glycoproteins. *Biochem J 245*, 1.

[36] Finne J (1982) Occurrence of unique polysialosyl carbohydrate units in glycoproteins of developing brain. *J Biol Chem 257*, 11966.

[37] Finne J, Leinonen M & Mäkelä PH (1983) Antigenic similarities between brain components causing meningitis. Implications for vaccine development and pathogenesis. *Lancet II*, 355.

[38] Finne J & Mäkelä PH (1985) Cleavage of the polysialosyl units of brain glycoproteins by bacteriophage endosialidase. Involvement of a long polysialic acid segment in molecular interactions of polysialic acid. *J Biol Chem 260*, 1265.

[39] Finne J, Bitter-Suermann D, Goridis C & Finne U (1987) An IgG monoclonal antibody to group B meningococci crossreacts with developmentally regulated polysialic acid units of glycoproteins in neural and extraneural tissues. *J Immunol 138*, 4402.

[40] Frasch CE, Zahradnik JM, Wang LY, Mocca LF & Tsai C-M (1988) Antibody response of adults to an aluminium hydroxide adsorbed *Neisseria meningitidis* serotype 2b protein group B-polysaccharide vaccine. *J Infect Dis 158*, 700.

[41] Frasch CE (1990) Production and control of *Neisseria meningitidis* vaccines. *Adv Biotechnol Processes 13*, 123.

[42] Frosch M, Görgen I, Boulnois GJ, Timmis KN & Bitter-Suermann D (1985) NZB mouse system for production of monoclonal antibodies to weak bacterial antigens: Isolation of an IgG antibody to the polysaccharide capsules of *Escherichia coli* K1 and group B meningococci. *Proc Natl Acad Sci USA 82*, 1194.

[43] Fukuda MN, Dell A, Oates JE & Fukuda M (1985) Embryonal lactosaminoglycan. The structure of branched lactosaminoglycans with novel disialosyl (sialyl alpha 2–9 sialyl) terminals isolated from PA1 human embryonal carcinoma cells. *J Biol Chem 260*, 6623.

[44] de Gans J & van de Beek D (2002) European Dexamethasone in Adulthood Bacterial Meningitis Study Investigators. Dexamethasone in adults with bacterial meningitis. *N Engl J Med. 347*, 1549.

[45] Gotschlich EC, Liu TY & Artenstein MS (1969) Human immunity to the meningococcus. III. Preparation and immunochemical properties of the group A, group B and group C meningococcal polysaccharides. *J Exp Med 129*, 1349.

[46] Gotschlich EC, Fraser BA, Nishimura O, Robbins JB & Liu TY (1981) Lipid on capsular polysaccharides of gram-negative bacteria. *J Biol Chem 256*, 8915.

[47] Granoff DM, Bartoloni A, Ricci S, Gallo E, Rosa D, Ravenscroft N, Guarnieri V, Seid RC, Shan A, Usinger WR, Tan S, McHugh YE & Moe GR (1998) Bactericidal monoclonal antibodies that define unique meningococcal B polysaccharide epitopes that do not cross-react with human polysialic acid. *J Immunol 160*, 5028.

[48] Grifantini R, Bartolini E, Muzzi A, Draghi M, Frigimelica E, Berger J, Ratti G, Petracca R, Galli G, Agnusdei M, Giuliani MM, Santini L, Brunelli B, Tettelin H, Rappuoli R, Randazzo F & Grandi G (2002) Previously unrecognized vaccine candidates against group B meningococcus identified by DNA microarrays. *Nature Biotech 20*, 914.

[49] Haneberg B, Dalseg R, Wedege E, Høiby EA, Haugen IL, Oftung F, Andersen SR, Meyer Næss L, Aase A, Michaelsen TE & Holst J (1998) Intranasal Administration of a Meningococcal Outer Membrane Vesicle Vaccine Induces Persistent Local Mucosal Antibodies and Serum Antibodies with Strong Bactericidal Activity in Humans. *Infect Immun 66*, 1334.

[50] Harrison LH (1995) The worldwide prevention of meningococcal infection: Still an elusive goal. *J Am Med Assoc 273*, 419.

[51] He HT, Finne J & Goridis C (1987) Biosynthesis, membrane association, and release of N-CAM-120, a phosphatidylinositol-linked form of the neural cell adhesion molecule. *J Cell Biol 105*, 2489.

[52] Hoffman S & Edelman GM (1983) Kinetics of homophilic binding by E and A forms of the neural cell adhesion molecule. *Proc Natl Acad Sci USA 80*, 5762.

[53] Häyrinen J, Bitter-Suermann D & Finne J (1989a) Interaction of meningococcal group B monoclonal antibody and its Fab fragment with α2–8 linked sialic acid polymers: Requirement of a long oligosaccharide segment for binding. *Mol Immunol 26*, 523.

[54] Häyrinen J, Pelkonen S & Finne J (1989b) Structural similarity of the type-specific group B streptococcal polysaccharides and the carbohydrate units of tissue glycoproteins: Evaluation of possible cross-reactivity. *Vaccine 7*, 217.

[55] Häyrinen J, Jennings H, Raff H, Rougon G, Hanai N, Gerardy-Schahn R & Finne J (1995) Antibodies to polysialic acid and its *N*-propyl derivative: Binding properties and interaction with human embryonal brain glycopeptides. *J Inf Dis 171*, 1481.

[56] Häyrinen J, Haseley S, Talaga P, Mühlenhoff M, Finne J & Vliegenthart JFG (2002) High affinity binding of long-chain polysialic acid to antibody, and modulation by divalent cations and polyamines. *Mol Immunol 39*, 399.

[57] Idänpään-Heikkilä I, Muttilainen S, Wahlström E, Saarinen L, Leinonen M, Sarvas M & Mäkelä PH (1995) the antibody response to a prototype liposome vaccine containing *Neisseria meningitidis* outer membrane protein P1 produced in *Bacillus subtilis*. *Vaccine 13*, 1501.

[58] Jaques LW, Brown EB, Barret JM, Brey WS Jr & Weltner W Jr (1976) Sialic acid: A calcium binding carbohydrate. *J Biol Chem 252*, 4533.

[59] Jennings HJ, Rosell K-G & Kasper DL (1980) Structure and serology of the native polysaccharide antigen of type Ia group B *Streptococcus*. *Proc Natl Acad Sci USA 77*, 2931.

[60] Jennings HJ & Lugowski C (1981) Immunochemistry of groups A, B and C meningococcal polysaccharide-tetanus toxoid conjugates. *J Immunol 127*, 1011.

[61] Jennings HJ (1983) Capsular polysaccharides as human vaccines. *Adv Carbohydr Chem Biochem 41*, 155.

[62] Jennings HJ, Katzenellenbogen E, Lugowski C, Michon F, Roy R & Kasper DL (1984) Structure, conformation and immunology of sialic acid-containing polysaccharides of human pathogenic bacteria. *Pure Appl Chem 56*, 893.

[63] Jennings HJ, Roy R & Michon F (1985) Determinant specificities of the groups B and C polysaccharides of *Neisseria meningitidis*. *J Immunol 134*, 2651.

[64] Jennings HJ, Roy R & Gamian A (1986) Induction of meningococcal group B polysaccharide-specific IgG antibodies in mice by using an *N*-propionylated B polysaccharide-tetanus toxoid conjugate vaccine. *J Immunol 137*, 1708.

[65] Jennings HJ, Gamian A, Ashton FE (1987) *N*-Propionylated group B meningococcal polysaccharide mimics a unique epitope on group B *Neisseria meningitidis*. *J Exp Med 165*, 1207.

[66] Jennings HJ (1988) Chemically modified capsular polysaccharides as vaccines. *Adv Exp Med Biol 228*, 495.

[67] Jennings HJ (1989) The capsular polysaccharide of group B *Neisseria meningitidis* as a vehicle for vaccine development. *In: Cruse JM & Lewis RE Jr (eds.) Conjugate vaccines. Contrib Microbiol Immunol, Karger, Basel, Switzerland*, 151.

[68] Jennings HJ & Kasper DL (1992) Group B *Streptococcus* type II and type V polysaccharide-protein conjugate vaccines. US Patent Application no 07/949970.

[69] Jennings HJ (1994) Presented at the Workshop on Potential for Group B Meningococcal Polysaccharide Conjugate Vaccine, Bethesda, ML, USA.

[70] Jodar L, Feavers IM, Salisbury D, Granoff DM (2002) Development of vaccines against meningococcal disease. *Lancet 359*, 1499.

[71] Kabat EA (1960) The upper limit for the size of the human antidextran combining site. *J Immunol 84*, 82.

[72] Kabat EA, Liao J, Osserman EF, Gamian A, Michon F & Jennings HJ (1988) The epitope associated with the binding of the capsular polysaccharide of the group B meningococcus and of *Escherichia coli* K1 to a human monoclonal macroglobulin, IgM^{NOV}. *J Exp Med 168*, 699.

[73] Kasper DL (1986) Bacterial capsule - old dogmas and new tricks. *J Infect Dis 153*, 407.

[74] Kay R, Cheng AF & Tse CY (1995) *Streptococcus suis* infection in Hong Kong. QJM Month *J Assoc Physicians 88*, 39.

[75] Kiss, JZ (1998) Polysialic acid: Biochemistry, Cell biology and Diseases, October 2–6, Ile des Embiez, France.

[76] Kiss JZ, Wang C, Olive S, Rougon G, Lang J, Baetens D, Harry D & Pralong WF (1994) Activity-dependent mobilization of the adhesion molecule polysialic NCAM to the cell surface of neurons and endocrine cells. *EMBO J 13*, 5284.

[77] Koch C, Staffler G, Huttinger R, Hilgert I, Prager E, Cerny J, Steinlein P, Majdic O, Horejsi V& Stockinger H (1999) T cell activation-associated epitopes of CD147 in regulation of the T cell response, and their definition by antibody affinity and antigen density. *Int Immunol 11*, 777.

[78] Kornelisse RF, de Groot R & Neijens HJ (1995) Bacterial meningitis: Mechanisms of disease and therapy. *Eur J Pediatr 154*, 85.

[79] Krug LM, Ragupathi G, Ng KK, Hood C, Jennings HJ, Guo Z, Kris MG, Miller V, Pizzo B, Tyson L, Baez V & Livingston PO (2004) Vaccination of Small Cell Lung Cancer Patients with Polysialic Acid or *N*-Propionylated Polysialic Acid Conjugated to Keyhole Limpet Hemocyanin. *Clin Cancer Res 10*, 916.

[80] Krusius T, Finne J & Rauvala H (1978) The poly(glycosyl) chains of glycoproteins. *Eur J Biochem 92*, 289.

[81] Käyhty H, Karanko V, Peltola H & Mäkelä P (1984) Serum antibodies after vaccination with *Hemophilus influenzae* type b capsular polysaccharide and responses to reimmunization: No evidence of immunological tolerance or memory. *Pediatrics 74*, 857.

[82] Käyhty H, Åhman H, Rönnberg P-R, Tiilikainen R & Eskola J (1995) Pneumococcal polysaccharide–meningococcal outer membrabne protein complex conjugate vaccine is immunogenic in infants and children. *J Infect Dis 172*, 1273.

[83] Kyaw MH, Clarke SC, Christie P, Jones IG & Campbell H (2002) Invasive meningococcal disease in Scotland, 1994 to 1999, with emphasis on group B meningococcal disease. *J Clin Microbiol 40*, 1834.

[84] Lackie P, Zuber C & Roth J (1993) Expression patterns of polysialic acid during vertebrate organogenesis. *In: Roth J, Rutishauser U & Troy II FA (eds.) Polysialic acid: From microbes to man. Birkhäuser Verlag, Basel, Switzerland*, 263.

[85] Lafeber AB, van Limpt CJP, Berbers GAM, Labadie J, de Kleijn ED, de Groot R, Rumke HC & van Alphen AJW (2000) Immunogenicity and safety of monovalent RIVM meningococcal B OMP vesicle F91 vaccine administered to children that received hexavalent meningococcal B vaccine 2.5 years ago. *RIVM Rapport* 000012002.

[86] Lagergard T, Shiloach J, Robbins J & Schneerson R (1990) Synthesis and immunological properties of conjugates composed of group B *Streptococcus* type III capsular polysaccharide covalently bound to tetanus toxoid. *Infect Immun 58*, 687.

[87] Lepow ML & Hughes PA (2003) Control of serogroup A disease in sub-Saharan Africa is a major challenge. *Immunol Allergy Clin North Am 23*, 769.

[88] Lesinski GB & Westerink MA (2001) Vaccines against polysaccharide antigens. *Curr Drug Targets Infect Disord 1*, 325.

[89] Leying H, Suerbaum S, Kroll H-P, Stahl D & Opferkuch W (1990) The capsular polysaccharide is a major determinant of serum resistance in K-1-positive blood culture isolates of *Escherichia coli*. *Infect Immun 58*, 222.

[90] Li Y-T, Månsson J-E, Vanier M-T & Svennerholm L (1973) Structure of the major glucosamine-containing ganglioside of human tissues. *J Biol Chem 248*, 2634.

[91] Li Y, Sun YH, Ison C, Levine MM & Tang CM (2004) Vaccination with attenuated Neisseria meningitidis strains protects against challenge with live Meningococci. *Infect Immun 72*, 345.

[92] Lifely MR & Moreno C (1986) Vaccine against meningococcal group B disease. *Lancet I*, 214.

[93] Lifely MR, Moreno C & Lindon JC (1987) An integrated molecular and immunological approach towards a meningococcal group B vaccine. *Vaccine 5,* 11.

[94] Lifely MR, Esdaile J & Moreno C (1989) Passive transfer of meningococcal group B polysaccharide antibodies to the offspring of pregnant rabbits and their protective role against infection with *Escherichia coli* K1. *Vaccine 7*, 17.

[95] Lifely MR & Esdaile J (1991) Specificity of the immune response to the group B polysaccharide of *Neisseria meningitidis*. *Immunology 74*, 490.

[96] Lifely MR, Roberts S, Shepherd WM, Esdaile J, Wang Z Cleverly A, Aulaqi AA & Moreno C (1991) Immunogenicity in adult males of a *Neisseria meningitidis* group B

vaccine composed of polysaccharide complexed with outer membrane proteins. *Vaccine 9*, 60.

[97] Liu TY, Gotsclich EC, Jonessen EK & Wysocki JR (1971) Studies on the meningococcal polysaccharides. I. Composition and chemical properties of the group A polysaccharide. *J Biol Chem 246*, 2849.

[98] Liukkonen J, Haataja S, Tikkanen K, Kelm S & Finne J (1992) Identification of *N*-acetylneuraminyl alpha 2→3 poly-*N*-acetyllactosamine glycans as the receptors of sialic acid-binding *Streptococcus suis* strains. *J Biol Chem 267*, 21105.

[99] Lookene A, Chevreuil O, Østergaard P & Olivecrona G (1996) Interaction of lipoprotein lipase with heparin fragments and with heparan sulfate: Stoichiometry, stabilization and kinetics. *Biochemistry 35*, 12155.

[100] MacKenzie CR & Jennings HJ (2003) Characterization of polysaccharide conformational epitopes by surface plasmon resonance. *Methods Enzymol 363*, 340.

[101] Mandrell RE & Zollinger WD (1987) Measurement of antibodies to meningococcal group B polysaccharide: Low avidity binding and equilibrium binding constants. *J Immunol 129,* 2172.

[102] Mandrell RE, Azmi FH & Granoff DM (1995) Complement-mediated bactericidal activity of human antibodies to poly α2→8 *N*-acetylneuraminic acid, the capsular polysaccharide of *Neisseria meningitidis* serogroup B. *J Inf Dis 172*, 1279.

[103] Marques MB, Kasper DL, Shroff A, Michon F, Jennings HJ & Wessels MR (1994) Functional activity of antibodies to the group B polysaccharide of group B streptococci elicited by a polysaccharide-protein conjugate vaccine. *Infect Immun 62*, 1593.

[104] Marwick C (1991) Vaccine for meningococcal meningitis tested. *J Am Med Assoc 266*, 2052.

[105] Michon F, Brisson JR & Jennings HJ (1987) Conformational differences between linear α(2–8)-linked homosialooligosaccharides and the epitope of the group B meningococcal polysaccharide. *Biochemistry 26*, 8399.

[106] Moe GR & Granoff DM (2001) Molecular mimetics of Neisseria meningitidis serogroup B polysaccharide. *Int Rev Immunol 20*, 201.

[107] Moreno C, Lifely MR & Esdaile J (1985) Effect of aluminium ions on the chemical and immunochemical properties of meningococcal group B polysaccharide. *Infect Immun 49*, 587.

[108] Munson PJ (1983) LIGAND: A computerized analysis of ligand binding data. *Methods Enzymol 92*, 543.

[109] Mölling P, Jacobsson S, Bäckman A, & Olcén P (2002) Direct and Rapid Identification and Genogrouping of Meningococci and porA Amplification by LightCycler PCR. *J Clin Microbiol 40*, 4531.

[110] Nassif X (2002) Genomics of Neisseria meningitidis. *Int J Med Microbiol 291*,419.

[111] Nedelec J, Boucraut J, Garnier JM, Bernard D & Rougon G (1990) Evidence for autoimmune antibodies directed against embryonic neural cell adhesion molecules (N-CAM) in patients with group-B meningitis. *J Neuroimmunol 29*, 45.

[112] Nelson D, Neill W & Poxton IR (1990) A comparison of immunoblotting, flow cytometry and ELISA to monitor the binding of anti-lipopolysaccharide monoclonal antibodies. *J Immunol Methods 133*, 227.

[113] Paoletti LC, Wessels MR, Michon F, DiFabio J, Jennings HJ & Kasper DL (1992) Group B *Streptococcus* type II polysaccharide-tetanus toxoid conjugate vaccine. *Infect Immun 60*, 4009.

[114] Paoletti LC, Wessels MR, Rodewald AK, Shroff AA, Jennings HJ & Kasper DL (1994) Neonatal mouse protection against infection with multiple group B streptococcal (GBS) serotypes by maternal immunization with a tetravalent GBS polysaccharide-tetanus toxoid conjugate vaccine. *Infect Immun 62*, 3236.

[115] Paoletti LC & Kasper DL (2002) Conjugate vaccines against group B *Streptococcus* types IV and VII. *J Infect Dis 186*, 123.

[116] Paoletti LC & Madoff LC (2002) Vaccines to prevent neonatal GBS infection. *Semin Neonatol 7*, 315.

[117] Patel K, Rossell RJ, Pemberton LF, Cheung NK, Walsh FS, Moore SE, Sugimoto T & Kemshead JT (1989) Monoclonal antibody 3F8 recognises the neural cell adhesion molecule (NCAM) in addition to the ganglioside GD2. *Br J Cancer 60*, 861.

[118] Pelkonen S, Häyrinen J & Finne J (1988) Polyacrylamide gel electrophoresis of the capsular polysaccharides of Escherichia coli K1 and other bacteria. *J Bacteriol 170*, 2646.

[119] Peltola H, Mäkelä PH, Käyhty H, Jousimies H, Hera E, Hällström K, Sivonen A, Renkonen O-V, Pettay O, Karanko V, Ahvonen, P & Sarna S (1977) Clinical efficacy of meningococcus group A capsular polysaccharide vaccine in children three months to five years of age. *N Engl J Med 297*, 686.

[120] Peltola H (1983) Meningococcal disease: Still with us. *Rev Infect Dis 5*, 71.

[121] Peltola H, Käyhty H, Virtanen M & Mäkelä PH (1984) Prevention of *Hemophilus influenzae* type b bacteremic infections with the capsular polysaccharide vaccine. *N Engl J Med 310,* 1561.

[122] Pon RA, Lussier M, Yang QL & Jennings HJ (1997) *N*-Propionylated group B meningococcal polysaccharide mimics a unique bactericidal capsular epitope in group B Neisseria meningitidis. *J Exp Med 185*, 1929.

[123] Poolman JT (1995) Development of a meningococcal vaccine. *Infect Agents Dis 4*, 13.

[124] Raff HV, Bradley C, Brady W, Donaldson K, Lipsich L, Maloney G, Shuford W, Walls M, Ward P, Wolff E & Harris L (1991) Comparison of functional antibodies between IgG1 and IgM class-switched human monoclonal antibodies reactive with group B streptococci or *Escherichia coli* K1. *J Infect Dis 163*, 346.

[125] Rafuse F & Landmesser L (1996) Contractile activity regulates isoform expression and polysialylation of NCAM in cultured myotubes: Involvement of Ca2+ and protein kinase C. *J Cell Biol 132*, 969.

[126] Rauvala H & Finne J (1979) Structural similarity of the terminal carbohydrate sequences of glycoproteins and glycolipids. *FEBS Lett 97*, 1.

[127] Regan C (1993) Regulation of NCAM polysialylation state during information processing in the adult rodent. *In: Roth J, Rutishauser U & Troy II FA (eds.) Polysialic acid: From microbes to man. Birkhäuser Verlag, Basel, Switzerland*, 313.

[128] Remsen LG, Strain GM, Newman MJ, Satterlee N & Daniloff JK (1990) Antibodies to the neural cell adhesion molecule disrupt functional recovery in injured nerves. *Exp Neurology 110*, 268.

[129] Robbins J (1978) Vaccines for the prevention of encapsulated bacterial diseases: Current status, problems and prospects for the future. *Immunochemistry 15*, 839.

[130] Rodríguez-Aparicio LB, Luengo JM, Ferrero MA & Reglero A (1993) Comparative analysis of the antibodies against capsular polysaccharides of *Escherichia coli* K-92 and K-235: An immunochemical method for the identification of polysialic acids. *Int J Biochem 25*, 427.
[131] Rouiller DG, Cirulli V & Halban PA (1990) Differences in aggregation properties and levels of the neural cell adhesion molecule, NCAM between islet cell types. *Exp Cell Res 191*, 305.
[132] Sato C, Kitajima K, Inoue S, Seki T, Troy II FA & Inoue Y (1995) Characterization of the antigenic specificity of four different anti-(α2→8-linked polysialic acid) antibodies using lipid-conjugated oligo/polysialic acids. *J Biol Chem 270*, 18923.
[133] Saukkonen K, Leinonen M, Abdillahi H & Poolman JT (1989) Comparative evaluation of potential components for group B meningococcal vaccine by passive protection in the infant rat and *in vitro* bactericidical assay. *Vaccine 7*, 325.
[134] Segal S & Pollard AJ (2003) The future of meningitis vaccines. *Hosp Med 64*, 161.
[135] Sela M & Mozes E (1966) Dependence of the chemical nature of antibodies on the net electrical charge of antigens. *Proc Natl Acad Sci USA 55*, 445.
[136] Shapiro ED, Capobianco LA, Berg AT & Zitt MQ (1989) The immunogenicity of *Hemophilus influenzae* type B Polysaccharide–*Neisseria meningitidis* group B outer membrane protein complex vaccine in infants and young children. *J Inf Dis 160*, 1064.
[137] Shimoda Y, Kitajima K, Inoue S & Inoue Y (1994) Calcium ion binding of three different types of oligo/ polysialic acids as studied by equilibrium dialysis and circular dichroic methods. *Biochemistry 33*, 1202.
[138] Shin JS, Lin JS, Anderson PW, Insel RA & Nahm MH (2001) Monoclonal antibodies specific for Neisseria meningitidis group B polysaccharide and their peptide mimotopes *Infect Immun 69*, 3335.
[139] Stacy JE, Kausmally L, Simonsen B, Nordgard SH, Alsoe L, Michaelsen TE & Brekke OH (2003) Direct isolation of recombinant human antibodies against group B *Neisseria meningitidis* from scFv expression libraries. *J Immunol Methods 283*, 247.
[140] Suri M, Kabra M, Singh S, Rattan A & Verma IC (1994) Group B meningococcal meningitis in India. *Scand J Inf Dis 26*, 771.
[141] Tabor CW & Tabor H (1984) Polyamines. *Annu Rev Biochem 53*, 749.
[142] Tikkanen K, Häyrinen J, Pelkonen S & Finne J (1995) Immunoblot analysis of bacterial polysaccharides: Application to the the type-specific polysaccharides of *Streptococcus suis* and *Streptococcus agalactiae*. *J Immunol Meth 187*, 233.
[143] Toikka J, Aalto J, Häyrinen J, Pelliniemi LJ & Finne J (1998) The polysialic acid units of the neural cell adhesion molecule N-CAM form filament bundle networks. *J Biol Chem. 273*, 28557.
[144] Troy FA (1992) Polysialylation: From bacteria to brains. *Glycobiology 2*, 5.
[145] Tsang RS, Squires SG & Tam TW (2001) Characterization of Neisseria meningitidis strains isolated from invasive meningococcal disease cases in Canada in 2001. *Can J Microbiol 49*, 633.
[146] Watanabe K, Hakomori S, Childs RA & Feizi T (1979) Characterization of a blood group I-active ganglioside. *J Biol Chem 254*, 3221.
[147] Warren HS Jr, Gonzalez RG & Tian D (2003) Case records of the Massachusetts General Hospital. Weekly clinicopathological exercises. Case 38-2003. *N Engl J Med, 349*, 2341.

[148] Welsch JA, Moe GR, Rossi R, Adu-Bobie J, Rappuoli R & Granoff DM (2003) Antibody to genome-derived neisserial antigen 2132, a Neisseria meningitidis candidate vaccine, confers protection against bacteremia in the absence of complement-mediated bactericidal activity. *J Infect Dis 188*, 1730.

[149] Wessels MR, Muñoz A & Kasper DL (1987) A model of high-affinity antibody binding to type III group B *Streptococcus* capsular polysaccharide. *Proc Natl Acad Sci USA 84*, 9170.

[150] Wessels MR, DiFabio JL, Benedi V-J, Kasper DL, Michon F, Brisson JR, Jelinková J & Jennings HJ (1991) Structural determination and immunochemical characterization of the type V group B *Streptococcus* capsular polysaccharide. *J Biol Chem 266*, 6714.

[151] Wessels MR, Paoletti LC, Rodewald AK, Michon F, DiFabio J, Jennings HJ & Kasper DL (1993) Stimulation of protective antibodies against type Ia and Ib group B streptococci by a type Ia polysaccharide-tetanus toxoid conjugate vaccine. *Infect Immun 61*, 4760.

[152] World Health Organization (2003) Meningogoccal meningitis. *Indian J Med Sci 57*,369.

[153] Zollinger WD, Boslego JE, Frasch CE & Frøholm LO (1984) Safety of vaccines containing meningococcal group B polysaccharide. *Lancet II*, 166.

[154] Zuber C, Lackie P & Roth J (1993) Polysialic acid in adult brain: Its presence on the neural cell adhesion molecule and Na^+-channels. *In: Roth J, Rutishauser U & Troy II FA (eds.) Polysialic acid: From microbes to man. Birkhäuser Verlag, Basel, Switzerland*, 299.

In: Vaccinations: Types, Potential Complications… ISBN: 978-1-60692-969-8
Editors: D. B. Steen and H. L. Dyson

Chapter VII

Replication-Incompetent Adenoviral Vectors for Vaccination*

Angelique A. C. Lemckert[1,*], Ronald Vogels[1], Katarina Radošević[1], Dan H. Barouch[2], Jaap Goudsmit[1,3] and Menzo J. E. Havenga[1]

[1]Crucell Holland BV, P.O. Box 2048, 2301 CA, Leiden, The Netherlands;
[2]Beth Israel Deaconess Medical Center, Harvard Medical School, Boston, USA;
[3]Center of Poverty-related Communicable Diseases, Academic Medical Center, Amsterdam, The Netherlands.

Abstract

Recombinant viral vectors are being developed as vaccine carriers since they have been shown to induce strong antigen specific T-lymphocyte responses, which will likely prove important for effective vaccination against diseases such as HIV, malaria and tuberculosis. Of the many different viral vectors under development, replication-incompetent adenovirus vectors are particularly promising. These vectors have excellent safety records in vaccine and gene therapy trials, a mature production platform resulting in high yields, and excellent transgene-specific immune responses in both pre-clinical and early clinical studies. Of the 51 known human adenoviruses, adenovirus serotype 5 (Ad5) was first characterized and completely sequenced and therefore Ad5 has been used in the vast majority of gene therapy and vaccination studies. However, the high prevalence and neutralizing antibody titer against Ad5 in human populations worldwide, coupled to data from both pre-clinical and clinical studies demonstrating significant reduction of Ad5 based vaccination potency in presence of anti-Ad5 immunity, indicates a serious potential limitation for the clinical utility of Ad5 vectors. To overcome this limitation, the development of alternative adenoviral vectors with low seroprevalence is currently an area of active investigation. Alternative vectors under investigation generally group into three categories: (1) human adenovirus serotypes other than Ad5, (2) non-human

* * A version of this chapter was also published in *Genetic Vectors Research Focus*, edited by Pablo S. Ruiz published by Nova Science Publishers, Inc. It was submitted for appropriate modifications in an effort to encourage wider dissemination of research.

* Correspondence concerning this article should be addressed to: Angelique Lemckert, Phone: +31 (0)71 5199239; Fax: +31 (0)71 5199800; Email: Angelique.Lemckert@crucell.com.

adenoviruses, and (3) Ad5-based chimeric vectors. In this chapter, we will review recent advances in our understanding of adenoviral biology and progress in the development of alternative adenoviral vectors for vaccination.

Introduction

Traditional vaccine approaches consist of live attenuated organisms, whole killed pathogens, or protein subunits. Licensed vaccines based on these technologies are safe and protect millions of lives each year, and in general they function by inducing neutralizing antibodies. However, these traditional vaccine modalities often induce poor $CD8^+$ cytotoxic T lymphocytes (CTL) [1,2]. Induction of a strong CTL response is thought to be important for the control of a number of important human pathogens including human immunodeficiency virus (HIV), *Plasmodium falciparum* (malaria), and *Mycobacterium tuberculosis* (TB) [3-6]. Developing novel vaccine approaches is therefore an important research objective. One of the most exciting and promising vaccine modalities for this purpose are genetic vector-based vaccines. These types of vaccines consist of either naked DNA-based vectors or live recombinant viral/ bacterial-based vectors. In all cases the vaccines are genetically engineered to express proteins derived from human pathogens that elicit immune responses when presented to the host immune system. The use of naked DNA-based vaccine approaches has shown great promise in rodents (reviewed in [7]). However in humans, the level of CTLs induced has thus far been disappointing [8-11]. Considerable effort is therefore being spent currently on improving the immunogenicity of these carriers. Research focuses on improving the level of expression in eukaryotic cells through codon optimization and on identification of cytokines or costimulatory molecules that further prime the host immune system. Alternatively, combinations of naked DNA-based vectors with either live recombinant viral- or bacterial-based vectors is being studied intensively (reviewed in [12]).

In addition to naked DNA-based vaccines, a large panel of live recombinant vectors is being investigated. Live recombinant vector-based vaccines comprise either viral vectors predominantly derived from poxviruses, adenoviruses, alphaviruses, rhabdoviruses, myxoviruses, paramyxoviruses and picornaviruses (reviewed in [13-15]) or bacterial vectors mainly derived from Bacillus Calmette & Guérin (BCG), Salmonella, Shigella or Listeria (reviewed in [16,17]). Although many live recombinant vector-based vaccines are being explored, most pre-clinical and clinical experience has been obtained with live recombinant viral vectors based on poxviruses or adenoviruses.

The first poxvirus-based vaccinations, utilizing vaccinia virus, aimed to protect humans against smallpox. This vaccination was discontinued upon the successful eradication of smallpox from the human population but has resumed in certain first responder populations due to bioterrorism concerns. Vaccinia virus-based vaccination has also continued in the form of recombinant vaccinia virus-vectors expressing proteins derived from other pathogens. Nevertheless, safety concerns were already raised during the use of vaccinia virus to eradicate smallpox. The safety concerns were due to vaccine-related adverse events including eczema and encephalitis and spread of vaccinia virus from vaccinees to close contacts [18]. This led to the development of recombinant attenuated poxvirus vectors, including modified vaccinia virus Ankara (MVA), New York vaccine strain (NYVAC), canarypox (ALVAC) and fowlpox strain 9 (FP9). To date, several clinical phase I/ II trials have demonstrated excellent safety of such further attenuated poxvirus vectors, either as stand alone vaccines or in prime-boost vaccination studies [19-29]. Stand-alone vaccinations demonstrated the induction of only moderate frequencies of antigen specific CTLs. In contrast, heterologous prime-boost vaccine regimens, consisting of two serotypically distinct poxvirus vectors or a poxvirus vector in combination with a naked DNA vector or protein, have shown a marked improved immunogenicity as compared to single modality vaccine regimen. A phase III clinical HIV vaccine trial evaluating a replication-defective ALVAC vector prime with an alum-adjuvated gp120 protein boost is currently ongoing in Thailand [30].

The adenoviral vector has been tested as vaccine carrier against a variety of both veterinary and human pathogens and the number of diseases targeted via an adenovirus-based vaccine approach is rapidly growing. The use of the replication-incompetent adenoviral vector as vaccine carrier is most intensively studied within the HIV field. Two clinical phase I studies using replication incompetent adenovirus serotype 5 (Ad5) have been completed [31,32]. These phase I clinical trials have clearly illustrated the ability of Ad5-based vaccine vectors to induce potent T lymphocyte mediated immune responses, which warranted further testing of these candidate vaccines in phase II clinical trials [32,33]. However, these trials also demonstrated that pre-existing immunity against Ad5, which is highly prevalent among human populations, might interfere with vaccine potency and dose control. This chapter details the knowledge accumulated over two decades of basic adenovirus research and the generation of safe replication incompetent adenoviral vectors. Moreover, recent insights in adenovirus-vector based vaccine potency in relation to host neutralizing activity will be described as well as exciting novel strategies to circumvent this vector neutralization.

Adenovirus Biology

Classification, Disease Association, Particle Structure and Life Cycle

Human adenovirus (Ad) was first isolated from adenoidal tissues in 1953 [34], hence the name adenovirus. To date, 51 human adenovirus serotypes are identified [35] and classified into 6 subgroups A to F (table 1). Classification of adenovirus serotypes is based on (1) the ability of the adenovirus serotype to either or not hemagglutinate with erythrocytes from different animal species, (2) an unique antigenic fingerprint which means that sera raised in animals against one serotype do not cross-react with any other adenovirus serotype, and (3) DNA restriction analysis on the double stranded adenoviral DNA genome [36]. Clinical disease associations have been identified for many of the 51 human adenovirus serotypes (see also table 1). Adenoviral infections are normally self-limiting and do not require specific antiviral therapy. However, in immunocompromised hosts, such as HIV patients or transplant recipients, adenoviruses can cause severe illness which upon disseminated disease can become fatal [37-40].

Table 1. Classification of human adenoviruses and possible disease association

Subgroup	Serotypes	Possible disease association
A	12, 18, 31	Central nervous system (CNS) disease, Febrile respiratory disease
B	3, 7, 11, 14, 16, 21, 34, 35, 50	Hemorrhagic cystitis, Febrile respiratory disease
C	1, 2, 5, 6	Febrile respiratory disease, Hepatitis, CNS disease
D	8, 9, 10, 13, 15, 17, 19, 20, 22, 23, 24, 25, 26, 27, 28, 29, 30, 32, 33, 36, 37, 38, 39, 42, 43, 44, 45, 46, 47, 48, 49, 51	Keratoconjunctivitis, Febrile respiratory disease, CNS disease, Gastroenteritis
E	4	Febrile respiratory disease
F	40, 41	Gastroenteritis

The adenoviral genome ranges from 25 to 36 kilobases (kb) depending on the serotype and is remarkably conserved among the adenoviridae. The adenoviral genome is always flanked on both ends by inverted terminal repeats (ITR), which are essential for DNA replication. Attached to the ITRs at both ends of the viral genome is the so-called terminal protein (TP), which is considered to be essential to ensure early transcription and onset of DNA replication [41]. Three other viral proteins are directly associated with the viral DNA and are called, V, VII and X (also called mu [42]) [43]. These core proteins are essential for folding the DNA genome such that it can be packaged into the adenoviral particle. Adenoviruses are non-enveloped viruses with an icosahedral capsid (see figure 1), which is predominantly made up from three proteins: hexon (in total 240 trimeric proteins), penton-base (in total 12 pentameric proteins) and fiber (in total 12 trimeric proteins and associated with penton base). So-called minor capsid proteins, called IIIa and IX are located near the outer surface of the particle and interact with the hexon protein thereby increasing the strengths of the particle. Likewise, minor capsid proteins called VI and VIII which are located more at the interior, ensure DNA genome binding to the capsid and regulate particle size by interacting with hexon respectively [44,45].

The life cycle of adenovirus (figure 2) is both fascinating and complex starting with binding of the adenovirus particle to a specific cellular receptor. Thereafter the adenovirus particle is internalized via coated pits and escapes from the cellular endosome. Subsequently the adenoviral particle is transported to the nucleus (see paragraph *Tropism and internalization*). Once the adenoviral DNA is delivered to the nucleus a tightly controlled process of adenoviral transcription, replication and particle assembly follows. During this process the adenovirus takes complete control of the cellular transcription and translation machinery. Eventually, this leads to cell death and subsequent escape of hundreds of thousands of newly synthesized adenoviral particles (see paragraph *replication cycle*). Since the first adenoviruses studies were based on serotypes 2 and 5 most of the knowledge regarding the adenovirus life cycle is based on these two viruses. It is therefore that the processes described below are based predominantly on these viruses unless indicated otherwise.

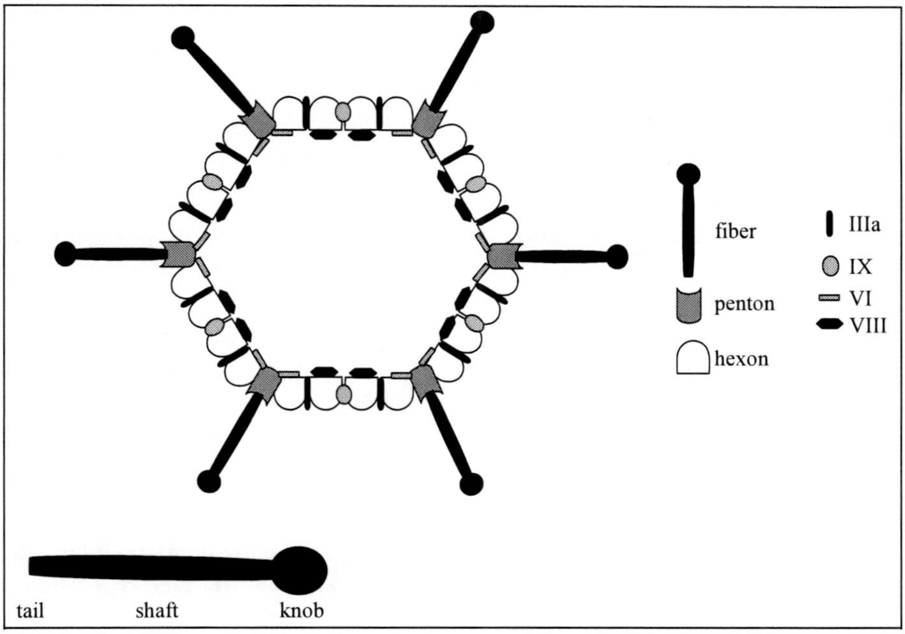

Figure 1. Schematic representation of the adenoviral capsid, showing the major capsid proteins (hexon, penton and fiber) and minor capsid proteins, polypeptides IIIa, IX, VI and VIII.

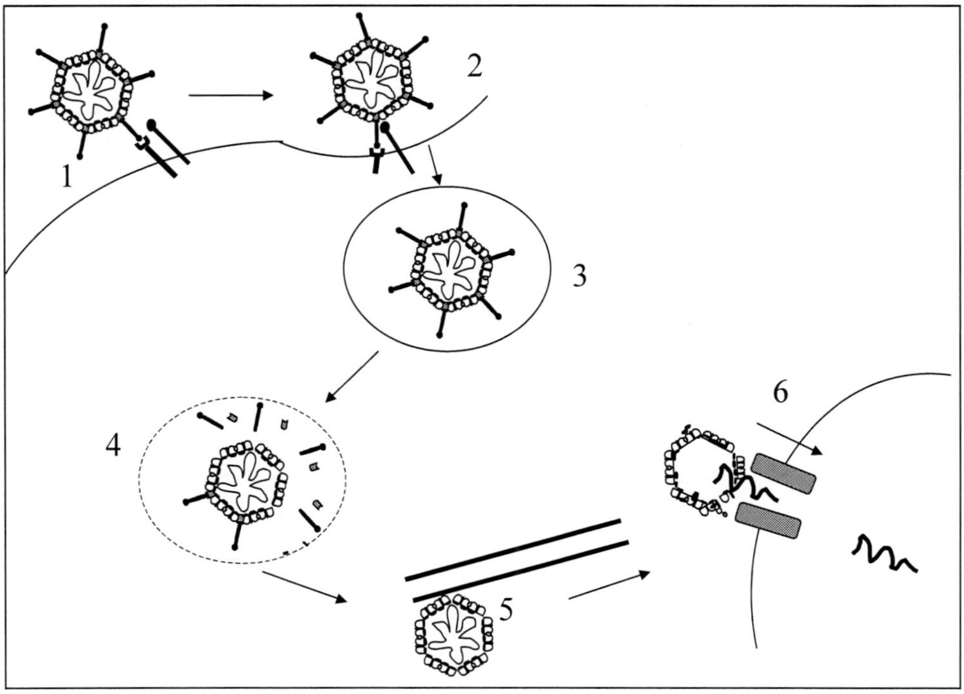

Figure 2. Adenovirus life-cycle: 1) Receptor-mediated binding to a cell, 2) Upon integrin binding, endocytosis, 3) Adenovirus particle in early endosome, 4) pH drop in endosome leads to particle destabilization and endosome membrane disruption through protein VI, 5) Destabilized particle is transported to the nucleus through dynein- and microtubule-mediated transport, 6) Adenoviral DNA enters the nucleus through the NPC.

Tropism and Internalization

The fiber protein has a characteristic structure, which consists of a tail domain located at the N-terminus, a central shaft and a knob domain at the C-terminus (figure 1). The first thirty amino acids of the fiber-tail are pivotal for the attachment of the fiber to the penton base [46]. The fiber and penton base are necessary for both cellular attachment and internalization of the adenovirus particle during infection. The fiber knob interacts with a specific cellular receptor to initiate cellular attachment. To date, several cellular receptors are identified that are employed by adenoviruses for cellular attachment. The coxsackievirus-adenovirus receptor (CAR) is used by most serotypes [47,48], except for those from subgroup B and some from subgroup D. The serotypes from subgroup B and some from subgroup D can utilize the membrane cofactor protein CD46 as primary receptor [49-54]. However, several other molecules like sialic acid [55], dipalmitoyl phosphatidylcholines (DPPC) [56], vascular cell adhesion molecule 1 (VCAM1) [57], CD80 and CD86 [58], heparan sulfate glycosaminoglycans [59], αMβ2 and αLβ2 integrins [60], major histocompatability complex I (MHC-I) [61] and lactoferrin [62] may also function as adenoviral cellular attachment molecules for certain serotypes. Despite the knowledge gathered to date, it is likely that the list of adenoviral receptors is to increase over time since for some adenoviral serotypes the cellular receptor has not yet been identified.

After initial adenoviral attachment to its cellular receptor, particle internalization via clathrin-mediated endocytosis occurs (figure 2). This is facilitated through binding of the penton base to cellular integrins. Essential for the binding to cellular integrins are three amino acids (Arg-Gly-Asp) that are located within the penton base and together are called the RGD motif [63-65]. Once in the endosome the adenovirus particle destabilizes due to a decrease in pH. This destabilization leads to dissociation of the fiber, penton base and minor capsid proteins IIIa, VI, VIII and IX from the adenovirus particle [66]. The dissociation of these proteins liberates protein VI, which is normally located on the inner surface of the adenovirus particle where it connects the bases of the hexon proteins adjacent to the penton base [67]. Once protein VI is liberated from the particle it exerts its membrane lytic activity, leading to endosomal membrane disruption [68]. This process finally results in the release of the destabilized adenovirus particle into the cytosol. From here it is transported to the nuclear pore complex (NPC) through a dynein- and microtubule-mediated transportation [69]. At the NPC the destabilized adenovirus particle docks to the NPC-filament protein CAN/Nup214, after which the viral DNA is released to enter the nucleus through a process that requires binding of the CAN/Nup214 docked capsids to nuclear histone H1 [70]. Once the adenoviral DNA is located within the nucleus the processes of transcription, replication and assembly of new adenoviral particles will take place.

The route of cellular internalization described above is predominantly determined for Ad5 and Ad2. Through recent knowledge on other human adenovirus serotypes and fiber chimeric adenoviral vectors, some exceptions have become apparent. The RGD motif needed for the cellular integrin binding, is absent in serotypes Ad40 and Ad41 that belong to subgroup F indicating an alternative entry route [71,72]. The cellular internalization of Ad41 proves to be delayed in comparison to other human adenovirus serotypes, which is attributed to the lack of the RGD motif and the consequential inability to bind to the cellular integrins [72]. In addition, Ad40 and Ad41 differ from other human adenoviruses in that their genome codes for two distinct fiber proteins that are both expressed and displayed on the viral particle, a short and a long fiber [73,74]. It has been convincingly shown that the long fiber of Ad41 is able to bind CAR, but the short fiber cannot [48]. Although poorly understood at present, the role of the short fiber is considered to lie in alternative routes of cellular internalization.

The viral escape from the endosome upon cellular internalization, resulting in release of the adenoviral particle into the cytosol and the subsequent transport to the NPC, is also not a conserved process among human adenoviridae. For instance, Ad7 which is a member of subgroup B does not escape the endosome but instead ends up in late endosomes and lysosomes [75]. Given the observation that an Ad5 vector containing only the fiber protein of Ad7 (Ad5fib7) also ends up in late endosomes and lysosomes, it has been speculated that the fiber protein is predominantly involved in determining the postinternalization trafficking route [76]. This finding was further supported by data demonstrating that an Ad5 vector carrying only the fiber knob of a B-group adenovirus, Ad35, ended up in late endosomes and lysosomes [77]. Since the fiber knob interacts with a specific cellular receptor and both Ad7 and Ad35 do not bind to CAR [48], it can be envisioned that specific receptor binding of the adenoviral particle determines the trafficking pathway towards the nucleus.

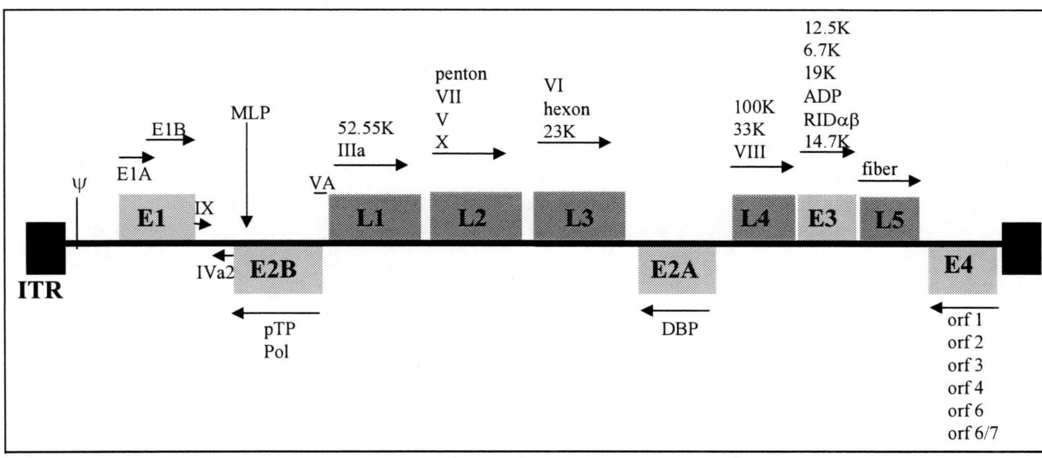

Figure 3. Schematic representation of the adenoviral genome, showing locations of the early (E) and late (L) transcription regions and the proteins derived thereoff. The packaging domain is indicated by Ψ.

Adenoviral Replication Cycle

The adenoviral transcription can be clearly distinguished in two phases, an early and a late phase. In the early transcription phase, proteins derived from six different genomic regions (E1A, E1B, E2A, E2B, E3 and E4; figure 3) are highly expressed. Most of these genomic regions produce multiple messenger RNAs (mRNA) and protein products through differential mRNA processing. In the late transcription phase proteins derived from five different genomic regions are expressed (L1 to L5; figure 3) and, like for the early regions, multiple transcripts and proteins can be derived per region. The start of DNA replication defines the transition between the early- and late transcription phase, sometimes also designated as the intermediate phase. Given the complexity of the replication system and vast amount of knowledge gathered on the diverse proteins and their role in replication, the early and late phase as well the different proteins will be discussed in separate headings below.

Early Phase of Adenoviral Replication

E1 -Proteins

Proteins derived from region E1A (289R and 243R) are known to trans-activate all other early regions and activate the infected cell by pushing the cell into the active DNA replication state (S-phase). By doing so, they create an environment that is optimal for adenoviral replication [78]. The cell activation by E1A-derived proteins occurs through interference with cellular proteins from the retinoblastoma (Rb) family (pRB, p107 and p130) resulting in free E2F [79,80]. In turn, E2F is a transcriptional activator that promotes expression of genes necessary to push cells into the S phase [81]. However, a downside of this mechanism of E1A-derived proteins is that the cells are forced into apoptosis via up-regulation of the tumor suppressor p53 levels [82]. To counteract this phenomenon, proteins of the E1B region are required. One of the products of the E1B region, 55K, is able to block the p53-dependent apoptosis by direct binding to p53 [83,84] and in cooperation with E4-orf6 [85-87]. Alternatively, E1A-derived proteins also induce a p53-independent cellular apoptosis pathway, mediated by the tumor necrosis factor α (TNFα) [88]. This pathway is effectively inhibited by another protein of the E1B region called 19K. The 19K protein binds to the Bak protein thereby preventing the interaction between the Bak and Bax proteins that would otherwise ensure triggering of the caspase induced apoptosis pathway [89].

E2-Proteins

The E2A region produces one transcript resulting in expression of the protein called adenoviral DNA binding protein (DBP). This protein is involved in several processes regarding adenovirus DNA replication such as initiation, elongation (reviewed in [90]), transcription control, DNA recombination, adenovirus particle assembly and mRNA stability (reviewed in [91,92]). The two transcripts of the E2B region called precursor terminal protein (pTP) and DNA polymerase (pol), together with DBP and two cellular transcription factors (Nuclear Factor (NF) I and III) form a complex that is required for forming adenovirus progeny genomes (reviewed in [93]).

E3-Proteins

From the E3 region seven transcripts are derived encoding for proteins called 12.5K, 6.7K, 19K, Adenovirus Death Protein (ADP), RIDα, RIDβ and 14.7K. Some of these proteins (RIDα and RIDβ) are involved in down-regulating cellular immunological response mechanisms in an attempt of the adenovirus to escape the host immune system (reviewed in [94]). For instance, the RIDα and RIDβ proteins (formerly known as E3-10.4K and E3-14.5K respectively) are both type I integral membrane proteins and together form the RID (receptor internalization and degradation) complex. The RID complex inhibits cellular apoptosis triggered by death ligands through down-regulation of their receptors [95-99]. Well known death ligands include TNF-related apoptosis-inducing ligand (TRAIL), TNFα and Fas ligand and they are launched by the host in defence against virus-infected cells. In addition, the RID complex hampers the TNF-mediated apoptosis and inflammatory responses by blocking of arachidonic acid release and by down regulating NF-κB activation [100,101]. Another protein of the E3 region (6.7K) is a type III integral membrane protein, localized in the endoplasmic reticulum (ER) [102], and known to suppress apoptosis by maintaining the cytosolic Ca^{2+} homeostasis [103]. Protein 6.7K can also be found in the plasma membrane, where it forms a complex with the RIDα and RIDβ proteins to down-regulate the TNF-related apoptosis-inducing ligand (TRAIL) receptor 2 [96,104]. Yet another protein of the E3 region (19K) is a type I integral membrane protein located mainly in the ER. In the ER 19K binds to major histocompatibility complex I molecules (MHC-I), resulting in inhibition of the transport of MHC-I molecules to the cell surface [105]. Normally, MHC-I molecules are relocated to the cell surface to present foreing antigens to the immune system. To further elucidate the mechanism of action of the 19K protein, mutants of this protein have been constructed and studied. It has been shown using a 19K protein deleted for the ER-retention motif in the C-terminus of the protein that, even though the protein was unable to block the transport of MHC-I to the cell surface, only a portion of the MHC-I molecules reached the cell surface. The latter finding indicates an additional interference of the 19K protein on the MHC-I pathway, which by now is known to be caused by the inhibition of MHC-I/ complex formation with TAP [106]. This inhibition results in obstruction of normal MHC-I maturation, which also results in reduction of the CTL-mediated cellular killing upon adenoviral infection. The last protein of the E3 region involved in immune escape is the 14.7K protein. In contrast to the other E3 derived proteins, 14.7K is not an integral membrane protein but is located in the cytoplasm and nucleus [107]. Like the RID complex and the 6.7K protein, 14.7K inhibits TNF-mediated apoptosis. However, unlike the other proteins described, 14.7K exerts its action by inhibiting the internalization of TNF receptor 1 [108]. Normally, the internalization of TNF receptor 1 leads to cellular apoptosis through so-called death inducing signaling complex (DISC) formation. The former last protein of the E3 region called ADP and formerly known as E3-11.6K is not involved in immune escape mechanisms. This protein is essential for the release of newly assembled adenoviral particles from the infected cell since absence of ADP proved to significantly delay the release of adenoviral progeny from the cell [109]. As a result of its function, ADP is predominantly expressed in the late phase of adenovirus replication in contrast to the other E3 proteins [110]. The last protein derived from the E3 region is called 12.5K and despite several investigations no function could as yet be attributed to this protein. Again, several exceptions exist to the number of proteins described from the E3 region derived from different adenoviridae. For instance the organization of the E3 region of the other adenoviral subgroups is not identical to those of subgroup C (reviewed in [111]). The only conserved E3-proteins throughout all subgroups are the proteins that form the RID complex and E3-14.7K indicating their importance. Some subgroups have E3 proteins that are unique to their own subgroup, like for example E3-20.3K and E3-20.6K for subgroup B [112] and E3-49K for subgroup D [113]. Studying the function of these E3 proteins derived from alternative serotypes is in its infancy.

E4-Proteins

The last early region (E4) codes for a number of proteins called open reading frame (orf) 1, 2, 3, 4, 6, and 6/7 that exert a variety of functions. The orf1 protein is related to dUTP pyrophosphatase (dUTPase) enzymes of viral and animal origin, however it does not appear to exert any enzymatic activity [114] and the precise function of the orf1 protein remains currently a mistery. Likewise, the function of orf2, has not yet been elucidated.

The orf3 protein shares several properties with orf6, including the interruption of the cellular double-stranded (ds) DNA repair mechanisms [115,116] and they both mediate efficient transportation of adenoviral mRNA from the nucleus to the cytoplasm in order to increase late adenoviral protein synthesis [117,118]. Interference with ds DNA repair is based on the inhibition of adenoviral DNA concatamer formation, which otherwise would block adenoviral DNA replication and adenoviral packaging [115,119]. Both orf3 and orf6 bind to and inhibit the function of DNA damage-activated DNA-dependent protein kinase (DNA-PK) [116]. Also, orf3 and orf6 both inactivate the Mre11 DNA repair complex [115] albeit through different mechanisms. For instance orf6 inactivates the Mre11 complex together with E1B-55K by proteasome-mediated degradation [115], while orf3 inactivates the Mre11 complex by directing the Mre11 complex from sites of DNA replication into large nuclear and cytoplasmic accumulations [115] consisting of aggregates of misfolded proteins [120]. The function of orf3 to relocate the Mre11 complex appeared not to be conserved between all human adenovirus serotypes, since it was found that the orf3 proteins of Ad4 and Ad12 are not able to relocalize the Mre11 complex [121]. The second shared property of orf3 and orf6 i.e. the efficient transportation of adenoviral mRNA from the nucleus to the cytoplasm [117,118] is poorly understood, although it is known that orf6, in contrast to orf3, forms a complex with E1B-55K to exert this function [122-124].

Besides the shared properties of orf3 and orf6, the proteins also display several unique functions. For example, orf3 has the ability to reorganize the promyelocytic leukemia protein (PML) nuclear body (also called PML oncogenic domain (POD), PODs/ND10 or ND10) [125,126], through interaction with PML isoform II (PMLII) [126]. The PML nuclear body structures are thought to be involved in DNA replication, DNA repair, transcriptional regulation, post-translational modifications, apoptosis and IFN-induced antiviral state [127-130]. Likewise, recently it has been demonstrated that the orf3 protein interacts with transcriptional intermediary factor 1α (TIF1α) which, like PML, is a member of the tripartite motif (TRIM) protein family [131]. Although the function of binding of orf3 to either PML or TIF1α is not completely understood, it has been postulated that the reorganization of the PML nuclear body by orf3 results in the inhibition of an IFN-induced antiviral response [132]. In contrast to orf3, unique functions provided by orf6 are almost exclusively performed after complexing with E1B-55K. For instance, the E1B-55K/E4-orf6 complex is involved in the shut-off of host cell protein synthesis, through inhibition of the transport of host cell mRNA to the cytoplasm. The latter finding contrasts with the finding that the E1B-55K/E4-orf6 complex mediates the efficient transport of the adenoviral mRNA to the cytoplasm. The mechanism by which the distinction between adenoviral mRNA and cellular mRNA is made has not yet been elucidated [133]. In addition, the E1B-55K/orf6 complex is also involved in the inhibition of p53-mediated apoptosis, as has been described before in the *E1-proteins* section.

The next E4-derived protein called orf4 is not essential for adenoviral growth [134], but is able to block transcription activation induced by E1A [135-137], auto-regulates its own transcription [137], regulates adenovirus alternative RNA splicing [138], induces hypophosphorylation of a variety of both viral and cellular proteins [135,138], induces p53-independent apoptosis [139,140], and induces cell cycle arrest [141]. Protein orf4 exhibits all these functions by its binding to serine/threonine specific protein phosphatase 2A (PP2A) [136].

The last protein derived from the E4 region is called protein orf6/7 since it exists as a fusion protein obtained through alternative splicing. This protein is known to interact with the cellular transcription factor E2F [142]. As mentioned before E2F is an important protein involved in the cell cycle [143]. Through the interaction with E2F, orf6/7 activates the adenovirus E2 promoter and the E2F-1 promoter itself [144,145] that is considered crucial in the adenoviral life-cycle.

Intermediate Phase

The start of DNA replication initiates the expression of two intermediate phase proteins called IVa2 and IX. Both proteins activate the major late promoter (MLP) [146,147], which is essential for expression of the late genes (see below). For IVa2 it has been demonstrated that activation of MLP is achieved only when IVa2 properly interacts with protein 33K derived from L4 [146,148]. Besides this primary role, protein IVa2 is part of a multi-protein complex that is involved in the packaging of adenoviral DNA [149-151] through binding to the packaging domain. The latter could be mediated by IVa2, since it has been demonstrated to interact with packaging sequences [152-154], possibly in conjunction with the proposed 22K protein derived from L4 [155]. Also for protein IX multiple distinct functions have been proposed next to its role as MLP activator, such as involvement in nuclear reorganization induced by adenovirus [156], full length viral DNA packaging [157] and ensurening proper interaction between hexon proteins [67,158].

Late Phase of Adenoviral Replication

The late phase proteins are transcribed from one single promoter, the major late promoter (MLP) (figure 3). The proteins produced in the late transcription phase are the structural proteins that together form the adenovirus particle (minor and major capsid proteins) or are proteins that are essential for the encapsidation and maturation of the adenovirus particle. In the early phase of infection the MLP is already active albeit at low level, leading to transciption only up to L3 and a mRNA production of L1-52.55K [159]. The MLP becomes fully activated upon adenovirus DNA replication, which is accomplished as described by protein IX [147] and protein IVa2 together with protein L4-33K [146,148]. In the late phase the MLP transcription proceeds up to L5, leading to a very large primary RNA transcript from which multiple mRNAs are produced through alternative 3'splice sites and five different poly(A) sites [160]. All mRNAs contain the tripartite leader (TPL) sequence, which is important for nuclear export, and translation of the mRNAs [161,162].

L1-Proteins

Late region-1 (L1) codes for 2 proteins called 52.55K and the minor capsid protein IIIa. Protein IIIa is a monomer that is in contact with four hexon proteins on the edge between facets (figure 1). In this way, IIIa stabilizes the interfaces between the facets in the adenoviral capsid [45,67]. The other L1 protein 52.55K plays an important role in adenoviral DNA packaging and virus particle assembly [163,164]. The precise mechanism of action is not determined yet. Nonetheless, it has been shown that 52.55K is able to bind to protein IVa2 [165] and that it is associated with the packaging domain [153]. However, further studies illustrated that the binding of 52.55K to the packaging domain is not associated with protein IVa2 but dependent of another yet unknown protein [154,166].

L2- Proteins

The four proteins derived from the L2 region are called penton base, VII, V and X. The penton base has been described before and is an important structural protein of the capsid situated at the twelve vertices and anchors the fiber protein to the capsid (figure 1). Protein VII, one of the core proteins, associates with the adenovirus DNA inside the capsid together with protein V and protein X [43]. Protein VII has been shown to interact with protein IVa2, protein 52.55K and unpackaged adenoviral DNA, suggesting a role for VII in an adenoviral DNA packaging complex [167]. In addition, protein VII is involved in the nuclear entry of the adenoviral DNA upon infection [168]. Protein V is one of the minor capsid proteins and forms a connection between protein VI and protein VII or the DNA [43,169], thereby connecting the adenovirus DNA to the capsid. In additon, a recent study using an adenovirus 5 vector deleted for protein V suggested that this protein may be important for correct viral particle assembly and that it could play a regulatory role in adenovirus-infected cells [170]. For protein X (mu), besides being one of the core proteins, not much is known. Although it has been hypothesized that it may has a role in the condensation of the adenovirus DNA [42].

L3- Proteins

The L3 region expresses three proteins called protein VI, hexon and the protease (23K). Hexon is the major component of the adenovirus particle as described earlier. The hexon appears to be the major target of the immune system of the host, proven by the identification of epitopes for neutralizing antibodies [171,172], $CD8^+$ T lymphocytes [173] and $CD4^+$ T lymphocytes [174] in the hexon protein. Minor capsid protein VI is, as most of the adenoviral proteins, a multi-functional protein. In the capsid it is positioned near the penton bases, where it connects the bases of the peripentonal hexons and connects the capsid to the DNA core through its connection with protein V [67]. During cellular internalization upon infection, VI has a role in the endosomal escape of the viral particle by working as a membrane lytic factor [68]. Near the end of the infection phase, protein VI plays a role in recruiting the hexon protein to the nucleus for assembly of the adenoviral particle [175]. Finally, VI works as a stimulant for 23K protease activity [176]. The last protein derived from L3 called 23K, is a protease [177] that is packaged within each viral particle released [178] and is essential for the adenoviral un-coating process that makes the cellular infection successful [179]. The activity of the protease is upregulated by the adenovirus DNA and protein VI [176]. In addition, the protease cleaves several minor capsid and core proteins during viral maturation, which is crucial for the stability of the adenovirus particle [180].

L4- Proteins

The L4 region expresses three proteins, which are called 100K, 33K and protein VIII. The 100K protein is involved in hexon trimer formation [181], ribosome shunting, and preference of the translation of viral mRNA in the late phase of infection through specific binding to adenoviral tripartite leader mRNAs [182]. Finally protein 100K is involved in inhibition of granzyme B-mediated cell death [183]. Protein 33K is derived from a spliced version of a L4 transcript [184]. The 33K protein has been reported to be involved in the adenoviral particle' assembly [185,186]. Additionally, 33K plays together with protein IVa2 a role in MLP activation [148] and is required to turn on full late gene expression [187], indicating that 33K is involved in both transcriptional and posttranscriptional mechanisms. Recently it has been found that at the start site of the 33K transcript, an alternative 22K transcript also initiates [155]. The proposed 22K protein is found to bind the packaging domain together with IVa2 and truncation of 22K blocks the production of infectious virus [155]. The last protein derived from the L4 region called protein VIII is one of the minor capsid proteins shown to interact with the inner surface of the hexon proteins in the particle [45]. It is further hypothesized that VIII works as a "tape measure" determining the viral particle size [188] and that it is involved in the particle stability [189].

L5- Proteins

The only protein derived from L5 is the adenovirus fiber. The fiber protein is involved in binding to the cellular receptor as described earlier. The fiber protein determines the adenoviral tropism through fiber knob mediated binding to a specific cellular receptor. Additionally not only the fiber knob determines the transduction of cell, but also the fiber shaft domain plays a role [190]. The fiber shaft is composed of several pseudo-repeats of which the amount varies between serotypes. It was illlustrated that by using different fiber shaft length the CAR-dependent transduction of cells could be altered; by using a long fiber shaft the transduction was more efficient in comparison to the use of a short fiber shaft [190]. This indicates the role of the fiber shaft in adenoviral cell transduction.

Virus-Associated RNAs

Besides all the proteins described above with clear time dependent expression, a number of viral RNAs are produced in the infected cells that exert important roles in the adenovirus replication cycle. These RNAs are called virus-associated (VA) RNA genes I and II and are transcribed first in the early phase and more abundantly in the late phase of the adenoviral infection. The genes encoding for the VA RNAs are the only genes in the adenoviral genome that are transcribed by RNA polymerase III [191]. VA RNA I is required for the relocation of adenoviral mRNA from the nucleus to the cytoplasm [192], for efficient initiation of translation of the adenoviral mRNAs in the late phase [193], and in the defense against the host immune response evoked by dsRNA through inhibition of protein kinase R (PKR) [194] and the RNAi pathway [195]. Little is known about the activity of VA RNA II. It has been demonstrated that VA RNA II is able to inhibit RNA helicase A [196] and that, like VA RNA I, VA RNA II interferes with the RNAi pathway [195]. Not all human adenoviruses express two VA RNAs. Subgroup A, B2 and F adenoviruses express only one VA RNA [197]. Whether this VA RNA gene has the same function as VA RNA I and II of the others is not known.

Adenoviral Vectors and the Host Immune Response

There are several features of adenoviruses that make them promising vectors for gene therapy and vaccination. First, adenoviruses are able to infect a wide range of tissues, and expression occurs regardless of the cell cycle status. Second, the genomes of Ad5, Ad2, and a variety of other serotypes are fully sequenced and well characterized, and these viruses have not been associated with severe disease. Third, initiation of the adenovirus replication cycle is tightly controlled by expression of E1 proteins. Therefore the generation of E1-deleted replication deficient vectors has easily been achieved using cell lines expressing the E1 protein *in trans* in order to complement the lack of E1 in the vector. Fourth, expression of foreign DNA under the control of heterologous promoters located in the former E1 region has been extremely succesful, resulting in high levels of transcription and protein expression of foreign genes. Finally, mammalian cell lines have been constructed that can support large-scale generation of adenoviral vectors for clinical applications.

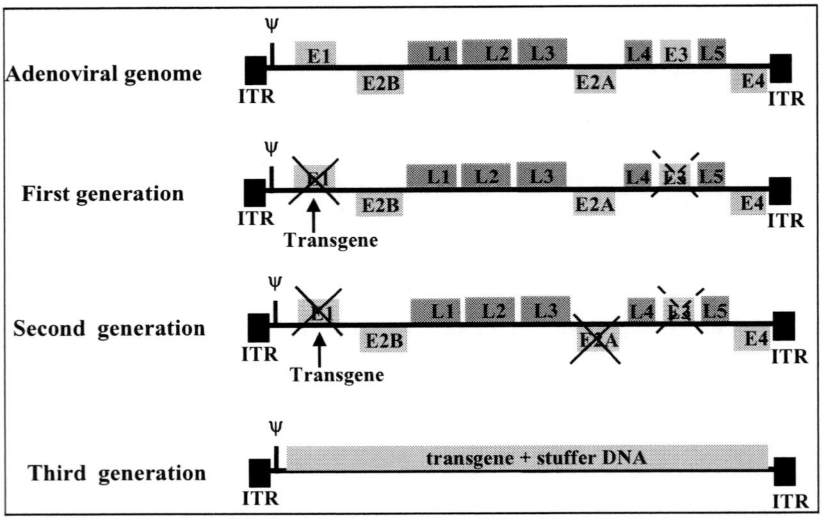

Figure 4. Schematic representation of the first, second and third generation of Ad5-based vectors. The deletion of certain early transcription regions is indicated by a cross. The deletion of the E3 region is optional for the first and second generation vectors.

First generation adenoviral vectors are deleted for the E1 region, or the E1 plus E3 regions (figure 4). Subsequently, vectors have been constructed in which an additional early transcription region, E2A, was deleted, and these vectors are commonly known as second generation vectors (figure 4). Finally, vectors have been constructed for which essentially the entire adenovirus genome was deleted except for the ITRs and packaging domain (figure 4). These crippled or "gutless" vectors, also called third generation vectors, are completely dependent on helper viruses in order to replicate. The advantages and disadvantages of each generation of vectors are described below.

First Generation Adenoviral Vectors

The first generation of Ad5 based vectors contains deletions in the E1 (E1A and E1B) region. This deletion renders them replication incompetent, since the activation of the E2 region required for DNA replication is strictly dependent on E1, as described above. The deletion of the E1 region, which encompasses approximately 5kb of genomic viral DNA, can subsequently be used for the insertion of a foreign DNA expression cassette. This expression cassette in general consists of a heterologous promoter such as the cytomegalovirus promoter (CMV), a foreign DNA insert coding for a protein of interest (transgene) and a heterologous transcription termination signal (typically derived from SV40). For propagation and production of these E1-deleted vectors, E1 has to be provided *in trans* and therefore specific mammalian packaging cells expressing the Ad5 E1 proteins have been generated. The first of such cell lines became known as HEK 293 cells [198]. These cells contain approximately 4300 bp of the left end of Ad5 genome including the E1 coding domain as well as the left ITR, the packaging domain, and DNA coding for protein IX [199]. This cell line allows efficient propagation of E1-deleted Ad5 vectors, however HEK 293 cells also allow the generation of replication-competent adenoviruses (RCA) [200]. RCA can emerge from HEK 293 cells through a recombination event between overlapping sequences in the adenoviral vector and the E1 region sequences present in the cellular HEK 293 DNA. The presence of RCA in an adenoviral batch represents a potential safety risk. For this reason, a new E1-complementing cell line has been developed referred to as PER.C6® cells [201]. PER.C6® cells do not result in RCA since no sequences other than the strict Ad5 E1 region are present. This has proven to avoid homologous recombination between the E1-deleted adenoviral vector and sequences within the cell line and thus the generation of RCA is prevented.

In addition to the E1 deletion in first generation adenoviral vectors, the E3 region can also be deleted. This has the advantage that it allows the insertion of larger expression cassettes (up to 8 kb). Since the E3 region is not essential for adenoviral growth, as described above, the loss of E3 does not have to be compensated. Therefore, the double E1/E3-deleted adenoviral vectors can also be propagated and produced on E1-complementing cell lines. In general, given the known functions of the E3-derived proteins, the E3 region is present in vectors used in gene therapy where long-term expression of the transgene is desired. In contrast, vectors are deleted for the E3 region when the vectors are used for vaccination where strong immune responses are desired. Since adenoviral vectors do not integrate into the cellular host genome, expression of a transgene is transient [202-204], which represents a serious limitation for gene therapy against inherited genetic disorders or other targets that require long-term transgene expression. The rapid loss of transgene expression, i.e. within two weeks after administration, is in part explained by the vigorous host immune response raised against the vector [205-208]. Confirmation of the importance of the immune system in eradicting transgene expression came from *in vivo* experiments using first generation adenoviral vectors in immune-compromised mice which demonstrated that transgene expression in these mice could be obtained for a long period of time [209,210]. This host immune response could theoretically be elicited simply by exposure of the administered adenoviral capsids to the immune system, or could be provoked by *de novo* sythesis of adenoviral proteins. The reason for considering both options was the observation that, even in the absence of the E1 region, low background expression of both early and late proteins could be readily detected in infected cells [205,207]. Since at the time both options seemed valid, the field moved into improving adenoviral vectors by deleting more adenoviral genes, which resulted in the second generation vectors.

Second and third Generation Adenoviral Vectors

To eradicate expression of either early or late proteins in infected cells upon exposure to an adenoviral vector, an additional deletion of the E2A gene was performed. This resulted in second generation adenoviral vectors. Since the E2A region is essential for adenoviral replication, an additional cell line had to be generated that complemented the E2A gene function *in trans* [211]. At first, the need for such a novel E1-E2A trans-complementing cell line was avoided by the use of a heat sensitive mutation (H5*ts*125) in the E2A gene [212]. This mutation allows for growth and production of the adenoviral vector at the permissive temperature of 32°C, but not at 39°C. Initial results with this vector were encouraging, demonstrating less *de novo* production of adenoviral proteins in cell culture experiments and prolonged transgene expression in mice [213-216]. However, risk of virus reversion to the E2A wild type coupled to leaky E2A expression at 37°C of the H5*ts*125 mutation, further stimulated the development of adenoviral vectors carrying a complete E2A deletion. Surprisingly, this second generation vector did not meet the expectation raised by the H5*ts*125 mutant vector [217] for reasons poorly understood. One plausible explanation was offered by finding that with the H5*ts*125 mutation low- level DBP was still produced in infected cells. The DBP down regulates expression of the E4 gene products 6 hours post infection [218,219]. Therefore, it was hypothesized that complete lack of DBP could result in prolonged expression of E4-derived proteins with possible negative impact on host immune responses launched against vector infected cells, resulting in diminished transgene expression [220]. This hypothesis resulted in further attenuation by deleting the E4 region. Our own unpublished results using an Ad5 vector deleted for E1 and E2A as well as E4 failed to demonstrate prolonged transgene expression in mice. Furthermore, this vector failed to show any advantage in vector mediated toxicity as compared to a first generation vector in rats, as measured by identical dose dependent liver pathology, reduced platelet counts and liver enzyme levels (alanine transaminase) measured in blood that is indicative for liver damage (unpublished results).

Third generation vectors (also called helper-dependent or "gutless" vectors) are deleted for almost the complete adenoviral genome, except for the ITRs and the packaging domain. Consequently, an expression cassette of up to 37 kb can be inserted. This in itself poses challenges since it is known that an adenoviral genome smaller than 27 kb poorly replicates [221]. Thus in order to obtain a insert of the proper size, stuffer DNA must be used which does not influence transgene expression but also does not encode for any other protein [222]. Another point of concern for third generation adenoviral vectors is the need for a helper virus during manufacture and the inability to eradicate this helper virus post production [223,224]. Potentially the helper virus may than induce an immune response. A strategy developed to reduce helper virus contamination is the use of the Cre-lox system. In this system loxP-sites are inserted around the packaging domain of the helper virus to prevent helper virus packaging through Cre-recombinase [225]. However, complete loss of contamination with helper virus is not yet achieved, since CRE escape, inversion and packaging domain recombination can all occur (figure 5). Several *in vivo* studies have demonstrated encouraging results in that both expression and detection of the transgene DNA was prolonged in pre-clinical models [226-228]. However, other resports demonstrated that third generation adenoviral vectors still induce adenoviral-specific T lymphocyte responses [229,230].

The lack of convincing data demonstrating the advantage of further attenuated second and third generation vectors in escaping the immune response turned the focus of the field in investigating the antigenicity of the adenoviral particle itself. A convincing study administrating biologically inactivated adenoviral vectors in mice [231], together with the anti-vector responses observed for the third generation vectors [229,230], demonstrated that the adenoviral particle itself plays an important role in the elicited immune response.

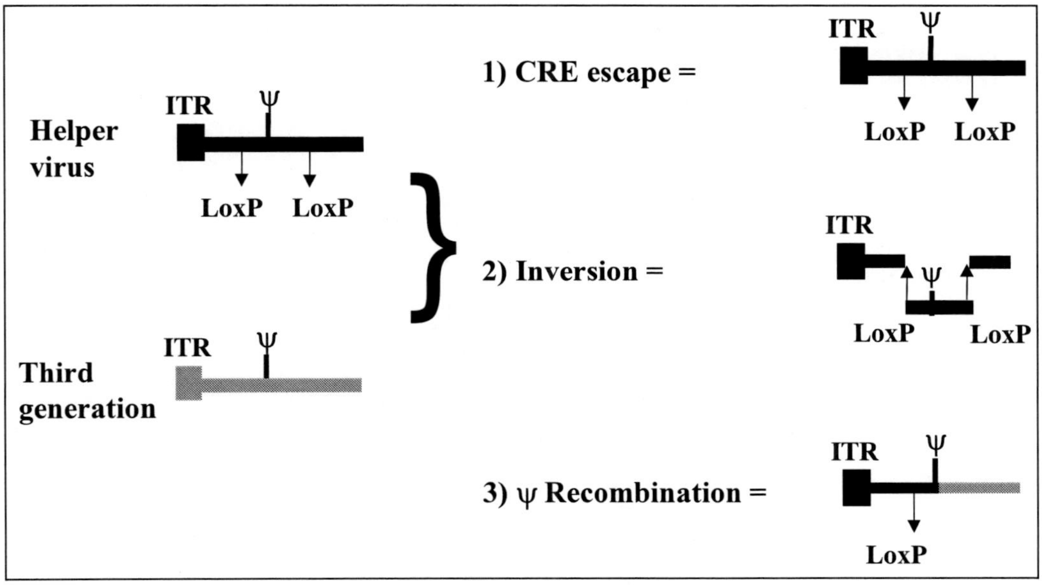

Figure 5. Cre-lox system for third generation vector growth. In this system loxP-sites are inserted around the packaging domain of the helper virus to prevent helper virus packaging through Cre-recombinase. CRE escape (1), inversion (2) and packaging domain recombination (3) can however still occur.

Immune Responses against Adenovirus Vectors and the Transgene

Further detailed investigations of the antigenicity of adenoviral vectors revealed that the adenoviral particle induced anti-vector cellular immune response through mediation of the innate immune response [232-234]. The importance of the adenoviral capsid for induction of an innate immune reponse was exemplified by a study which showed that the hexon protein alone has adjuvant-like qualities since it was capable of inducing a cell mediated immunity (CMI) [235]. Cells exposed to adenovirus react by releasing pro-inflammatory cytokines and chemokines including TNFα, IL-6, IL-8, IL-12, IFNγ, MIP-2, MIP-1β, IP-10 and RANTES [232,233,236,237]. These cytokines and chemokines ensure that the infection remains local by inhibiting viral protein synthesis and ensure attraction and activation of effector cells (e.g. granulocytes, natural killer (NK) cells, dendritic cells (DC) and macrophages) [238]. The effector cells do not only execute cytolytic functions at the site of infection but also secrete additional cytokines and chemokines that aid the adaptive immune response. In addition, uptake of adenoviral particles by DC and macrophages and subsequent antigen presentation results in activation of $CD8^+$ CTL and $CD4^+$ T-lymphocytes (figure 6) [237].

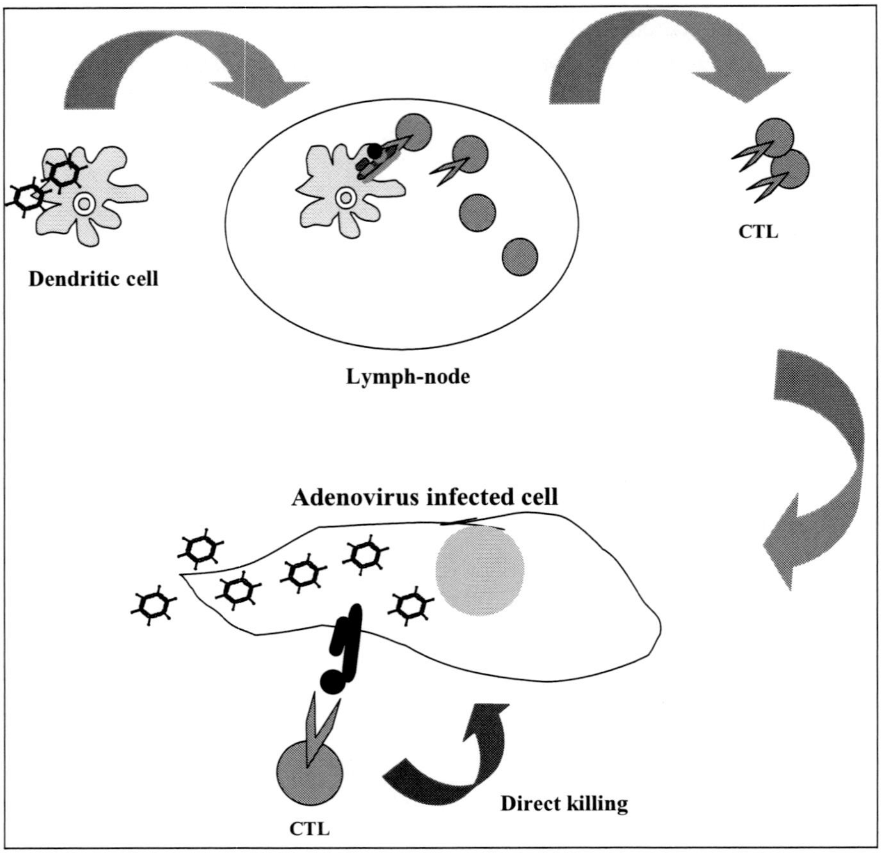

Figure 6. Uptake of adenoviral particles by DC and subsequent antigen presentation in the lymphnode results in activation of $CD8^+$ CTL. The CTL than directly kills adenovirus infected cells upon antigen presentation.

The first evidence that an immune response can be obtained against an inserted antigen was demonstrated by showing prolonged expression in mice of a mouse antigen as compare to the same vector carrying the human equivalent [239]. Another elegant study demonstrating the immunogenicity of the transgene utilized adenoviral vectors carrying human factor IX (FIX) that were administrated to mouse strains with different genetic backgrounds. This study proved that expression of FIX depended on the type of immune reponse elicited (humoral versus cellular) and on the tolerance of the mouse strain to the transgene [210].

The induction of an innate immune response and the capability of inducing a transgene-specific immune response are clearly serious limitations for the use of these vectors for gene therapy purposes. However, these studies triggered interest in the adenovirus vector system for vaccination, since the induction of vigorous immune responses are desirable features of a vaccine carrier. The potential of adenoviral vectors as vaccines has raised enormous interest in a variety of disease models. Most of these studies employ Ad5 since this vector system was readily available. The remainder of this chapter will describe the scientific findings thus far on the use of adenoviral vectors for vaccination purposes, in particular in the field of infectious diseases.

Adenoviral Vectors for Vaccination

The rationale for using adenoviral vectors as vaccine carriers is based on the many observations demonstrating the vigorous host immune response upon adenoviral vector administration. This section will review the advantages and disadvantages of Ad-based vectors as vaccine carriers.

Pre-Clinical and Clinical Studies using Ad5 Based Vaccines

As mentioned above, many vaccine studies have been performed using adenovirus 5 (Ad5)-based vaccine vectors. An overview of such studies is provided in table 2. A common denominator of these studies is that they target human pathogens that require induction of cell-mediated immunity (CMI) as well as antibodies. Ad5-based vaccines are potent inducers of transgene-specific $CD8^+$ T lymphocytes. In addition to transgene-specific $CD8^+$ T lymphocytes, Ad5-based vaccines also induce transgene-specific antibodies and $CD4^+$ T lymphocytes.

Several landmark studies have been reported demonstrating the potency of Ad5-based vaccines. For instance, a single administration with Ad5 vectors has proven to protect either mice and monkeys upon challenge against various infectious pathogens [240-248]. As candidate AIDS vaccines, Ad5 vectors have achieved partial protection against SHIV and SIV in the non-human primate model [249]. Based on these promising pre-clinical studies, a number of Ad5-based vaccines have entered human clinical trials (a partial list is shown in table 3). Recently, the first two phase I clinical trials for Ad5 based vectors have been finalized. The first included an Ad5-based vector expressing HIV clade B Gag or a combination of Ad5-based vector expressing clade B Gag, Pol and Nef [32]. The Ad5-based vaccines proved well-tolerated, safe and transgene-specific T cell responses were readily detected in approximately 70% of the participants. Following this phase I clinical study a phase IIb proof-of-concept study was launched with the Ad5-based vector expressing clade B Gag, Pol and Nef. This study aims to answer the pivotal question regarding whether cell-mediated immunity will prevent or control HIV in humans [33]. The other phase I clinical trial completed utilized a vaccine consisting of a 3:1:1:1 ratio of Ad5-based vectors expressing HIV clade B Gag-Pol fusion protein, HIV clade A Env, HIV clade B Env and HIV clade C Env [31]. This study demonstrated induction of transgene-specific $CD4^+$ and $CD8^+$ T lymphocytes with 93.3% and 60% response rates respectively. Additional studies are evaluating whether priming with a DNA vaccine can further potentiate immune responses obtained with Ad5-based vectors. This DNA prime, Ad5 boost regimen is expected to enter phase IIb testing later this year.

Table 2. Infectious agents to which Ad5-based vaccine vectors are developed

INFECTIOUS AGENT	GENE OF INTEREST	REFERENCES
Human/simian immunodeficiency virus	Gag, Env, Pol	[249-252, 259, 269]
Malaria	CS	[240, 254, 258, 312]
Ebola	GP, NP	[241, 257, 313]
Marburg virus	GP	[314]
Dengue virus	E, prM	[315-317]
Influenza	HA	[242]
SARS	spike, membrane, nucleocapsid protein	[318-320]
Rabies virus	glycoprotein	[243, 244]
Hepatitis C	NS3, core, E2	[255, 321, 322]
Herpes simplex 2 virus	gB	[245, 246]
Tuberculosis	Ag85A	[253]
Bacillus anthracis	PA	[247, 256, 323]
Yersinia pestis	V antigen	[248]

Table 3. Ad5-based vaccine vectors currently in clinical trials

IMMUNOGEN	REGIMEN	PHASE	SPONSOR
HIV-1 clade B Gag, Pol and Nef and clades A, B and C Env	p: DNA b: Ad5 vector	I	NIH VRC
Ebola Zaire and Sudan-Gulu GP	p: Ad5 vector	I	NIH VRC
P. falciparum CSP and AMA1	p: Ad5 vector	I/IIa	USAID, CDMRP, MIDRP
HIV-1 clade B Gag, Pol and Nef	p: Ad5 vector	IIb	Merck
HIV-1 clade B Gag, Pol and Nef and clades A, B and C Env	p: DNA b: Ad5 vector	IIa	NIH VRC

prime (p), boost (b), National Institutes of Health Vaccine Research Center (NIH VRC), United States Agency for International Development (USAID), Congressionally Directed Medical Research Programs (CDMRP), Military Infectious Diseases Research Program (MIDRP).

The use of prime-boost regimens is a strategy to increase the immunogenicity of Ad5-based vectors. In pre-clinical studies it was shown that heterologous prime-boost regimens, either Ad5-vector in combination with DNA vaccines or poxvirus vectors, were substantially more potent than homologous prime-boost regimens (Ad5-vector prime and Ad5-vector boost) [249-256] and achieved and/or improved protection against a variety of pathogens [249,254,256-259]. Although these studies with prime-boost regimens have shown improvement on immune induction, from a product perspective the combined use of two different vaccine components poses challenges to the vaccine industry. However, results obtained with homologous Ad5 prime-boost regimens have thus far been disappointing. Reason for the latter are the very high and potent neutralizing antibody response induced against the Ad5 vector after the initial priming vaccination that largely prevent effective homologous boosting with the same vector. These findings have propelled investigation into the worldwide seroprevalence of Ad5 in human populations. The detrimental effects of anti-

Ad5 immunity on Ad5 vaccine potency and current strategies to circumvent the high titered and prevalent anti-Ad5 immunity in human populations will be discussed in the next section.

The Problem of Ad5 Pre-Existing Immunity and Possible Solutions

Pre-clinical studies using both mice and non-human primates have shown that pre-existing anti-Ad5 immunity blunts the immunogenicity (figure 7) of Ad5-based vaccine vectors [250,260,261]. These findings have been confirmed by results obtained from the completed phase I human trials as described earlier [31,32]. In mice, it has been demonstrated that both Ad5-specific neutralizing antibodies (NAbs) and T lymphocytes play a role in the anti-Ad5 immunity, with the Ad5-specific antibodies being the most important component [262,263]. In humans, Ad5-specific NAbs are highly prevalent and in certain regions (e.g. sub-Saharan Africa) NAb titers are very high [53,54,264-267] (figure 6). Ad-specific $CD4^+$ and $CD8^+$ T lymphocytes have been found in humans [173,268], although the importance of Ad-specific T lymphocyte responses remains unclear. The high prevalence of anti-Ad5 immunity in the human population is a potential major limitation to the utility of Ad5-based vaccine vectors. Pre-existing anti-Ad5 immunity could reduce the immunogenicity and protective efficacy of Ad5-based vaccines as well as prevent accurate dose control.

Currently several research strategies are being pursued to tackle the problem of Ad5 pre-existing immunity. One strategy is exploring the possibility that Ad5-based vaccines may still be effective as a boosting agent following an efficient alternative priming agent. Therefore, a combination of a DNA vaccine prime and Ad5 vector boost is being investigated [260,261,269]. Other strategies to circumvent anti-Ad5 immunity are based on adenoviral vectors that at least are devoid of key regions of the hexon protein of Ad5 given the importance of hexon as a target for NAbs [171,172]. Two strategies include the generation of replication incompetent adenoviral vectors derived from either alternative human adenoviruses or non-human adenoviruses. A third strategy encompasses the generation of chimeric Ad5-based vectors in which key regions of the hexon have been replaced by corresponding regions from rare human adenoviruses. The advantages and disadvantages of these diverse strategies will be discussed in more detail below.

Alternative Human Serotype Adenoviral-based Vaccines

To identify human adenoviruses with low seroprevalence among human populations, our lab and others have conducted worldwide seroprevalence surveys using sera derived from healthy adults [53,264-266,270]. These studies helped identify a panel of human adenoviruses that have a low seroprevalence worldwide and that also have low NAb titers in individuals who are seropositive, including human serotypes Ad11, Ad26, Ad35, Ad48, Ad49 and Ad50. Most importantly, many of these serotypes do not only display low seroprevalence in developed countries but also in developing countries (see figure 8), which are important target regions for vaccines. From these and other serotypes, replication-incompetent vector systems have been generated (table 4). Initially it was found that these particular vector systems grew poorly on A5-E1 complementing cell lines [53,264,265,271]. The exchange of the native E4-orf6 gene for the Ad5 E4-orf6 gene in this systems, resulted in efficient propagation of these replication-deficient vector systems on an A5-E1 complementing cell line [53,54,271]. This phenomenon confirms the importance of the formation of E1B-55K/E4-orf6 complex for efficient transport of viral mRNAs from the nucleus to the cytoplasm and subsequent progeny viruses.

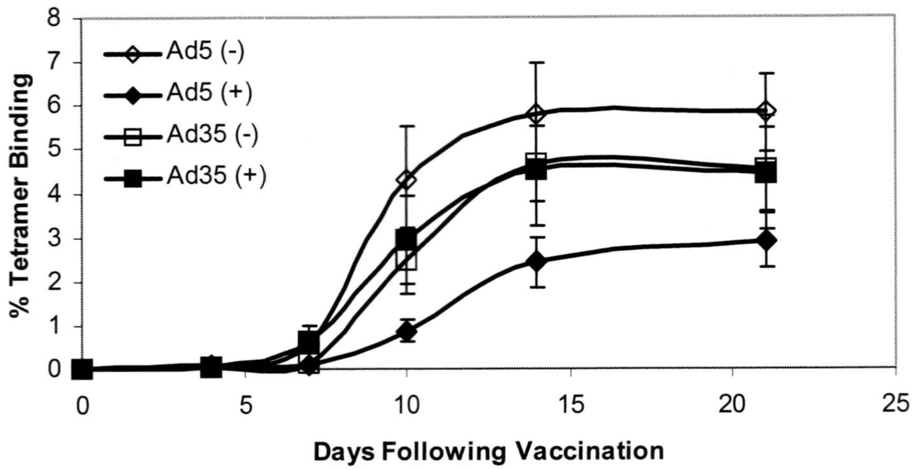

Figure 7. Naïve mice (-) and mice with anti-Ad5 immunity (+) were vaccinated with Ad5.SIVGag or Ad35.SIVGag and transgen-specific T lymphocyte responses were assessed by tetramer-bining assays at different timepoints post vaccination.

Human adenovirus 35 (Ad35) has proven to be rare in human populations [264,266,267] and is the first rare serotype adenovirus to enter phase I clinical trials. Ad35-based vectors are being studied as vaccine carriers for HIV/SIV [272,273], malaria [274] and tuberculosis [271,275]. Pre-clinical studies in mice [272] and non-human primates [273,276] have demonstrated that an Ad35-based vaccine is capable of inducing potent antigen-specific $CD4^+$ and $CD8^+$ T lymphocyte reponses against SIV Gag and HIV Env. Furthermore, an Ad35-based vector expressing the *Plasmodium yoelii* circumsporozoite (PyCS) protein resulted in a 96% inhibition of liver infection upon high *Plasmodium yoelii* sporozoite challenge [274]. In addition, a tuberculosis challenge model demonstrated the potency of an Ad35-based vector expressing the tuberculosis antigens Ag85A, Ag85B and TB10.4 as a fusion protein (Ad35.TBS) and protective efficacy against challenge with *Mycobacterium tuberculosis* [275]. These studies also demonstrated that in contrast to Ad5, an Ad35-based vaccine retained its full potency in presence of experimentally induced high levels of anti-Ad5 immunity (see figure 7). Interestingly, the potency and breath of vaccine-elicited immune responses appears to be dependent on the transgene used. For instance, in mice antibodies against SIV Gag could not be detected [272], whereas antibodies against HIV Env were readily detected (unpublished data). Likewise, antibodies against the circumsporozoite protein derived from the *Plasmodium yoelii* were clearly detect upon rAd35 vaccine administration [274]. This phenomenon is currently poorly understood but likely is related to both antigen-specific and vector-specific effects.

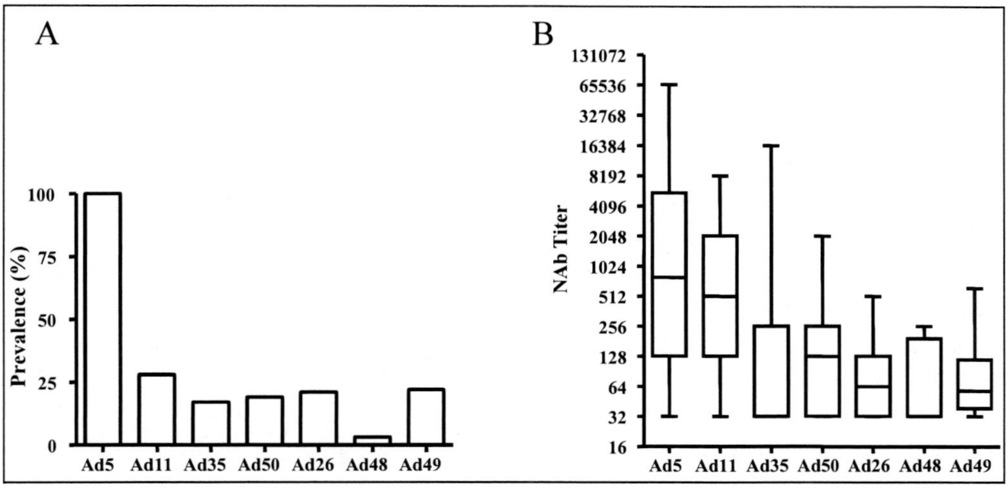

Figure 8. Human sera from Sub-Saharan Africa were analyzed for A) percentage positive (prevalence) human sera to the adenoviral vectors tested and B) Adenovirus-specific neutralizing antibody (NAb) titers are presented in Box-and-whisker plots.

Table 4. Alternative human adenoviruses from which vaccine vectors are derived

HUMAN ADENOVIRAL SEROTYPE	SUBGROUP	REFERENCE
Ad6	C	[324]
Ad11	B	[265, 325]
Ad24	D	[279]
Ad26	D	[54]
Ad34	B	[279]
Ad35	B	[264]
Ad41	F	[281]
Ad48	D	[54]
Ad49	D	[53]
Ad50	B	[54]

Like the Ad35 vector, Ad11-based vectors have been developed and tested for their immunogenic potential in an SIV Gag mouse model and proved to induce potent antigen specific cellular immune reponses [277]. This vector was developed initially as a possible booster for an Ad35 based vaccine, with the idea that Ad11 may be sufficiently serologically distinct from Ad35. In mice with high levels of anti-Ad5 immunity, an Ad35/Ad11 prime-boost regimen proved superior to Ad11/Ad5 or Ad35/Ad5 vaccine modalities. However, these studies also clearly indicated that Ad11/Ad5 and Ad35/Ad5 vaccine combinations induced more potent immune responses in naïve mice than Ad11/Ad35 vaccine regimens. Further investigations revealed the presence of cross-reactive NAbs between Ad35 and Ad11. These cross-reactive NAbs played a critical role in the diminished immunogenicity of the Ad35/Ad11 prime-boost regimen [277].

Since Ad35 and Ad11 are derived from the same human adenoviral subgroup (table 1), it was hypothesized that more distantly related adenoviruses may be required. However, an Ad6-based vaccine vector was capable of overcoming anti-Ad5 immunity, despite the fact that both Ad5 and Ad5 are from subgroup C [278]. This suggests that subgroup C viruses may not be as immunologically related as the Ad35 and Ad11 members of subgroup B.

Notwithstanding the latter finding, further development of replication-incompetent adenoviral vectors derived from other subgroups was further pursued to define improved prime-boost combinations. These efforts have led to extensive reports whereby stand-alone and prime-boost combinations of vectors derived from different subgroups were tested. In one report the stand-alone immunogenicity of both Ad24 and Ad34 was tested in a non-human primate model, and both proved to be immunogenic [279]. The Ad24-based vector has been further used as a boost to an Ad6-based vector prime in non-human primates demonstrating that this vaccine only marginally improved antigen-specific $CD8^+$ T lymphocytes but not antigen-specific $CD4^+$ T lymphocytes [280]. In another report, seven different human adenovirus vaccine vectors, based on Ad5, Ad11, Ad26, Ad35, Ad48, Ad49 and Ad50 were tested, and again all proved capable of inducing potent antigen specific cellular immune reponses in mice as well as circumvention of anti-Ad5 immunity [54]. An interesting finding in this study was the high immunogenicity of an Ad26-based vector, which proved more potent than any of the other non-Ad5 based vectors in the generation of SIV Gag-specific T lymphocyte responses in both mice and non-human primates [54]. The Ad26-based vector proved also successful in heterologous prime-boost regimens, including those also involving another human adenovirus subgroup D member, i.e. Ad48 or Ad49 [54]. The latter corroborates with the Ad5-Ad6 findings and indicated that, like subgroup C adenoviruses, members of the human subgroup D adenoviridae might be less immunologically cross-reactive than subgroup B members. The last addition to the growing panel of human replication-deficient vectors is based on Ad41 [281]. Human adenovirus serotype 41 is one of the two members of subgroup F (table 1). This vaccine vector is, as demonstrated for all vectors, capable of inducing antigen immune reponses and is not suppressed by previous immunization with an Ad5-based vector [281].

Although pre-clinical studies have thus far shown encouraging results with alternative serotype human replication deficient vectors, human clinical trials are required to assess their safety and potency profile. In this respect, Ad35-based malaria- and an Ad35-based tuberculosis phase I clinical trials, which have recently been initiated, will undoubtly provide valuable insides into the value of these vectors derived from rare human adenovirus serotypes.

Chimeric Adenoviral Vector-based Vaccines

The exact knowledge regarding the Ad5 genomic structure and gene location have provided the know how to exchange DNA coding for the major capsid proteins. Using this knowledge, chimeric Ad5 vectors have been constructed that contained fiber molecules derived from alternative serotypes. These vectors have been successfully generated to improve vector tropism for cells and tissues that are important for different medical applications [282]. One such vector, carrying the fiber of Ad35 proved to infect many cell types of interest but also proved to be hampered still by anti-Ad5 immunity [283]. Likewise, Ad5 vectors carrying both the fiber and penton of Ad35 proved to be neutralized by anti-Ad5 immunity [171]. With the absence of any neutralization against a full Ad35 vector with the sera used in these studies it could be concluded that the hexon capsid protein is the major determinant for anti-vector immunity [171,172]. With this finding, many attempts were subsequently made to construct Ad5 chimeric vectors carrying hexon proteins derived from rare adenoviruses. This has proven to be a major challenge and many attempts have failed [284]. Reason for the latter likely reflects the lack of structural compatability between the newly introduced hexon proteins and the other Ad5 capsid proteins e.g. penton base, protein IX, protein IIIa, protein VI. Despite this challenge, several hexon chimeric vectors, based on the hexon of 1, 2, 3, 6 and 12 have been successfully constructed [284,285]. With at least two of these vectors, i.e. Ad5-Hex6 and Ad5-Hex3, succesful escape of anti-Ad5 immmunity was demonstrated [284,285]. However since many of these vectors proved poorly viable, an alternative strategy was employed in which not the entire hexon coding domain was exchanged but only the short amino acid stretches called hypervariable regions (HVRs), which are considered to contain the major NAb determinants. Seven HVRs are present in all adenoviral hexon sequences known to date [286]. These HVRs are predicted to be exposed on the surface of the viral particle [287]. The importance of the HVRs as NAb epitopes was confirmed by the finding that an Ad5-chimeric vector, in which all the Ad5 hexon HVRs were replaced by Ad48 derived HVRs (Ad5HVR48), was successful in escaping anti-Ad5 immunity in both mice and non-human primates [287]. This vector proved to be as immunogenic as the parental Ad5-based vector [287], making it a prime candidate vector for clinical evaluation.

Non-Human Adenoviral-based Vaccines

Since replication of most non-human adenoviruses occurs in cells or tissues from species that present the natural host for the adenovirus or closely related species, cell lines to trans-complement for the E1-deficiency in the vector are usually derived from diverse species as well. Such complementary cell lines have been developed based on Bovine adenovirus 3 (BAd3) [288-290], Canine adenovirus 2 (CAV2) [291,292], Ovine adenovirus 7 (OAd7) [293], Porcine adenovirus 3 (PAd3) [294,295] and Fowl adenovirus 1 (CELO) [296,297]. To date many successful pre-clinical vaccination studies have been conducted with these non-human Ad vectors (reviewed in [298,299]), resulting ultimately in the protection of vaccinated animals against for instance bovine herpesvirus 1 (using BAd3) [300], canine distemper virus (using CAV2) [301], classical swine fever (using PAd3) [302] and infectious bursal disease virus (using CELO) [303]. In most of these veterinary vaccine studies either an E1-deleted vector was used as carrier or the vector still contained the E1 region but the E3 region was removed. In the latter case, the vaccine carrier is still able to replicate in the host but has been made more immunogenic by deletion of the E3 region. These non-human adenoviruses have not been associated with severe illness in their natural hosts and have proven that they can induce insert-specific immunity upon vaccination in animals. Furthermore, since humans do not represent a natural host, one can expect that pre-existing immunity in humans will be low. Several research groups are therefore evaluating safety and potency aspects of these non-human adenovirus derived carriers for human vaccine development. One of the furthest studies pursued in this context are adenoviruses derived from chimpanzees. Vectors systems from chimpanzee adenovirus serotypes C68 [304], C6 [305], C7 [305] and the chimeric C5/C1 vector [306] have been successfully prepared. The chimpanzee adenoviruses are genetically very similar to human adenoviruses both in genome organization as well as protein conservation. Serotype C68 for example has an approximately 90% sequence homology to human Ad4 (subgroup E) and it also utilises CAR, which also is highly conserved among primates, as its primary cellular receptor [307]. Moreover, chimpanzee adenoviruses C68, C6 and C7 deleted for the E1 region can be successfully propagated to high titers on human Ad5 E1-complementing cell lines such as HEK293. The latter demonstrates that the Ad5 E1 proteins are able to trans-complement for the deficiency of the chimpanzee adenovirus E1 proteins. The latter was less obvious using chimpanzee adenovirus serotype C1, which proved to grow very poorly on Ad5-E1 complementing cell lines. This observation corroborates with the finding that human subgroup B adenoviruses like Ad35 also grow poorly on A5-E1 complementing cell lines without for example E4 alterations [271], given the close relationship of C1 with human subgroup B adenoviruses. An elegant solution to this propagation problem was introduced by exchanging both the ITRs and several regions in the C1 genome coding for early phase proteins from chimpanzee serotype C5 [306] which readily grows on Ad5-E1 complementing cells [306]. The similarity between chimpanzee adenovirus C1 and human B-group adenoviruses was further strengthened by the finding that all these adenovirus serotypes utilize CD46 as their primary cellular receptor [306,308].

Although these chimpanzee adenoviruses are prevalent within their species and thus highly antigenic, the close similarity with human adenoviruses has not resulted in cross reactivity with anti-adenovirus antibodies in humans. As expected, chimpanzee viruses are able to ccircumvent anti-Ad5 immunity. In a head-to-head vaccination study, the C68-based vector encoding the rabies glycoprotein induced comparable levels of antigen-specific antibodies in mice after intranasal immunization as the Ad5-based vector [309]. The antigen-specific antibody levels proved somewhat lower in mice after subcutaneous immunization in comparison with the Ad5-based vaccine. The difference in the potency of immune induction mediated by the vaccine carrier related to the route of administration is seen with all different vector strategies and is currently poorly understood. As with the rare human and chimeric vectors, the C68-based vaccine carrier was not hampered in its induction of antigen specific immune responses by anti-Ad5 immunity [309]. Also, as described for other strategies, the C68-based vector induced a strong antigen-specific CD8$^+$ T lymphocytes [304]. Another chimpanzee vector based on serotype C7 encoding the envelope glycoprotein from Ebola also was able to induce potent anti-glycoprotein humoral and cellular immune reponses in mice and guinea pigs resulting in protection upon otherwise fatal Ebola challenge [310]. The C1/C5-based vector, which can be propagated to high titers on Ad5-E1 complementing cells lines (see above), also proved to induce strong anti-glycoprotein antibody and T-lymphocyte reponses and to induce protection upon Ebola challenge in mice [306]. A third human pathogen for which chimpanzee adenovirus based vaccines are being investigated is HIV. In one of these studies, the C68-based vector induced anti-HIV Gag CD8$^+$ T-lymphocyte reponses [304]. Likewise, a heterologous prime-boost regimen using a C6-based vaccine prime and C68-based vaccine boost, was shown to efficiently improve the HIV Gag-specific CD8$^+$ T lymphocytes response in mice [311]. Together these studies demonstrate that the use of non-human adenoviral vectors for vaccination is feasible and safe and affords protection in a variety of pre-clinical models. Results showing that these non-human vectors can be propagated to high titers on well–established human Ad5-E1 complementing cell lines will aid the manufacture of such vaccines to the scale required. Understanding the potency of these non-human vectors as well as their safety profile awaits the initiation of human clinical trials. Regulatory issues associated with the clinical development of chimpanzee adenovirus vectors will likely prove more complex than rare human serotype adenovirus vectors.

Conclusion

The last two decades have spurred the search for safe and effective methods to introduce genes into human subjects. The enormous interest stems from the possibility that such technologies may prove effective in gene therapy for inherited or congenital diseases as well as vaccination for cancer or infectious pathogens. Although a wide variety of strategies are actively being explored, one of the most promising technologies for these purposes is replication incompetent adenoviruses. The tremendous knowledge gathered on the basic biology of adenoviridae has proven pivotal to develop and to improve adenoviral vectors. This knowledge has been critical in the efforts to make safe and efficient vectors that can be produced at scale. Within the field of vaccination, tremendous advances has been made in the last decade culminating in recent demonstrations of protective efficacy in a variety of pre-clinical models and early promising data from Ad5 vectors in clinical trials. The near future will also demonstrate the utility of vectors based on rare human serotype adenoviruses, Ad5-chimeric vectors and non-human adenoviruses. It is expected that many of these promising vaccine carriers will very soon be advanced into human clinical trials.

References

[1] Orentas, R. J.; Hildreth, J. E.; Obah, E.; Polydefkis, M.; Smith, G. E.; Clements, M. L. &Siliciano, R. F. (1990). Induction of CD4+ human cytolytic T cells specific for HIV-infected cells by a gp160 subunit vaccine. *Science, 248,* 1234-7.

[2] Clark, T. G. &Cassidy-Hanley, D. (2005). Recombinant subunit vaccines: potentials and constraints. *Dev Biol (Basel), 121,* 153-63.

[3] Borrow, P.; Lewicki, H.; Hahn, B. H.; Shaw, G. M. &Oldstone, M. B. (1994). Virus-specific CD8+ cytotoxic T-lymphocyte activity associated with control of viremia in primary human immunodeficiency virus type 1 infection. *J Virol, 68,* 6103-10.

[4] Schmitz, J. E.; Kuroda, M. J.; Santra, S.; Sasseville, V. G.; Simon, M. A.; Lifton, M. A.; Racz, P.; Tenner-Racz, K.; Dalesandro, M.; Scallon, B. J.; Ghrayeb, J.; Forman, M. A.; Montefiori, D. C.; Rieber, E. P.; Letvin, N. L. &Reimann, K. A. (1999). Control of viremia in simian immunodeficiency virus infection by CD8+ lymphocytes. *Science, 283,* 857-60.

[5] Smith, S. M. &Dockrell, H. M. (2000). Role of CD8 T cells in mycobacterial infections. *Immunol Cell Biol, 78,* 325-33.

[6] Hafalla, J. C.; Cockburn, I. A. &Zavala, F. (2006). Protective and pathogenic roles of CD8+ T cells during malaria infection. *Parasite Immunol, 28,* 15-24.

[7] Donnelly, J. J.; Ulmer, J. B.; Shiver, J. W. &Liu, M. A. (1997). DNA vaccines. *Annu Rev Immunol, 15,* 617-48.

[8] Wang, R.; Doolan, D. L.; Le, T. P.; Hedstrom, R. C.; Coonan, K. M.; Charoenvit, Y.; Jones, T. R.; Hobart, P.; Margalith, M.; Ng, J.; Weiss, W. R.; Sedegah, M.; de Taisne, C.; Norman, J. A. &Hoffman, S. L. (1998). Induction of antigen-specific cytotoxic T lymphocytes in humans by a malaria DNA vaccine. *Science, 282,* 476-80.

[9] Calarota, S.; Bratt, G.; Nordlund, S.; Hinkula, J.; Leandersson, A. C.; Sandstrom, E. &Wahren, B. (1998). Cellular cytotoxic response induced by DNA vaccination in HIV-1-infected patients. *Lancet, 351,* 1320-5.

[10] MacGregor, R. R.; Boyer, J. D.; Ugen, K. E.; Lacy, K. E.; Gluckman, S. J.; Bagarazzi, M. L.; Chattergoon, M. A.; Baine, Y.; Higgins, T. J.; Ciccarelli, R. B.; Coney, L. R.; Ginsberg, R. S. &Weiner, D. B. (1998). First human trial of a DNA-based vaccine for treatment of human immunodeficiency virus type 1 infection: safety and host response. *J Infect Dis, 178,* 92-100.

[11] Le, T. P.; Coonan, K. M.; Hedstrom, R. C.; Charoenvit, Y.; Sedegah, M.; Epstein, J. E.; Kumar, S.; Wang, R.; Doolan, D. L.; Maguire, J. D.; Parker, S. E.; Hobart, P.; Norman, J. &Hoffman, S. L. (2000). Safety, tolerability and humoral immune responses after intramuscular administration of a malaria DNA vaccine to healthy adult volunteers. *Vaccine, 18,* 1893-901.

[12] Gurunathan, S.; Klinman, D. M. &Seder, R. A. (2000). DNA vaccines: immunology, application, and optimization*. *Annu Rev Immunol, 18,* 927-74.

[13] Rocha, C. D.; Caetano, B. C.; Machado, A. V. &Bruna-Romero, O. (2004). Recombinant viruses as tools to induce protective cellular immunity against infectious diseases. *Int Microbiol, 7,* 83-94.

[14] Souza, A. P.; Haut, L.; Reyes-Sandoval, A. &Pinto, A. R. (2005). Recombinant viruses as vaccines against viral diseases. *Braz J Med Biol Res, 38,* 509-22.

[15] Bukreyev, A.; Skiadopoulos, M. H.; Murphy, B. R. &Collins, P. L. (2006). Nonsegmented negative-strand viruses as vaccine vectors. *J Virol, 80,* 10293-306.

[16] Schoen, C.; Stritzker, J.; Goebel, W. &Pilgrim, S. (2004). Bacteria as DNA vaccine carriers for genetic immunization. *Int J Med Microbiol, 294,* 319-35.

[17] Shata, M. T.; Stevceva, L.; Agwale, S.; Lewis, G. K. &Hone, D. M. (2000). Recent advances with recombinant bacterial vaccine vectors. *Mol Med Today, 6,* 66-71.

[18] Fulginiti, V. A.; Papier, A.; Lane, J. M.; Neff, J. M. &Henderson, D. A. (2003). Smallpox vaccination: a review, part II. Adverse events. *Clin Infect Dis, 37,* 251-71.

[19] Moorthy, V. S.; Pinder, M.; Reece, W. H.; Watkins, K.; Atabani, S.; Hannan, C.; Bojang, K.; McAdam, K. P.; Schneider, J.; Gilbert, S. &Hill, A. V. (2003). Safety and immunogenicity of DNA/modified vaccinia virus ankara malaria vaccination in African adults. *J Infect Dis, 188,* 1239-44.

[20] Moorthy, V. S.; Imoukhuede, E. B.; Keating, S.; Pinder, M.; Webster, D.; Skinner, M. A.; Gilbert, S. C.; Walraven, G. &Hill, A. V. (2004). Phase 1 evaluation of 3 highly immunogenic prime-boost regimens, including a 12-month reboosting vaccination, for malaria vaccination in Gambian men. *J Infect Dis, 189,* 2213-9.

[21] McShane, H.; Pathan, A. A.; Sander, C. R.; Keating, S. M.; Gilbert, S. C.; Huygen, K.; Fletcher, H. A. &Hill, A. V. (2004). Recombinant modified vaccinia virus Ankara expressing antigen 85A boosts BCG-primed and naturally acquired antimycobacterial immunity in humans. *Nat Med, 10,* 1240-4.

[22] Mwau, M.; Cebere, I.; Sutton, J.; Chikoti, P.; Winstone, N.; Wee, E. G.; Beattie, T.; Chen, Y. H.; Dorrell, L.; McShane, H.; Schmidt, C.; Brooks, M.; Patel, S.; Roberts, J.; Conlon, C.; Rowland-Jones, S. L.; Bwayo, J. J.; McMichael, A. J. &Hanke, T. (2004). A human immunodeficiency virus 1 (HIV-1) clade A vaccine in clinical trials: stimulation of HIV-specific T-cell responses by DNA and recombinant modified vaccinia virus Ankara (MVA) vaccines in humans. *J Gen Virol, 85,* 911-9.

[23] Goonetilleke, N.; Moore, S.; Dally, L.; Winstone, N.; Cebere, I.; Mahmoud, A.; Pinheiro, S.; Gillespie, G.; Brown, D.; Loach, V.; Roberts, J.; Guimaraes-Walker, A.; Hayes, P.; Loughran, K.; Smith, C.; De Bont, J.; Verlinde, C.; Vooijs, D.; Schmidt, C.; Boaz, M.; Gilmour, J.; Fast, P.; Dorrell, L.; Hanke, T. &McMichael, A. J. (2006). Induction of multifunctional human immunodeficiency virus type 1 (HIV-1)-specific T cells capable of proliferation in healthy subjects by using a prime-boost regimen of DNA- and modified vaccinia virus Ankara-vectored vaccines expressing HIV-1 Gag coupled to CD8+ T-cell epitopes. *J Virol, 80,* 4717-28.

[24] Evans, T. G.; Keefer, M. C.; Weinhold, K. J.; Wolff, M.; Montefiori, D.; Gorse, G. J.; Graham, B. S.; McElrath, M. J.; Clements-Mann, M. L.; Mulligan, M. J.; Fast, P.; Walker, M. C.; Excler, J. L.; Duliege, A. M. &Tartaglia, J. (1999). A canarypox vaccine expressing multiple human immunodeficiency virus type 1 genes given alone or with rgp120 elicits broad and durable CD8+ cytotoxic T lymphocyte responses in seronegative volunteers. *J Infect Dis, 180,* 290-8.

[25] Belshe, R. B.; Stevens, C.; Gorse, G. J.; Buchbinder, S.; Weinhold, K.; Sheppard, H.; Stablein, D.; Self, S.; McNamara, J.; Frey, S.; Flores, J.; Excler, J. L.; Klein, M.; Habib, R. E.; Duliege, A. M.; Harro, C.; Corey, L.; Keefer, M.; Mulligan, M.; Wright, P.; Celum, C.; Judson, F.; Mayer, K.; McKirnan, D.; Marmor, M. &Woody, G. (2001). Safety and immunogenicity of a canarypox-vectored human immunodeficiency virus Type 1 vaccine with or without gp120: a phase 2 study in higher- and lower-risk volunteers. *J Infect Dis, 183,* 1343-52.

[26] Cao, H.; Kaleebu, P.; Hom, D.; Flores, J.; Agrawal, D.; Jones, N.; Serwanga, J.; Okello, M.; Walker, C.; Sheppard, H.; El-Habib, R.; Klein, M.; Mbidde, E.; Mugyenyi, P.; Walker, B.; Ellner, J. &Mugerwa, R. (2003). Immunogenicity of a recombinant human immunodeficiency virus (HIV)-canarypox vaccine in HIV-seronegative Ugandan volunteers: results of the HIV Network for Prevention Trials 007 Vaccine Study. *J Infect Dis, 187,* 887-95.

[27] Bejon, P.; Mwacharo, J.; Kai, O. K.; Todryk, S.; Keating, S.; Lang, T.; Gilbert, S. C.; Peshu, N.; Marsh, K. &Hill, A. V. (2006). Immunogenicity of the candidate malaria vaccines FP9 and modified vaccinia virus Ankara encoding the pre-erythrocytic antigen ME-TRAP in 1-6 year old children in a malaria endemic area. *Vaccine, 24,* 4709-15.

[28] Ockenhouse, C. F.; Sun, P. F.; Lanar, D. E.; Wellde, B. T.; Hall, B. T.; Kester, K.; Stoute, J. A.; Magill, A.; Krzych, U.; Farley, L.; Wirtz, R. A.; Sadoff, J. C.; Kaslow, D. C.; Kumar, S.; Church, L. W.; Crutcher, J. M.; Wizel, B.; Hoffman, S.; Lalvani, A.; Hill, A. V.; Tine, J. A.; Guito, K. P.; de Taisne, C.; Anders, R.; Ballou, W. R. &et al. (1998). Phase I/IIa safety, immunogenicity, and efficacy trial of NYVAC-Pf7, a pox-vectored, multiantigen, multistage vaccine candidate for Plasmodium falciparum malaria. *J Infect Dis, 177,* 1664-73.

[29] Konishi, E.; Kurane, I.; Mason, P. W.; Shope, R. E.; Kanesa-Thasan, N.; Smucny, J. J.; Hoke, C. H., Jr. &Ennis, F. A. (1998). Induction of Japanese encephalitis virus-specific cytotoxic T lymphocytes in humans by poxvirus-based JE vaccine candidates. *Vaccine, 16,* 842-9.

[30] Cohen, J. (2002). Disappointing data scuttle plans for large-scale AIDS vaccine trial. *Science, 295,* 1616-7.

[31] Catanzaro, A. T.; Koup, R. A.; Roederer, M.; Bailer, R. T.; Enama, M. E.; Moodie, Z.; Gu, L.; Martin, J. E.; Novik, L.; Chakrabarti, B. K.; Butman, B. T.; Gall, J. G.; King, C.

R.; Andrews, C. A.; Sheets, R.; Gomez, P. L.; Mascola, J. R.; Nabel, G. J. &Graham, B. S. (2006). Phase 1 safety and immunogenicity evaluation of a multiclade HIV-1 candidate vaccine delivered by a replication-defective recombinant adenovirus vector. *J Infect Dis, 194,* 1638-49.

[32] Duerr, A.; Wasserheit, J. N. &Corey, L. (2006). HIV vaccines: new frontiers in vaccine development. *Clin Infect Dis, 43,* 500-11.

[33] Cohen, J. (2005). HIV/AIDS. Hedged bet: an unusual AIDS vaccine trial. *Science, 309,* 1003.

[34] Rowe, W. P.; Huebner, R. J.; Gilmore, L. K.; Parrott, R. H. &Ward, T. G. (1953). Isolation of a cytopathogenic agent from human adenoids undergoing spontaneous degeneration in tissue culture. *Proc Soc Exp Biol Med, 84,* 570-3.

[35] De Jong, J. C.; Wermenbol, A. G.; Verweij-Uijterwaal, M. W.; Slaterus, K. W.; Wertheim-Van Dillen, P.; Van Doornum, G. J.; Khoo, S. H. &Hierholzer, J. C. (1999). Adenoviruses from human immunodeficiency virus-infected individuals, including two strains that represent new candidate serotypes Ad50 and Ad51 of species B1 and D, respectively. *J Clin Microbiol, 37,* 3940-5.

[36] Francki, R.; Fauquet, C.; Knudson, L. &Brown, F. (1991). Classification and nomenclature of adenoviruses. Fifth report of the International Committee on Taxonomy of Viruses. *Arch Virol,* 140-144.

[37] Hierholzer, J. C. (1992). Adenoviruses in the immunocompromised host. *Clin Microbiol Rev, 5,* 262-74.

[38] Khoo, S. H.; Bailey, A. S.; de Jong, J. C. &Mandal, B. K. (1995). Adenovirus infections in human immunodeficiency virus-positive patients: clinical features and molecular epidemiology. *J Infect Dis, 172,* 629-37.

[39] Kojaoghlanian, T.; Flomenberg, P. &Horwitz, M. S. (2003). The impact of adenovirus infection on the immunocompromised host. *Rev Med Virol, 13,* 155-71.

[40] Hoffman, J. A. (2006). Adenoviral disease in pediatric solid organ transplant recipients. *Pediatr Transplant, 10,* 17-25.

[41] Webster, A.; Leith, I. R.; Nicholson, J.; Hounsell, J. &Hay, R. T. (1997). Role of preterminal protein processing in adenovirus replication. *J Virol, 71,* 6381-9.

[42] Anderson, C. W.; Young, M. E. &Flint, S. J. (1989). Characterization of the adenovirus 2 virion protein, mu. *Virology, 172,* 506-12.

[43] Chatterjee, P. K.; Vayda, M. E. &Flint, S. J. (1985). Interactions among the three adenovirus core proteins. *J Virol, 55,* 379-86.

[44] van Oostrum, J. &Burnett, R. M. (1985). Molecular composition of the adenovirus type 2 virion. *J Virol, 56,* 439-48.

[45] Vellinga, J.; Van der Heijdt, S. &Hoeben, R. C. (2005). The adenovirus capsid: major progress in minor proteins. *J Gen Virol, 86,* 1581-8.

[46] Chroboczek, J.; Ruigrok, R. W. H. &Cusack, S. (1995). Adenovirus fiber. In:W. Doerfler &P. Bohm, eds, *The Molecular Repertoire of Adenoviruses* 163-200). Berlin: Springer.

[47] Bergelson, J. M.; Cunningham, J. A.; Droguett, G.; Kurt-Jones, E. A.; Krithivas, A.; Hong, J. S.; Horwitz, M. S.; Crowell, R. L. &Finberg, R. W. (1997). Isolation of a common receptor for Coxsackie B viruses and adenoviruses 2 and 5. *Science, 275,* 1320-3.

[48] Roelvink, P. W.; Lizonova, A.; Lee, J. G.; Li, Y.; Bergelson, J. M.; Finberg, R. W.; Brough, D. E.; Kovesdi, I. &Wickham, T. J. (1998). The coxsackievirus-adenovirus receptor protein can function as a cellular attachment protein for adenovirus serotypes from subgroups A, C, D, E, and F. *J Virol, 72,* 7909-15.

[49] Gaggar, A.; Shayakhmetov, D. M. &Lieber, A. (2003). CD46 is a cellular receptor for group B adenoviruses. *Nat Med, 9,* 1408-12.

[50] Segerman, A.; Atkinson, J. P.; Marttila, M.; Dennerquist, V.; Wadell, G. &Arnberg, N. (2003). Adenovirus type 11 uses CD46 as a cellular receptor. *J Virol, 77,* 9183-91.

[51] Sirena, D.; Lilienfeld, B.; Eisenhut, M.; Kalin, S.; Boucke, K.; Beerli, R. R.; Vogt, L.; Ruedl, C.; Bachmann, M. F.; Greber, U. F. &Hemmi, S. (2004). The human membrane cofactor CD46 is a receptor for species B adenovirus serotype 3. *J Virol, 78,* 4454-62.

[52] Wu, E.; Trauger, S. A.; Pache, L.; Mullen, T. M.; von Seggern, D. J.; Siuzdak, G. &Nemerow, G. R. (2004). Membrane cofactor protein is a receptor for adenoviruses associated with epidemic keratoconjunctivitis. *J Virol, 78,* 3897-905.

[53] Lemckert, A. A.; Grimbergen, J.; Smits, S.; Hartkoorn, E.; Holterman, L.; Berkhout, B.; Barouch, D. H.; Vogels, R.; Quax, P.; Goudsmit, J. &Havenga, M. J. (2006). Generation of a novel replication-incompetent adenoviral vector derived from human adenovirus type 49: manufacture on PER.C6 cells, tropism and immunogenicity. *J Gen Virol, 87,* 2891-9.

[54] Abbink, P.; Lemckert, A. A.; Ewald, B. A.; Lynch, D. M.; Denholtz, M.; Smits, S.; Holterman, L.; Damen, I.; Vogels, R.; Thorner, A. R.; O'Brien, K. L.; Carville, A.; Mansfield, K. G.; Goudsmit, J.; Havenga, M. J. &Barouch, D. H. (2007). Comparative Seroprevalence and Immunogenicity of Six Rare Serotype Recombinant Adenovirus Vaccine Vectors from Subgroups B and D. *J Virol, 81,* 4654-63.

[55] Arnberg, N.; Edlund, K.; Kidd, A. H. &Wadell, G. (2000). Adenovirus type 37 uses sialic acid as a cellular receptor. *J Virol, 74,* 42-8.

[56] Balakireva, L.; Schoehn, G.; Thouvenin, E. &Chroboczek, J. (2003). Binding of adenovirus capsid to dipalmitoyl phosphatidylcholine provides a novel pathway for virus entry. *J Virol, 77,* 4858-66.

[57] Chu, Y.; Heistad, D.; Cybulsky, M. I. &Davidson, B. L. (2001). Vascular cell adhesion molecule-1 augments adenovirus-mediated gene transfer. *Arterioscler Thromb Vasc Biol, 21,* 238-42.

[58] Short, J. J.; Vasu, C.; Holterman, M. J.; Curiel, D. T. &Pereboev, A. (2006). Members of adenovirus species B utilize CD80 and CD86 as cellular attachment receptors. *Virus Res, 122,* 144-53.

[59] Dechecchi, M. C.; Melotti, P.; Bonizzato, A.; Santacatterina, M.; Chilosi, M. &Cabrini, G. (2001). Heparan sulfate glycosaminoglycans are receptors sufficient to mediate the initial binding of adenovirus types 2 and 5. *J Virol, 75,* 8772-80.

[60] Huang, S.; Kamata, T.; Takada, Y.; Ruggeri, Z. M. &Nemerow, G. R. (1996). Adenovirus interaction with distinct integrins mediates separate events in cell entry and gene delivery to hematopoietic cells. *J Virol, 70,* 4502-8.

[61] Hong, S. S.; Karayan, L.; Tournier, J.; Curiel, D. T. &Boulanger, P. A. (1997). Adenovirus type 5 fiber knob binds to MHC class I alpha2 domain at the surface of human epithelial and B lymphoblastoid cells. *Embo J, 16,* 2294-306.

[62] Johansson, C.; Jonsson, M.; Marttila, M.; Persson, D.; Fan, X. L.; Skog, J.; Frangsmyr, L.; Wadell, G. &Arnberg, N. (2007). Adenoviruses use lactoferrin as a bridge for CAR-independent binding to and infection of epithelial cells. *J Virol, 81,* 954-63.
[63] Wickham, T. J.; Mathias, P.; Cheresh, D. A. &Nemerow, G. R. (1993). Integrins alpha v beta 3 and alpha v beta 5 promote adenovirus internalization but not virus attachment. *Cell, 73,* 309-19.
[64] Li, E.; Brown, S. L.; Stupack, D. G.; Puente, X. S.; Cheresh, D. A. &Nemerow, G. R. (2001). Integrin alpha(v)beta1 is an adenovirus coreceptor. *J Virol, 75,* 5405-9.
[65] Salone, B.; Martina, Y.; Piersanti, S.; Cundari, E.; Cherubini, G.; Franqueville, L.; Failla, C. M.; Boulanger, P. &Saggio, I. (2003). Integrin alpha3beta1 is an alternative cellular receptor for adenovirus serotype 5. *J Virol, 77,* 13448-54.
[66] Greber, U. F.; Willetts, M.; Webster, P. &Helenius, A. (1993). Stepwise dismantling of adenovirus 2 during entry into cells. *Cell, 75,* 477-86.
[67] Stewart, P. L.; Fuller, S. D. &Burnett, R. M. (1993). Difference imaging of adenovirus: bridging the resolution gap between X- ray crystallography and electron microscopy. *Embo J, 12,* 2589-99.
[68] Wiethoff, C. M.; Wodrich, H.; Gerace, L. &Nemerow, G. R. (2005). Adenovirus protein VI mediates membrane disruption following capsid disassembly. *J Virol, 79,* 1992-2000.
[69] Leopold, P. L.; Kreitzer, G.; Miyazawa, N.; Rempel, S.; Pfister, K. K.; Rodriguez-Boulan, E. &Crystal, R. G. (2000). Dynein- and microtubule-mediated translocation of adenovirus serotype 5 occurs after endosomal lysis. *Hum Gene Ther, 11,* 151-65.
[70] Trotman, L. C.; Mosberger, N.; Fornerod, M.; Stidwill, R. P. &Greber, U. F. (2001). Import of adenovirus DNA involves the nuclear pore complex receptor CAN/Nup214 and histone H1. *Nat Cell Biol, 3,* 1092-100.
[71] Davison, A. J.; Telford, E. A.; Watson, M. S.; McBride, K. &Mautner, V. (1993). The DNA sequence of adenovirus type 40. *J Mol Biol, 234,* 1308-16.
[72] Albinsson, B. &Kidd, A. H. (1999). Adenovirus type 41 lacks an RGD alpha(v)-integrin binding motif on the penton base and undergoes delayed uptake in A549 cells. *Virus Res, 64,* 125-36.
[73] Kidd, A. H.; Chroboczek, J.; Cusack, S. &Ruigrok, R. W. (1993). Adenovirus type 40 virions contain two distinct fibers. *Virology, 192,* 73-84.
[74] Yeh, H. Y.; Pieniazek, N.; Pieniazek, D.; Gelderblom, H. &Luftig, R. B. (1994). Human adenovirus type 41 contains two fibers. *Virus Res, 33,* 179-98.
[75] Miyazawa, N.; Crystal, R. G. &Leopold, P. L. (2001). Adenovirus serotype 7 retention in a late endosomal compartment prior to cytosol escape is modulated by fiber protein. *J Virol, 75,* 1387-400.
[76] Miyazawa, N.; Leopold, P. L.; Hackett, N. R.; Ferris, B.; Worgall, S.; Falck-Pedersen, E. &Crystal, R. G. (1999). Fiber swap between adenovirus subgroups B and C alters intracellular trafficking of adenovirus gene transfer vectors. *J Virol, 73,* 6056-65.
[77] Shayakhmetov, D. M.; Li, Z. Y.; Ternovoi, V.; Gaggar, A.; Gharwan, H. &Lieber, A. (2003). The interaction between the fiber knob domain and the cellular attachment receptor determines the intracellular trafficking route of adenoviruses. *J Virol, 77,* 3712-23.
[78] Flint, J. &Shenk, T. (1989). Adenovirus E1A protein paradigm viral transactivator. *Annu Rev Genet, 23,* 141-61.

[79] Howe, J. A.; Mymryk, J. S.; Egan, C.; Branton, P. E. &Bayley, S. T. (1990). Retinoblastoma growth suppressor and a 300-kDa protein appear to regulate cellular DNA synthesis. *Proc Natl Acad Sci U S A, 87,* 5883-7.

[80] Ikeda, M. A. &Nevins, J. R. (1993). Identification of distinct roles for separate E1A domains in disruption of E2F complexes. *Mol Cell Biol, 13,* 7029-35.

[81] Johnson, D. G.; Schwarz, J. K.; Cress, W. D. &Nevins, J. R. (1993). Expression of transcription factor E2F1 induces quiescent cells to enter S phase. *Nature, 365,* 349-52.

[82] Debbas, M. &White, E. (1993). Wild-type p53 mediates apoptosis by E1A, which is inhibited by E1B. *Genes Dev, 7,* 546-54.

[83] Kao, C. C.; Yew, P. R. &Berk, A. J. (1990). Domains required for in vitro association between the cellular p53 and the adenovirus 2 E1B 55K proteins. *Virology, 179,* 806-14.

[84] Martin, M. E. &Berk, A. J. (1998). Adenovirus E1B 55K represses p53 activation in vitro. *J Virol, 72,* 3146-54.

[85] Querido, E.; Blanchette, P.; Yan, Q.; Kamura, T.; Morrison, M.; Boivin, D.; Kaelin, W. G.; Conaway, R. C.; Conaway, J. W. &Branton, P. E. (2001). Degradation of p53 by adenovirus E4orf6 and E1B55K proteins occurs via a novel mechanism involving a Cullin-containing complex. *Genes Dev, 15,* 3104-17.

[86] Querido, E.; Morrison, M. R.; Chu-Pham-Dang, H.; Thirlwell, S. W.; Boivin, D. &Branton, P. E. (2001). Identification of three functions of the adenovirus e4orf6 protein that mediate p53 degradation by the E4orf6-E1B55K complex. *J Virol, 75,* 699-709.

[87] Konig, C.; Roth, J. &Dobbelstein, M. (1999). Adenovirus type 5 E4orf3 protein relieves p53 inhibition by E1B-55-kilodalton protein. *J Virol, 73,* 2253-62.

[88] Shao, R.; Hu, M. C.; Zhou, B. P.; Lin, S. Y.; Chiao, P. J.; von Lindern, R. H.; Spohn, B. &Hung, M. C. (1999). E1A sensitizes cells to tumor necrosis factor-induced apoptosis through inhibition of IkappaB kinases and nuclear factor kappaB activities. *J Biol Chem, 274,* 21495-8.

[89] Sundararajan, R.; Cuconati, A.; Nelson, D. &White, E. (2001). Tumor necrosis factor-alpha induces Bax-Bak interaction and apoptosis, which is inhibited by adenovirus E1B 19K. *J Biol Chem, 276,* 45120-7.

[90] de Jong, R. N.; van der Vliet, P. C. &Brenkman, A. B. (2003). Adenovirus DNA replication: protein priming, jumping back and the role of the DNA binding protein DBP. *Curr Top Microbiol Immunol, 272,* 187-211.

[91] Hay, R. T.; Freeman, A.; Leith, I.; Monaghan, A. &Webster, A. (1995). Molecular interactions during adenovirus DNA replication. *Curr Top Microbiol Immunol, 199 (Pt 2),* 31-48.

[92] Van der Vliet, P. C. (1995). Adenovirus DNA replication. *Curr Top Microbiol Immunol, 199 (Pt 2),* 1-30.

[93] Liu, H.; Naismith, J. H. &Hay, R. T. (2003). Adenovirus DNA replication. *Curr Top Microbiol Immunol, 272,* 131-64.

[94] Lichtenstein, D. L.; Toth, K.; Doronin, K.; Tollefson, A. E. &Wold, W. S. (2004). Functions and mechanisms of action of the adenovirus E3 proteins. *Int Rev Immunol, 23,* 75-111.

[95] Tollefson, A. E.; Toth, K.; Doronin, K.; Kuppuswamy, M.; Doronina, O. A.; Lichtenstein, D. L.; Hermiston, T. W.; Smith, C. A. &Wold, W. S. (2001). Inhibition of

TRAIL-induced apoptosis and forced internalization of TRAIL receptor 1 by adenovirus proteins. *J Virol, 75,* 8875-87.

[96] Lichtenstein, D. L.; Doronin, K.; Toth, K.; Kuppuswamy, M.; Wold, W. S. &Tollefson, A. E. (2004). Adenovirus E3-6.7K protein is required in conjunction with the E3-RID protein complex for the internalization and degradation of TRAIL receptor 2. *J Virol, 78,* 12297-307.

[97] Fessler, S. P.; Chin, Y. R. &Horwitz, M. S. (2004). Inhibition of tumor necrosis factor (TNF) signal transduction by the adenovirus group C RID complex involves downregulation of surface levels of TNF receptor 1. *J Virol, 78,* 13113-21.

[98] Shisler, J.; Yang, C.; Walter, B.; Ware, C. F. &Gooding, L. R. (1997). The adenovirus E3-10.4K/14.5K complex mediates loss of cell surface Fas (CD95) and resistance to Fas-induced apoptosis. *J Virol, 71,* 8299-306.

[99] Tollefson, A. E.; Hermiston, T. W.; Lichtenstein, D. L.; Colle, C. F.; Tripp, R. A.; Dimitrov, T.; Toth, K.; Wells, C. E.; Doherty, P. C. &Wold, W. S. (1998). Forced degradation of Fas inhibits apoptosis in adenovirus-infected cells. *Nature, 392,* 726-30.

[100] Krajcsi, P.; Dimitrov, T.; Hermiston, T. W.; Tollefson, A. E.; Ranheim, T. S.; Vande Pol, S. B.; Stephenson, A. H. &Wold, W. S. (1996). The adenovirus E3-14.7K protein and the E3-10.4K/14.5K complex of proteins, which independently inhibit tumor necrosis factor (TNF)-induced apoptosis, also independently inhibit TNF-induced release of arachidonic acid. *J Virol, 70,* 4904-13.

[101] Friedman, J. M. &Horwitz, M. S. (2002). Inhibition of tumor necrosis factor alpha-induced NF-kappa B activation by the adenovirus E3-10.4/14.5K complex. *J Virol, 76,* 5515-21.

[102] Wilson-Rawls, J. &Wold, W. S. (1993). The E3-6.7K protein of adenovirus is an Asn-linked integral membrane glycoprotein localized in the endoplasmic reticulum. *Virology, 195,* 6-15.

[103] Moise, A. R.; Grant, J. R.; Vitalis, T. Z. &Jefferies, W. A. (2002). Adenovirus E3-6.7K maintains calcium homeostasis and prevents apoptosis and arachidonic acid release. *J Virol, 76,* 1578-87.

[104] Benedict, C. A.; Norris, P. S.; Prigozy, T. I.; Bodmer, J. L.; Mahr, J. A.; Garnett, C. T.; Martinon, F.; Tschopp, J.; Gooding, L. R. &Ware, C. F. (2001). Three adenovirus E3 proteins cooperate to evade apoptosis by tumor necrosis factor-related apoptosis-inducing ligand receptor-1 and -2. *J Biol Chem, 276,* 3270-8.

[105] Andersson, M.; Paabo, S.; Nilsson, T. &Peterson, P. A. (1985). Impaired intracellular transport of class I MHC antigens as a possible means for adenoviruses to evade immune surveillance. *Cell, 43,* 215-22.

[106] Bennett, E. M.; Bennink, J. R.; Yewdell, J. W. &Brodsky, F. M. (1999). Cutting edge: adenovirus E19 has two mechanisms for affecting class I MHC expression. *J Immunol, 162,* 5049-52.

[107] Gooding, L. R.; Sofola, I. O.; Tollefson, A. E.; Duerksen-Hughes, P. &Wold, W. S. (1990). The adenovirus E3-14.7K protein is a general inhibitor of tumor necrosis factor-mediated cytolysis. *J Immunol, 145,* 3080-6.

[108] Schneider-Brachert, W.; Tchikov, V.; Merkel, O.; Jakob, M.; Hallas, C.; Kruse, M. L.; Groitl, P.; Lehn, A.; Hildt, E.; Held-Feindt, J.; Dobner, T.; Kabelitz, D.; Kronke, M. &Schutze, S. (2006). Inhibition of TNF receptor 1 internalization by adenovirus 14.7K as a novel immune escape mechanism. *J Clin Invest, 116,* 2901-13.

[109] Tollefson, A. E.; Scaria, A.; Hermiston, T. W.; Ryerse, J. S.; Wold, L. J. &Wold, W. S. (1996). The adenovirus death protein (E3-11.6K) is required at very late stages of infection for efficient cell lysis and release of adenovirus from infected cells. *J Virol, 70,* 2296-306.

[110] Tollefson, A. E.; Scaria, A.; Saha, S. K. &Wold, W. S. (1992). The 11,600-MW protein encoded by region E3 of adenovirus is expressed early but is greatly amplified at late stages of infection. *J Virol, 66,* 3633-42.

[111] Windheim, M.; Hilgendorf, A. &Burgert, H. G. (2004). Immune evasion by adenovirus E3 proteins: exploitation of intracellular trafficking pathways. *Curr Top Microbiol Immunol, 273,* 29-85.

[112] Basler, C. F. &Horwitz, M. S. (1996). Subgroup B adenovirus type 35 early region 3 mRNAs differ from those of the subgroup C adenoviruses. *Virology, 215,* 165-77.

[113] Windheim, M. &Burgert, H. G. (2002). Characterization of E3/49K, a novel, highly glycosylated E3 protein of the epidemic keratoconjunctivitis-causing adenovirus type 19a. *J Virol, 76,* 755-66.

[114] Weiss, R. S.; Lee, S. S.; Prasad, B. V. &Javier, R. T. (1997). Human adenovirus early region 4 open reading frame 1 genes encode growth-transforming proteins that may be distantly related to dUTP pyrophosphatase enzymes. *J Virol, 71,* 1857-70.

[115] Stracker, T. H.; Carson, C. T. &Weitzman, M. D. (2002). Adenovirus oncoproteins inactivate the Mre11-Rad50-NBS1 DNA repair complex. *Nature, 418,* 348-52.

[116] Boyer, J.; Rohleder, K. &Ketner, G. (1999). Adenovirus E4 34k and E4 11k inhibit double strand break repair and are physically associated with the cellular DNA-dependent protein kinase. *Virology, 263,* 307-12.

[117] Bridge, E. &Ketner, G. (1989). Redundant control of adenovirus late gene expression by early region 4. *J Virol, 63,* 631-8.

[118] Huang, M. M. &Hearing, P. (1989). Adenovirus early region 4 encodes two gene products with redundant effects in lytic infection. *J Virol, 63,* 2605-15.

[119] Weiden, M. D. &Ginsberg, H. S. (1994). Deletion of the E4 region of the genome produces adenovirus DNA concatemers. *Proc Natl Acad Sci U S A, 91,* 153-7.

[120] Araujo, F. D.; Stracker, T. H.; Carson, C. T.; Lee, D. V. &Weitzman, M. D. (2005). Adenovirus type 5 E4orf3 protein targets the Mre11 complex to cytoplasmic aggresomes. *J Virol, 79,* 11382-91.

[121] Stracker, T. H.; Lee, D. V.; Carson, C. T.; Araujo, F. D.; Ornelles, D. A. &Weitzman, M. D. (2005). Serotype-specific reorganization of the Mre11 complex by adenoviral E4orf3 proteins. *J Virol, 79,* 6664-73.

[122] Bridge, E. &Ketner, G. (1990). Interaction of adenoviral E4 and E1b products in late gene expression. *Virology, 174,* 345-53.

[123] Ornelles, D. A. &Shenk, T. (1991). Localization of the adenovirus early region 1B 55-kilodalton protein during lytic infection: association with nuclear viral inclusions requires the early region 4 34-kilodalton protein. *J Virol, 65,* 424-9.

[124] Goodrum, F. D.; Shenk, T. &Ornelles, D. A. (1996). Adenovirus early region 4 34-kilodalton protein directs the nuclear localization of the early region 1B 55-kilodalton protein in primate cells. *J Virol, 70,* 6323-35.

[125] Doucas, V.; Ishov, A. M.; Romo, A.; Juguilon, H.; Weitzman, M. D.; Evans, R. M. &Maul, G. G. (1996). Adenovirus replication is coupled with the dynamic properties of the PML nuclear structure. *Genes Dev, 10,* 196-207.

[126] Hoppe, A.; Beech, S. J.; Dimmock, J. &Leppard, K. N. (2006). Interaction of the adenovirus type 5 E4 Orf3 protein with promyelocytic leukemia protein isoform II is required for ND10 disruption. *J Virol, 80,* 3042-9.

[127] Zhong, S.; Salomoni, P. &Pandolfi, P. P. (2000). The transcriptional role of PML and the nuclear body. *Nat Cell Biol, 2,* E85-90.

[128] Borden, K. L. (2002). Pondering the promyelocytic leukemia protein (PML) puzzle: possible functions for PML nuclear bodies. *Mol Cell Biol, 22,* 5259-69.

[129] Hofmann, T. G. &Will, H. (2003). Body language: the function of PML nuclear bodies in apoptosis regulation. *Cell Death Differ, 10,* 1290-9.

[130] Regad, T. &Chelbi-Alix, M. K. (2001). Role and fate of PML nuclear bodies in response to interferon and viral infections. *Oncogene, 20,* 7274-86.

[131] Yondola, M. A. &Hearing, P. (2007). The Adenovirus E4 ORF3 Protein Binds and Reorganizes the TRIM Family Member Transcriptional Intermediary Factor 1 Alpha. *J Virol, 81,* 4264-71.

[132] Ullman, A. J.; Reich, N. C. &Hearing, P. (2007). The Adenovirus E4 ORF3 Protein Inhibits the Interferon-Mediated Antiviral Response. *J Virol, 81,* 4744-52.

[133] Flint, S. J. &Gonzalez, R. A. (2003). Regulation of mRNA production by the adenoviral E1B 55-kDa and E4 Orf6 proteins. *Curr Top Microbiol Immunol, 272,* 287-330.

[134] Halbert, D. N.; Cutt, J. R. &Shenk, T. (1985). Adenovirus early region 4 encodes functions required for efficient DNA replication, late gene expression, and host cell shutoff. *J Virol, 56,* 250-7.

[135] Muller, U.; Kleinberger, T. &Shenk, T. (1992). Adenovirus E4orf4 protein reduces phosphorylation of c-Fos and E1A proteins while simultaneously reducing the level of AP-1. *J Virol, 66,* 5867-78.

[136] Kleinberger, T. &Shenk, T. (1993). Adenovirus E4orf4 protein binds to protein phosphatase 2A, and the complex down regulates E1A-enhanced junB transcription. *J Virol, 67,* 7556-60.

[137] Bondesson, M.; Ohman, K.; Manervik, M.; Fan, S. &Akusjarvi, G. (1996). Adenovirus E4 open reading frame 4 protein autoregulates E4 transcription by inhibiting E1A transactivation of the E4 promoter. *J Virol, 70,* 3844-51.

[138] Kanopka, A.; Muhlemann, O.; Petersen-Mahrt, S.; Estmer, C.; Ohrmalm, C. &Akusjarvi, G. (1998). Regulation of adenovirus alternative RNA splicing by dephosphorylation of SR proteins. *Nature, 393,* 185-7.

[139] Marcellus, R. C.; Lavoie, J. N.; Boivin, D.; Shore, G. C.; Ketner, G. &Branton, P. E. (1998). The early region 4 orf4 protein of human adenovirus type 5 induces p53-independent cell death by apoptosis. *J Virol, 72,* 7144-53.

[140] Marcellus, R. C.; Chan, H.; Paquette, D.; Thirlwell, S.; Boivin, D. &Branton, P. E. (2000). Induction of p53-independent apoptosis by the adenovirus E4orf4 protein requires binding to the Balpha subunit of protein phosphatase 2A. *J Virol, 74,* 7869-77.

[141] Kornitzer, D.; Sharf, R. &Kleinberger, T. (2001). Adenovirus E4orf4 protein induces PP2A-dependent growth arrest in Saccharomyces cerevisiae and interacts with the anaphase-promoting complex/cyclosome. *J Cell Biol, 154,* 331-44.

[142] Huang, M. M. &Hearing, P. (1989). The adenovirus early region 4 open reading frame 6/7 protein regulates the DNA binding activity of the cellular transcription factor, E2F, through a direct complex. *Genes Dev, 3,* 1699-710.

[143] Nevins, J. R. (1995). Adenovirus E1A: transcription regulation and alteration of cell growth control. *Curr Top Microbiol Immunol, 199 (Pt 3),* 25-32.

[144] Reichel, R.; Neill, S. D.; Kovesdi, I.; Simon, M. C.; Raychaudhuri, P. &Nevins, J. R. (1989). The adenovirus E4 gene, in addition to the E1A gene, is important for trans-activation of E2 transcription and for E2F activation. *J Virol, 63,* 3643-50.

[145] Schaley, J.; O'Connor, R. J.; Taylor, L. J.; Bar-Sagi, D. &Hearing, P. (2000). Induction of the cellular E2F-1 promoter by the adenovirus E4-6/7 protein. *J Virol, 74,* 2084-93.

[146] Lutz, P. &Kedinger, C. (1996). Properties of the adenovirus IVa2 gene product, an effector of late-phase-dependent activation of the major late promoter. *J Virol, 70,* 1396-405.

[147] Lutz, P.; Rosa-Calatrava, M. &Kedinger, C. (1997). The product of the adenovirus intermediate gene IX is a transcriptional activator. *J Virol, 71,* 5102-9.

[148] Ali, H.; Leroy, G.; Bridge, G. &Flint, S. J. (2007). The adenovirus L4 33-kilodalton protein binds to intragenic sequences of the major late promoter required for late phase-specific stimulation of transcription. *J Virol, 81,* 1327-38.

[149] Zhang, W.; Low, J. A.; Christensen, J. B. &Imperiale, M. J. (2001). Role for the adenovirus IVa2 protein in packaging of viral DNA. *J Virol, 75,* 10446-54.

[150] Zhang, W. &Imperiale, M. J. (2003). Requirement of the adenovirus IVa2 protein for virus assembly. *J Virol, 77,* 3586-94.

[151] Tyler, R. E.; Ewing, S. G. &Imperiale, M. J. (2007). Formation of a multiple protein complex on the adenovirus packaging sequence by the IVa2 protein. *J Virol, 81,* 3447–3454.

[152] Zhang, W. &Imperiale, M. J. (2000). Interaction of the adenovirus IVa2 protein with viral packaging sequences. *J Virol, 74,* 2687-93.

[153] Ostapchuk, P.; Yang, J.; Auffarth, E. &Hearing, P. (2005). Functional interaction of the adenovirus IVa2 protein with adenovirus type 5 packaging sequences. *J Virol, 79,* 2831-8.

[154] Perez-Romero, P.; Tyler, R. E.; Abend, J. R.; Dus, M. &Imperiale, M. J. (2005). Analysis of the interaction of the adenovirus L1 52/55-kilodalton and IVa2 proteins with the packaging sequence in vivo and in vitro. *J Virol, 79,* 2366-74.

[155] Ostapchuk, P.; Anderson, M. E.; Chandrasekhar, S. &Hearing, P. (2006). The L4 22-kilodalton protein plays a role in packaging of the adenovirus genome. *J Virol, 80,* 6973-81.

[156] Rosa-Calatrava, M.; Grave, L.; Puvion-Dutilleul, F.; Chatton, B. &Kedinger, C. (2001). Functional analysis of adenovirus protein IX identifies domains involved in capsid stability, transcriptional activity, and nuclear reorganization. *J Virol, 75,* 7131-41.

[157] Ghosh-Choudhury, G.; Haj-Ahmad, Y. &Graham, F. L. (1987). Protein IX, a minor component of the human adenovirus capsid, is essential for the packaging of full length genomes. *Embo J, 6,* 1733-9.

[158] Furcinitti, P. S.; van Oostrum, J. &Burnett, R. M. (1989). Adenovirus polypeptide IX revealed as capsid cement by difference images from electron microscopy and crystallography. *Embo J, 8,* 3563-70.

[159] Nevins, J. R. &Wilson, M. C. (1981). Regulation of adenovirus-2 gene expression at the level of transcriptional termination and RNA processing. *Nature, 290,* 113-8.

[160] Shaw, A. R. &Ziff, E. B. (1980). Transcripts from the adenovirus-2 major late promoter yield a single early family of 3' coterminal mRNAs and five late families. *Cell, 22,* 905-16.

[161] Huang, W. &Flint, S. J. (1998). The tripartite leader sequence of subgroup C adenovirus major late mRNAs can increase the efficiency of mRNA export. *J Virol, 72,* 225-35.

[162] Logan, J. &Shenk, T. (1984). Adenovirus tripartite leader sequence enhances translation of mRNAs late after infection. *Proc Natl Acad Sci U S A, 81,* 3655-9.

[163] Gustin, K. E. &Imperiale, M. J. (1998). Encapsidation of viral DNA requires the adenovirus L1 52/55-kilodalton protein. *J Virol, 72,* 7860-70.

[164] Hasson, T. B.; Soloway, P. D.; Ornelles, D. A.; Doerfler, W. &Shenk, T. (1989). Adenovirus L1 52- and 55-kilodalton proteins are required for assembly of virions. *J Virol, 63,* 3612-21.

[165] Gustin, K. E.; Lutz, P. &Imperiale, M. J. (1996). Interaction of the adenovirus L1 52/55-kilodalton protein with the IVa2 gene product during infection. *J Virol, 70,* 6463-7.

[166] Perez-Romero, P.; Gustin, K. E. &Imperiale, M. J. (2006). Dependence of the encapsidation function of the adenovirus L1 52/55-kilodalton protein on its ability to bind the packaging sequence. *J Virol, 80,* 1965-71.

[167] Zhang, W. &Arcos, R. (2005). Interaction of the adenovirus major core protein precursor, pVII, with the viral DNA packaging machinery. *Virology, 334,* 194-202.

[168] Wodrich, H.; Cassany, A.; D'Angelo, M. A.; Guan, T.; Nemerow, G. &Gerace, L. (2006). Adenovirus core protein pVII is translocated into the nucleus by multiple import receptor pathways. *J Virol, 80,* 9608-18.

[169] Matthews, D. A. &Russell, W. C. (1998). Adenovirus core protein V is delivered by the invading virus to the nucleus of the infected cell and later in infection is associated with nucleoli. *J Gen Virol, 79 (Pt 7),* 1671-5.

[170] Ugai, H.; Borovjagin, A. V.; Le, L. P.; Wang, M. &Curiel, D. T. (2007). Thermostability/Infectivity Defect Caused by Deletion of the Core Protein V Gene in Human Adenovirus Type 5 Is Rescued by Thermo-selectable Mutations in the Core Protein X Precursor. *J Mol Biol, 366,* 1142-60.

[171] Sumida, S. M.; Truitt, D. M.; Lemckert, A. A.; Vogels, R.; Custers, J. H.; Addo, M. M.; Lockman, S.; Peter, T.; Peyerl, F. W.; Kishko, M. G.; Jackson, S. S.; Gorgone, D. A.; Lifton, M. A.; Essex, M.; Walker, B. D.; Goudsmit, J.; Havenga, M. J. &Barouch, D. H. (2005). Neutralizing antibodies to adenovirus serotype 5 vaccine vectors are directed primarily against the adenovirus hexon protein. *J Immunol, 174,* 7179-85.

[172] Pichla-Gollon, S. L.; Drinker, M.; Zhou, X.; Xue, F.; Rux, J. J.; Gao, G. P.; Wilson, J. M.; Ertl, H. C.; Burnett, R. M. &Bergelson, J. M. (2007). Structure-Based Identification of a Major Neutralizing Site in an Adenovirus Hexon. *J Virol, 81,* 1680-9.

[173] Tang, J.; Olive, M.; Pulmanausahakul, R.; Schnell, M.; Flomenberg, N.; Eisenlohr, L. &Flomenberg, P. (2006). Human CD8+ cytotoxic T cell responses to adenovirus capsid proteins. *Virology, 350,* 312-22.

[174] Heemskerk, B.; van Vreeswijk, T.; Veltrop-Duits, L. A.; Sombroek, C. C.; Franken, K.; Verhoosel, R. M.; Hiemstra, P. S.; van Leeuwen, D.; Ressing, M. E.; Toes, R. E.; van Tol, M. J. &Schilham, M. W. (2006). Adenovirus-specific CD4+ T cell clones

recognizing endogenous antigen inhibit viral replication in vitro through cognate interaction. *J Immunol, 177,* 8851-9.

[175] Wodrich, H.; Guan, T.; Cingolani, G.; Von Seggern, D.; Nemerow, G. &Gerace, L. (2003). Switch from capsid protein import to adenovirus assembly by cleavage of nuclear transport signals. *Embo J, 22,* 6245-55.

[176] Mangel, W. F.; McGrath, W. J.; Toledo, D. L. &Anderson, C. W. (1993). Viral DNA and a viral peptide can act as cofactors of adenovirus virion proteinase activity. *Nature, 361,* 274-5.

[177] Webster, A. &Kemp, G. (1993). The active adenovirus protease is the intact L3 23K protein. *J Gen Virol, 74 (Pt 7),* 1415-20.

[178] Chatterjee, P. K. &Flint, S. J. (1987). Adenovirus type 2 endopeptidase: an unusual phosphoprotein enzyme matured by autocatalysis. *Proc Natl Acad Sci U S A, 84,* 714-8.

[179] Greber, U. F.; Webster, P.; Weber, J. &Helenius, A. (1996). The role of the adenovirus protease on virus entry into cells. *Embo J, 15,* 1766-77.

[180] Matthews, D. A. &Russell, W. C. (1995). Adenovirus protein-protein interactions: molecular parameters governing the binding of protein VI to hexon and the activation of the adenovirus 23K protease. *J Gen Virol, 76 (Pt 8),* 1959-69.

[181] Cepko, C. L. &Sharp, P. A. (1982). Assembly of adenovirus major capsid protein is mediated by a nonvirion protein. *Cell, 31,* 407-15.

[182] Xi, Q.; Cuesta, R. &Schneider, R. J. (2005). Regulation of translation by ribosome shunting through phosphotyrosine-dependent coupling of adenovirus protein 100k to viral mRNAs. *J Virol, 79,* 5676-83.

[183] Andrade, F.; Bull, H. G.; Thornberry, N. A.; Ketner, G. W.; Casciola-Rosen, L. A. &Rosen, A. (2001). Adenovirus L4-100K assembly protein is a granzyme B substrate that potently inhibits granzyme B-mediated cell death. *Immunity, 14,* 751-61.

[184] Oosterom-Dragon, E. A. &Anderson, C. W. (1983). Polypeptide structure and encoding location of the adenovirus serotype 2 late, nonstructural 33K protein. *J Virol, 45,* 251-63.

[185] Fessler, S. P. &Young, C. S. (1999). The role of the L4 33K gene in adenovirus infection. *Virology, 263,* 507-16.

[186] Finnen, R. L.; Biddle, J. F. &Flint, J. (2001). Truncation of the human adenovirus type 5 L4 33-kDa protein: evidence for an essential role of the carboxy-terminus in the viral infectious cycle. *Virology, 289,* 388-99.

[187] Farley, D. C.; Brown, J. L. &Leppard, K. N. (2004). Activation of the early-late switch in adenovirus type 5 major late transcription unit expression by L4 gene products. *J Virol, 78,* 1782-91.

[188] Abrescia, N. G.; Cockburn, J. J.; Grimes, J. M.; Sutton, G. C.; Diprose, J. M.; Butcher, S. J.; Fuller, S. D.; San Martin, C.; Burnett, R. M.; Stuart, D. I.; Bamford, D. H. &Bamford, J. K. (2004). Insights into assembly from structural analysis of bacteriophage PRD1. *Nature, 432,* 68-74.

[189] Liu, G. Q.; Babiss, L. E.; Volkert, F. C.; Young, C. S. &Ginsberg, H. S. (1985). A thermolabile mutant of adenovirus 5 resulting from a substitution mutation in the protein VIII gene. *J Virol, 53,* 920-5.

[190] Shayakhmetov, D. M. &Lieber, A. (2000). Dependence of adenovirus infectivity on length of the fiber shaft domain. *J Virol, 74,* 10274-86.

[191] Mathews, M. B. &Shenk, T. (1991). Adenovirus virus-associated RNA and translation control. *J Virol, 65,* 5657-62.

[192] Svensson, C. &Akusjarvi, G. (1990). A novel effect of adenovirus VA RNA1 on cytoplasmic mRNA abundance. *Virology, 174,* 613-7.

[193] Thimmappaya, B.; Weinberger, C.; Schneider, R. J. &Shenk, T. (1982). Adenovirus VAI RNA is required for efficient translation of viral mRNAs at late times after infection. *Cell, 31,* 543-51.

[194] Kitajewski, J.; Schneider, R. J.; Safer, B.; Munemitsu, S. M.; Samuel, C. E.; Thimmappaya, B. &Shenk, T. (1986). Adenovirus VAI RNA antagonizes the antiviral action of interferon by preventing activation of the interferon-induced eIF-2 alpha kinase. *Cell, 45,* 195-200.

[195] Andersson, M. G.; Haasnoot, P. C.; Xu, N.; Berenjian, S.; Berkhout, B. &Akusjarvi, G. (2005). Suppression of RNA interference by adenovirus virus-associated RNA. *J Virol, 79,* 9556-65.

[196] Liao, H. J.; Kobayashi, R. &Mathews, M. B. (1998). Activities of adenovirus virus-associated RNAs: purification and characterization of RNA binding proteins. *Proc Natl Acad Sci U S A, 95,* 8514-9.

[197] Kidd, A. H.; Garwicz, D. &Oberg, M. (1995). Human and simian adenoviruses: phylogenetic inferences from analysis of VA RNA genes. *Virology, 207,* 32-45.

[198] Graham, F. L.; Smiley, J.; Russell, W. C. &Nairn, R. (1977). Characteristics of a human cell line transformed by DNA from human adenovirus type 5. *J Gen Virol, 36,* 59-74.

[199] Hehir, K. M.; Armentano, D.; Cardoza, L. M.; Choquette, T. L.; Berthelette, P. B.; White, G. A.; Couture, L. A.; Everton, M. B.; Keegan, J.; Martin, J. M.; Pratt, D. A.; Smith, M. P.; Smith, A. E. &Wadsworth, S. C. (1996). Molecular characterization of replication-competent variants of adenovirus vectors and genome modifications to prevent their occurrence. *J Virol, 70,* 8459-67.

[200] Lochmuller, H.; Jani, A.; Huard, J.; Prescott, S.; Simoneau, M.; Massie, B.; Karpati, G. &Acsadi, G. (1994). Emergence of early region 1-containing replication-competent adenovirus in stocks of replication-defective adenovirus recombinants (delta E1 + delta E3) during multiple passages in 293 cells. *Hum Gene Ther, 5,* 1485-91.

[201] Fallaux, F. J.; Bout, A.; van der Velde, I.; van den Wollenberg, D. J.; Hehir, K. M.; Keegan, J.; Auger, C.; Cramer, S. J.; van Ormondt, H.; van der Eb, A. J.; Valerio, D. &Hoeben, R. C. (1998). New helper cells and matched early region 1-deleted adenovirus vectors prevent generation of replication-competent adenoviruses. *Hum Gene Ther, 9,* 1909-17.

[202] Smith, T. A.; Mehaffey, M. G.; Kayda, D. B.; Saunders, J. M.; Yei, S.; Trapnell, B. C.; McClelland, A. &Kaleko, M. (1993). Adenovirus mediated expression of therapeutic plasma levels of human factor IX in mice. *Nat Genet, 5,* 397-402.

[203] Li, Q.; Kay, M. A.; Finegold, M.; Stratford-Perricaudet, L. D. &Woo, S. L. (1993). Assessment of recombinant adenoviral vectors for hepatic gene therapy. *Hum Gene Ther, 4,* 403-9.

[204] Kay, M. A.; Landen, C. N.; Rothenberg, S. R.; Taylor, L. A.; Leland, F.; Wiehle, S.; Fang, B.; Bellinger, D.; Finegold, M.; Thompson, A. R. &et al. (1994). In vivo hepatic gene therapy: complete albeit transient correction of factor IX deficiency in hemophilia B dogs. *Proc Natl Acad Sci U S A, 91,* 2353-7.

[205] Yang, Y.; Nunes, F. A.; Berencsi, K.; Furth, E. E.; Gonczol, E. &Wilson, J. M. (1994). Cellular immunity to viral antigens limits E1-deleted adenoviruses for gene therapy. *Proc Natl Acad Sci U S A, 91,* 4407-11.

[206] Yang, Y.; Li, Q.; Ertl, H. C. &Wilson, J. M. (1995). Cellular and humoral immune responses to viral antigens create barriers to lung-directed gene therapy with recombinant adenoviruses. *J Virol, 69,* 2004-15.

[207] Yang, Y.; Su, Q. &Wilson, J. M. (1996). Role of viral antigens in destructive cellular immune responses to adenovirus vector-transduced cells in mouse lungs. *J Virol, 70,* 7209-12.

[208] Dai, Y.; Schwarz, E. M.; Gu, D.; Zhang, W. W.; Sarvetnick, N. &Verma, I. M. (1995). Cellular and humoral immune responses to adenoviral vectors containing factor IX gene: tolerization of factor IX and vector antigens allows for long-term expression. *Proc Natl Acad Sci U S A, 92,* 1401-5.

[209] Barr, D.; Tubb, J.; Ferguson, D.; Scaria, A.; Lieber, A.; Wilson, C.; Perkins, J. &Kay, M. A. (1995). Strain related variations in adenovirally mediated transgene expression from mouse hepatocytes in vivo: comparisons between immunocompetent and immunodeficient inbred strains. *Gene Ther, 2,* 151-5.

[210] Michou, A. I.; Santoro, L.; Christ, M.; Julliard, V.; Pavirani, A. &Mehtali, M. (1997). Adenovirus-mediated gene transfer: influence of transgene, mouse strain and type of immune response on persistence of transgene expression. *Gene Ther, 4,* 473-82.

[211] Zhou, H.; O'Neal, W.; Morral, N. &Beaudet, A. L. (1996). Development of a complementing cell line and a system for construction of adenovirus vectors with E1 and E2a deleted. *J Virol, 70,* 7030-8.

[212] Schagen, F. H.; Ossevoort, M.; Toes, R. E. &Hoeben, R. C. (2004). Immune responses against adenoviral vectors and their transgene products: a review of strategies for evasion. *Crit Rev Oncol Hematol, 50,* 51-70.

[213] Yang, Y.; Nunes, F. A.; Berencsi, K.; Gonczol, E.; Engelhardt, J. F. &Wilson, J. M. (1994). Inactivation of E2a in recombinant adenoviruses improves the prospect for gene therapy in cystic fibrosis. *Nat Genet, 7,* 362-9.

[214] Engelhardt, J. F.; Litzky, L. &Wilson, J. M. (1994). Prolonged transgene expression in cotton rat lung with recombinant adenoviruses defective in E2a. *Hum Gene Ther, 5,* 1217-29.

[215] Engelhardt, J. F.; Ye, X.; Doranz, B. &Wilson, J. M. (1994). Ablation of E2A in recombinant adenoviruses improves transgene persistence and decreases inflammatory response in mouse liver. *Proc Natl Acad Sci U S A, 91,* 6196-200.

[216] Goldman, M. J.; Litzky, L. A.; Engelhardt, J. F. &Wilson, J. M. (1995). Transfer of the CFTR gene to the lung of nonhuman primates with E1-deleted, E2a-defective recombinant adenoviruses: a preclinical toxicology study. *Hum Gene Ther, 6,* 839-51.

[217] Lusky, M.; Christ, M.; Rittner, K.; Dieterle, A.; Dreyer, D.; Mourot, B.; Schultz, H.; Stoeckel, F.; Pavirani, A. &Mehtali, M. (1998). In vitro and in vivo biology of recombinant adenovirus vectors with E1, E1/E2A, or E1/E4 deleted. *J Virol, 72,* 2022-32.

[218] Nevins, J. R. &Winkler, J. J. (1980). Regulation of early adenovirus transcription: a protein product of early region 2 specifically represses region 4 transcription. *Proc Natl Acad Sci U S A, 77,* 1893-7.

[219] Handa, H.; Kingston, R. E. &Sharp, P. A. (1983). Inhibition of adenovirus early region IV transcription in vitro by a purified viral DNA binding protein. *Nature, 302,* 545-7.

[220] Gorziglia, M. I.; Lapcevich, C.; Roy, S.; Kang, Q.; Kadan, M.; Wu, V.; Pechan, P. &Kaleko, M. (1999). Generation of an adenovirus vector lacking E1, e2a, E3, and all of E4 except open reading frame 3. *J Virol, 73,* 6048-55.

[221] Parks, R. J. &Graham, F. L. (1997). A helper-dependent system for adenovirus vector production helps define a lower limit for efficient DNA packaging. *J Virol, 71,* 3293-8.

[222] Parks, R. J.; Bramson, J. L.; Wan, Y.; Addison, C. L. &Graham, F. L. (1999). Effects of stuffer DNA on transgene expression from helper-dependent adenovirus vectors. *J Virol, 73,* 8027-34.

[223] Fisher, K. J.; Choi, H.; Burda, J.; Chen, S. J. &Wilson, J. M. (1996). Recombinant adenovirus deleted of all viral genes for gene therapy of cystic fibrosis. *Virology, 217,* 11-22.

[224] Kochanek, S.; Clemens, P. R.; Mitani, K.; Chen, H. H.; Chan, S. &Caskey, C. T. (1996). A new adenoviral vector: Replacement of all viral coding sequences with 28 kb of DNA independently expressing both full-length dystrophin and beta-galactosidase. *Proc Natl Acad Sci U S A, 93,* 5731-6.

[225] Parks, R. J.; Chen, L.; Anton, M.; Sankar, U.; Rudnicki, M. A. &Graham, F. L. (1996). A helper-dependent adenovirus vector system: removal of helper virus by Cre-mediated excision of the viral packaging signal. *Proc Natl Acad Sci U S A, 93,* 13565-70.

[226] DelloRusso, C.; Scott, J. M.; Hartigan-O'Connor, D.; Salvatori, G.; Barjot, C.; Robinson, A. S.; Crawford, R. W.; Brooks, S. V. &Chamberlain, J. S. (2002). Functional correction of adult mdx mouse muscle using gutted adenoviral vectors expressing full-length dystrophin. *Proc Natl Acad Sci U S A, 99,* 12979-84.

[227] Ehrhardt, A. &Kay, M. A. (2002). A new adenoviral helper-dependent vector results in long-term therapeutic levels of human coagulation factor IX at low doses in vivo. *Blood, 99,* 3923-30.

[228] Mian, A.; McCormack, W. M., Jr.; Mane, V.; Kleppe, S.; Ng, P.; Finegold, M.; O'Brien, W. E.; Rodgers, J. R.; Beaudet, A. L. &Lee, B. (2004). Long-term correction of ornithine transcarbamylase deficiency by WPRE-mediated overexpression using a helper-dependent adenovirus. *Mol Ther, 10,* 492-9.

[229] Roth, M. D.; Cheng, Q.; Harui, A.; Basak, S. K.; Mitani, K.; Low, T. A. &Kiertscher, S. M. (2002). Helper-dependent adenoviral vectors efficiently express transgenes in human dendritic cells but still stimulate antiviral immune responses. *J Immunol, 169,* 4651-6.

[230] Muruve, D. A.; Cotter, M. J.; Zaiss, A. K.; White, L. R.; Liu, Q.; Chan, T.; Clark, S. A.; Ross, P. J.; Meulenbroek, R. A.; Maelandsmo, G. M. &Parks, R. J. (2004). Helper-dependent adenovirus vectors elicit intact innate but attenuated adaptive host immune responses in vivo. *J Virol, 78,* 5966-72.

[231] Kafri, T.; Morgan, D.; Krahl, T.; Sarvetnick, N.; Sherman, L. &Verma, I. (1998). Cellular immune response to adenoviral vector infected cells does not require de novo viral gene expression: implications for gene therapy. *Proc Natl Acad Sci U S A, 95,* 11377-82.

[232] Muruve, D. A.; Barnes, M. J.; Stillman, I. E. &Libermann, T. A. (1999). Adenoviral gene therapy leads to rapid induction of multiple chemokines and acute neutrophil-dependent hepatic injury in vivo. *Hum Gene Ther, 10,* 965-76.

[233] Schnell, M. A.; Zhang, Y.; Tazelaar, J.; Gao, G. P.; Yu, Q. C.; Qian, R.; Chen, S. J.; Varnavski, A. N.; LeClair, C.; Raper, S. E. &Wilson, J. M. (2001). Activation of innate immunity in nonhuman primates following intraportal administration of adenoviral vectors. *Mol Ther, 3,* 708-22.

[234] Muruve, D. A. (2004). The innate immune response to adenovirus vectors. *Hum Gene Ther, 15,* 1157-66.

[235] Molinier-Frenkel, V.; Lengagne, R.; Gaden, F.; Hong, S. S.; Choppin, J.; Gahery-Segard, H.; Boulanger, P. &Guillet, J. G. (2002). Adenovirus hexon protein is a potent adjuvant for activation of a cellular immune response. *J Virol, 76,* 127-35.

[236] Otake, K.; Ennist, D. L.; Harrod, K. &Trapnell, B. C. (1998). Nonspecific inflammation inhibits adenovirus-mediated pulmonary gene transfer and expression independent of specific acquired immune responses. *Hum Gene Ther, 9,* 2207-22.

[237] Zhang, Y.; Chirmule, N.; Gao, G. P.; Qian, R.; Croyle, M.; Joshi, B.; Tazelaar, J. &Wilson, J. M. (2001). Acute cytokine response to systemic adenoviral vectors in mice is mediated by dendritic cells and macrophages. *Mol Ther, 3,* 697-707.

[238] Guidotti, L. G. &Chisari, F. V. (2001). Noncytolytic control of viral infections by the innate and adaptive immune response. *Annu Rev Immunol, 19,* 65-91.

[239] Tripathy, S. K.; Black, H. B.; Goldwasser, E. &Leiden, J. M. (1996). Immune responses to transgene-encoded proteins limit the stability of gene expression after injection of replication-defective adenovirus vectors. *Nat Med, 2,* 545-50.

[240] Rodrigues, E. G.; Zavala, F.; Eichinger, D.; Wilson, J. M. &Tsuji, M. (1997). Single immunizing dose of recombinant adenovirus efficiently induces CD8+ T cell-mediated protective immunity against malaria. *J Immunol, 158,* 1268-74.

[241] Sullivan, N. J.; Geisbert, T. W.; Geisbert, J. B.; Xu, L.; Yang, Z. Y.; Roederer, M.; Koup, R. A.; Jahrling, P. B. &Nabel, G. J. (2003). Accelerated vaccination for Ebola virus haemorrhagic fever in non-human primates. *Nature, 424,* 681-4.

[242] Gao, W.; Soloff, A. C.; Lu, X.; Montecalvo, A.; Nguyen, D. C.; Matsuoka, Y.; Robbins, P. D.; Swayne, D. E.; Donis, R. O.; Katz, J. M.; Barratt-Boyes, S. M. &Gambotto, A. (2006). Protection of mice and poultry from lethal H5N1 avian influenza virus through adenovirus-based immunization. *J Virol, 80,* 1959-64.

[243] Prevec, L.; Campbell, J. B.; Christie, B. S.; Belbeck, L. &Graham, F. L. (1990). A recombinant human adenovirus vaccine against rabies. *J Infect Dis, 161,* 27-30.

[244] Xiang, Z. Q.; Yang, Y.; Wilson, J. M. &Ertl, H. C. (1996). A replication-defective human adenovirus recombinant serves as a highly efficacious vaccine carrier. *Virology, 219,* 220-7.

[245] Gallichan, W. S.; Johnson, D. C.; Graham, F. L. &Rosenthal, K. L. (1993). Mucosal immunity and protection after intranasal immunization with recombinant adenovirus expressing herpes simplex virus glycoprotein B. *J Infect Dis, 168,* 622-9.

[246] Gallichan, W. S. &Rosenthal, K. L. (1998). Long-term immunity and protection against herpes simplex virus type 2 in the murine female genital tract after mucosal but not systemic immunization. *J Infect Dis, 177,* 1155-61.

[247] Tan, Y.; Hackett, N. R.; Boyer, J. L. &Crystal, R. G. (2003). Protective immunity evoked against anthrax lethal toxin after a single intramuscular administration of an adenovirus-based vaccine encoding humanized protective antigen. *Hum Gene Ther, 14,* 1673-82.

[248] Chiuchiolo, M. J.; Boyer, J. L.; Krause, A.; Senina, S.; Hackett, N. R. &Crystal, R. G. (2006). Protective immunity against respiratory tract challenge with Yersinia pestis in mice immunized with an adenovirus-based vaccine vector expressing V antigen. *J Infect Dis, 194,* 1249-57.

[249] Shiver, J. W.; Fu, T. M.; Chen, L.; Casimiro, D. R.; Davies, M. E.; Evans, R. K.; Zhang, Z. Q.; Simon, A. J.; Trigona, W. L.; Dubey, S. A.; Huang, L.; Harris, V. A.; Long, R. S.; Liang, X.; Handt, L.; Schleif, W. A.; Zhu, L.; Freed, D. C.; Persaud, N. V.; Guan, L.; Punt, K. S.; Tang, A.; Chen, M.; Wilson, K. A.; Collins, K. B.; Heidecker, G. J.; Fernandez, V. R.; Perry, H. C.; Joyce, J. G.; Grimm, K. M.; Cook, J. C.; Keller, P. M.; Kresock, D. S.; Mach, H.; Troutman, R. D.; Isopi, L. A.; Williams, D. M.; Xu, Z.; Bohannon, K. E.; Volkin, D. B.; Montefiori, D. C.; Miura, A.; Krivulka, G. R.; Lifton, M. A.; Kuroda, M. J.; Schmitz, J. E.; Letvin, N. L.; Caulfield, M. J.; Bett, A. J.; Youil, R.; Kaslow, D. C. &Emini, E. A. (2002). Replication-incompetent adenoviral vaccine vector elicits effective anti-immunodeficiency-virus immunity. *Nature, 415,* 331-5.

[250] Casimiro, D. R.; Chen, L.; Fu, T. M.; Evans, R. K.; Caulfield, M. J.; Davies, M. E.; Tang, A.; Chen, M.; Huang, L.; Harris, V.; Freed, D. C.; Wilson, K. A.; Dubey, S.; Zhu, D. M.; Nawrocki, D.; Mach, H.; Troutman, R.; Isopi, L.; Williams, D.; Hurni, W.; Xu, Z.; Smith, J. G.; Wang, S.; Liu, X.; Guan, L.; Long, R.; Trigona, W.; Heidecker, G. J.; Perry, H. C.; Persaud, N.; Toner, T. J.; Su, Q.; Liang, X.; Youil, R.; Chastain, M.; Bett, A. J.; Volkin, D. B.; Emini, E. A. &Shiver, J. W. (2003). Comparative immunogenicity in rhesus monkeys of DNA plasmid, recombinant vaccinia virus, and replication-defective adenovirus vectors expressing a human immunodeficiency virus type 1 gag gene. *J Virol, 77,* 6305-13.

[251] Mascola, J. R.; Sambor, A.; Beaudry, K.; Santra, S.; Welcher, B.; Louder, M. K.; Vancott, T. C.; Huang, Y.; Chakrabarti, B. K.; Kong, W. P.; Yang, Z. Y.; Xu, L.; Montefiori, D. C.; Nabel, G. J. &Letvin, N. L. (2005). Neutralizing antibodies elicited by immunization of monkeys with DNA plasmids and recombinant adenoviral vectors expressing human immunodeficiency virus type 1 proteins. *J Virol, 79,* 771-9.

[252] Santra, S.; Seaman, M. S.; Xu, L.; Barouch, D. H.; Lord, C. I.; Lifton, M. A.; Gorgone, D. A.; Beaudry, K. R.; Svehla, K.; Welcher, B.; Chakrabarti, B. K.; Huang, Y.; Yang, Z. Y.; Mascola, J. R.; Nabel, G. J. &Letvin, N. L. (2005). Replication-defective adenovirus serotype 5 vectors elicit durable cellular and humoral immune responses in nonhuman primates. *J Virol, 79,* 6516-22.

[253] Wang, J.; Thorson, L.; Stokes, R. W.; Santosuosso, M.; Huygen, K.; Zganiacz, A.; Hitt, M. &Xing, Z. (2004). Single mucosal, but not parenteral, immunization with recombinant adenoviral-based vaccine provides potent protection from pulmonary tuberculosis. *J Immunol, 173,* 6357-65.

[254] Gilbert, S. C.; Schneider, J.; Hannan, C. M.; Hu, J. T.; Plebanski, M.; Sinden, R. &Hill, A. V. (2002). Enhanced CD8 T cell immunogenicity and protective efficacy in a mouse malaria model using a recombinant adenoviral vaccine in heterologous prime-boost immunisation regimes. *Vaccine, 20,* 1039-45.

[255] Park, S. H.; Yang, S. H.; Lee, C. G.; Youn, J. W.; Chang, J. &Sung, Y. C. (2003). Efficient induction of T helper 1 CD4+ T-cell responses to hepatitis C virus core and E2 by a DNA prime-adenovirus boost. *Vaccine, 21,* 4555-64.

[256] McConnell, M. J.; Hanna, P. C. &Imperiale, M. J. (2007). Adenovirus-based Prime-boost Immunization for Rapid Vaccination Against Anthrax. *Mol Ther, 15,* 203-10.

[257] Sullivan, N. J.; Sanchez, A.; Rollin, P. E.; Yang, Z. Y. &Nabel, G. J. (2000). Development of a preventive vaccine for Ebola virus infection in primates. *Nature, 408,* 605-9.

[258] Bruna-Romero, O.; Gonzalez-Aseguinolaza, G.; Hafalla, J. C.; Tsuji, M. &Nussenzweig, R. S. (2001). Complete, long-lasting protection against malaria of mice primed and boosted with two distinct viral vectors expressing the same plasmodial antigen. *Proc Natl Acad Sci U S A, 98,* 11491-6.

[259] Letvin, N. L.; Mascola, J. R.; Sun, Y.; Gorgone, D. A.; Buzby, A. P.; Xu, L.; Yang, Z. Y.; Chakrabarti, B.; Rao, S. S.; Schmitz, J. E.; Montefiori, D. C.; Barker, B. R.; Bookstein, F. L. &Nabel, G. J. (2006). Preserved CD4+ central memory T cells and survival in vaccinated SIV-challenged monkeys. *Science, 312,* 1530-3.

[260] Barouch, D. H.; McKay, P. F.; Sumida, S. M.; Santra, S.; Jackson, S. S.; Gorgone, D. A.; Lifton, M. A.; Chakrabarti, B. K.; Xu, L.; Nabel, G. J. &Letvin, N. L. (2003). Plasmid chemokines and colony-stimulating factors enhance the immunogenicity of DNA priming-viral vector boosting human immunodeficiency virus type 1 vaccines. *J Virol, 77,* 8729-35.

[261] Yang, Z. Y.; Wyatt, L. S.; Kong, W. P.; Moodie, Z.; Moss, B. &Nabel, G. J. (2003). Overcoming Immunity to a Viral Vaccine by DNA Priming before Vector Boosting. *J Virol, 77,* 799-803.

[262] McKelvey, T.; Tang, A.; Bett, A. J.; Casimiro, D. R. &Chastain, M. (2004). T-cell response to adenovirus hexon and DNA-binding protein in mice. *Gene Ther, 11,* 791-6.

[263] Sumida, S. M.; Truitt, D. M.; Kishko, M. G.; Arthur, J. C.; Jackson, S. S.; Gorgone, D. A.; Lifton, M. A.; Koudstaal, W.; Pau, M. G.; Kostense, S.; Havenga, M. J.; Goudsmit, J.; Letvin, N. L. &Barouch, D. H. (2004). Neutralizing antibodies and CD8+ T lymphocytes both contribute to immunity to adenovirus serotype 5 vaccine vectors. *J Virol, 78,* 2666-73.

[264] Vogels, R.; Zuijdgeest, D.; van Rijnsoever, R.; Hartkoorn, E.; Damen, I.; de Bethune, M. P.; Kostense, S.; Penders, G.; Helmus, N.; Koudstaal, W.; Cecchini, M.; Wetterwald, A.; Sprangers, M.; Lemckert, A.; Ophorst, O.; Koel, B.; van Meerendonk, M.; Quax, P.; Panitti, L.; Grimbergen, J.; Bout, A.; Goudsmit, J. &Havenga, M. (2003). Replication-deficient human adenovirus type 35 vectors for gene transfer and vaccination: efficient human cell infection and bypass of preexisting adenovirus immunity. *J Virol, 77,* 8263-71.

[265] Holterman, L.; Vogels, R.; van der Vlugt, R.; Sieuwerts, M.; Grimbergen, J.; Kaspers, J.; Geelen, E.; van der Helm, E.; Lemckert, A.; Gillissen, G.; Verhaagh, S.; Custers, J.; Zuijdgeest, D.; Berkhout, B.; Bakker, M.; Quax, P.; Goudsmit, J. &Havenga, M. (2004). Novel replication-incompetent vector derived from adenovirus type 11 (Ad11) for vaccination and gene therapy: low seroprevalence and non-cross-reactivity with Ad5. *J Virol, 78,* 13207-15.

[266] Nwanegbo, E.; Vardas, E.; Gao, W.; Whittle, H.; Sun, H.; Rowe, D.; Robbins, P. D. &Gambotto, A. (2004). Prevalence of neutralizing antibodies to adenoviral serotypes 5 and 35 in the adult populations of The Gambia, South Africa, and the United States. *Clin Diagn Lab Immunol, 11,* 351-7.

[267] Kostense, S.; Koudstaal, W.; Sprangers, M.; Weverling, G. J.; Penders, G.; Helmus, N.; Vogels, R.; Bakker, M.; Berkhout, B.; Havenga, M. &Goudsmit, J. (2004). Adenovirus

types 5 and 35 seroprevalence in AIDS risk groups supports type 35 as a vaccine vector. *AIDS, 18,* 1213-6.

[268] Heemskerk, B.; Veltrop-Duits, L. A.; van Vreeswijk, T.; ten Dam, M. M.; Heidt, S.; Toes, R. E.; van Tol, M. J. &Schilham, M. W. (2003). Extensive cross-reactivity of CD4+ adenovirus-specific T cells: implications for immunotherapy and gene therapy. *J Virol, 77,* 6562-6.

[269] Casimiro, D. R.; Tang, A.; Chen, L.; Fu, T. M.; Evans, R. K.; Davies, M. E.; Freed, D. C.; Hurni, W.; Aste-Amezaga, J. M.; Guan, L.; Long, R.; Huang, L.; Harris, V.; Nawrocki, D. K.; Mach, H.; Troutman, R. D.; Isopi, L. A.; Murthy, K. K.; Rice, K.; Wilson, K. A.; Volkin, D. B.; Emini, E. A. &Shiver, J. W. (2003). Vaccine-induced immunity in baboons by using DNA and replication-incompetent adenovirus type 5 vectors expressing a human immunodeficiency virus type 1 gag gene. *J Virol, 77,* 7663-8.

[270] Thorner, A. R.; Vogels, R.; Kaspers, J.; Weverling, G. J.; Holterman, L.; Lemckert, A. A.; Dilraj, A.; McNally, L. M.; Jeena, P. M.; Jepsen, S.; Abbink, P.; Nanda, A.; Swanson, P. E.; Bates, A. T.; O'Brien, K. L.; Havenga, M. J.; Goudsmit, J. &Barouch, D. H. (2006). Age dependence of adenovirus-specific neutralizing antibody titers in individuals from sub-Saharan Africa. *J Clin Microbiol, 44,* 3781-3.

[271] Havenga, M.; Vogels, R.; Zuijdgeest, D.; Radosevic, K.; Mueller, S.; Sieuwerts, M.; Weichold, F.; Damen, I.; Kaspers, J.; Lemckert, A.; van der Vlugt, R.; Holterman, L.; Hone, D.; Skeiky, Y.; Mintardjo, R.; Gillissen, G.; Barouch, D.; Sadoff, J. &Goudsmit, J. (2006). Novel replication-incompetent adenoviral B-group vectors: high vector stability and yield in PER.C6 cells. *J. Gen. Virol, 87,* 2135-2143.

[272] Barouch, D. H.; Pau, M. G.; Custers, J. H.; Koudstaal, W.; Kostense, S.; Havenga, M. J.; Truitt, D. M.; Sumida, S. M.; Kishko, M. G.; Arthur, J. C.; Korioth-Schmitz, B.; Newberg, M. H.; Gorgone, D. A.; Lifton, M. A.; Panicali, D. L.; Nabel, G. J.; Letvin, N. L. &Goudsmit, J. (2004). Immunogenicity of recombinant adenovirus serotype 35 vaccine in the presence of pre-existing anti-Ad5 immunity. *J Immunol, 172,* 6290-7.

[273] Barratt-Boyes, S. M.; Soloff, A. C.; Gao, W.; Nwanegbo, E.; Liu, X.; Rajakumar, P. A.; Brown, K. N.; Robbins, P. D.; Murphey-Corb, M.; Day, R. D. &Gambotto, A. (2006). Broad cellular immunity with robust memory responses to simian immunodeficiency virus following serial vaccination with adenovirus 5- and 35-based vectors. *J Gen Virol, 87,* 139-49.

[274] Ophorst, O. J. A. E.; Radosevic, K.; Havenga, M. J. E.; Pau, M. G.; Holterman, L.; Berkhout, B.; Goudsmit, J. &Tsuji, M. (2006). Immunogenicity and Protection of a Recombinant Human Adenovirus Serotype 35-Based Malaria Vaccine against *Plasmodium yoelii* in Mice. *Infect Immun, 74,* 313-320.

[275] Radoševic, K.; Wieland, C. W.; Rodriguez, A.; Weverling, G. J.; Mintardjo, R.; Gillissen, G.; Vogels, R.; Skeiky, Y. A. W.; Hone, D. M.; Sadoff, J.; van der Poll, T.; Havenga, M. &Goudsmit, J. (2007). Protective immune responses to a recombinant adenovirus type 35 tuberculosis vaccine in two mouse strains: CD4 and CD8 T-cell epitope mapping and role of gamma interferon. *Infect Immun, 75,* 4105-15.

[276] Nanda, A.; Lynch, D. M.; Goudsmit, J.; Lemckert, A. A.; Ewald, B. A.; Sumida, S. M.; Truitt, D. M.; Abbink, P.; Kishko, M. G.; Gorgone, D. A.; Lifton, M. A.; Shen, L.; Carville, A.; Mansfield, K. G.; Havenga, M. J. &Barouch, D. H. (2005).

Immunogenicity of recombinant fiber-chimeric adenovirus serotype 35 vector-based vaccines in mice and rhesus monkeys. *J Virol, 79,* 14161-8.

[277] Lemckert, A. A.; Sumida, S. M.; Holterman, L.; Vogels, R.; Truitt, D. M.; Lynch, D. M.; Nanda, A.; Ewald, B. A.; Gorgone, D. A.; Lifton, M. A.; Goudsmit, J.; Havenga, M. J. &Barouch, D. H. (2005). Immunogenicity of heterologous prime-boost regimens involving recombinant adenovirus serotype 11 (Ad11) and Ad35 vaccine vectors in the presence of anti-ad5 immunity. *J. Virol, 79,* 9694-701.

[278] Capone, S.; Meola, A.; Ercole, B. B.; Vitelli, A.; Pezzanera, M.; Ruggeri, L.; Davies, M. E.; Tafi, R.; Santini, C.; Luzzago, A.; Fu, T. M.; Bett, A.; Colloca, S.; Cortese, R.; Nicosia, A. &Folgori, A. (2006). A novel adenovirus type 6 (Ad6)-based hepatitis C virus vector that overcomes preexisting anti-ad5 immunity and induces potent and broad cellular immune responses in rhesus macaques. *J Virol, 80,* 1688-99.

[279] Shiver, J. W. &Emini, E. A. (2004). Recent advances in the development of HIV-1 vaccines using replication-incompetent adenovirus vectors. *Annu Rev Med, 55,* 355-72.

[280] Folgori, A.; Capone, S.; Ruggeri, L.; Meola, A.; Sporeno, E.; Ercole, B. B.; Pezzanera, M.; Tafi, R.; Arcuri, M.; Fattori, E.; Lahm, A.; Luzzago, A.; Vitelli, A.; Colloca, S.; Cortese, R. &Nicosia, A. (2006). A T-cell HCV vaccine eliciting effective immunity against heterologous virus challenge in chimpanzees. *Nat Med, 12,* 190-7.

[281] Lemiale, F.; Haddada, H.; Nabel, G. J.; Brough, D. E.; King, C. R. &Gall, J. G. (2007). Novel adenovirus vaccine vectors based on the enteric-tropic serotype 41. *Vaccine, 25,* 2074-84.

[282] Havenga, M. J.; Lemckert, A. A.; Ophorst, O. J.; van Meijer, M.; Germeraad, W. T.; Grimbergen, J.; van Den Doel, M. A.; Vogels, R.; van Deutekom, J.; Janson, A. A.; de Bruijn, J. D.; Uytdehaag, F.; Quax, P. H.; Logtenberg, T.; Mehtali, M. &Bout, A. (2002). Exploiting the natural diversity in adenovirus tropism for therapy and prevention of disease. *J Virol, 76,* 4612-20.

[283] Ophorst, O. J.; Kostense, S.; Goudsmit, J.; De Swart, R. L.; Verhaagh, S.; Zakhartchouk, A.; Van Meijer, M.; Sprangers, M.; Van Amerongen, G.; Yuksel, S.; Osterhaus, A. D. &Havenga, M. J. (2004). An adenoviral type 5 vector carrying a type 35 fiber as a vaccine vehicle: DC targeting, cross neutralization, and immunogenicity. *Vaccine, 22,* 3035-44.

[284] Youil, R.; Toner, T. J.; Su, Q.; Chen, M.; Tang, A.; Bett, A. J. &Casimiro, D. (2002). Hexon gene switch strategy for the generation of chimeric recombinant adenovirus. *Hum Gene Ther, 13,* 311-20.

[285] Wu, H.; Dmitriev, I.; Kashentseva, E.; Seki, T.; Wang, M. &Curiel, D. T. (2002). Construction and characterization of adenovirus serotype 5 packaged by serotype 3 hexon. *J Virol, 76,* 12775-82.

[286] Crawford-Miksza, L. &Schnurr, D. P. (1996). Analysis of 15 adenovirus hexon proteins reveals the location and structure of seven hypervariable regions containing serotype-specific residues. *J Virol, 70,* 1836-44.

[287] Roberts, D. M.; Nanda, A.; Havenga, M. J.; Abbink, P.; Lynch, D. M.; Ewald, B. A.; Liu, J.; Thorner, A. R.; Swanson, P. E.; Gorgone, D. A.; Lifton, M. A.; Lemckert, A. A.; Holterman, L.; Chen, B.; Dilraj, A.; Carville, A.; Mansfield, K. G.; Goudsmit, J. &Barouch, D. H. (2006). Hexon-chimaeric adenovirus serotype 5 vectors circumvent pre-existing anti-vector immunity. *Nature, 441,* 239-43.

[288] Reddy, P. S.; Idamakanti, N.; Chen, Y.; Whale, T.; Babiuk, L. A.; Mehtali, M. &Tikoo, S. K. (1999). Replication-defective bovine adenovirus type 3 as an expression vector. *J Virol, 73,* 9137-44.

[289] van Olphen, A. L. &Mittal, S. K. (1999). Generation of infectious genome of bovine adenovirus type 3 by homologous recombination in bacteria. *J Virol Methods, 77,* 125-9.

[290] van Olphen, A. L.; Tikoo, S. K. &Mittal, S. K. (2002). Characterization of bovine adenovirus type 3 E1 proteins and isolation of E1-expressing cell lines. *Virology, 295,* 108-18.

[291] Morrison, M. D.; Reid, D.; Onions, D.; Spibey, N. &Nicolson, L. (2002). Generation of E3-deleted canine adenoviruses expressing canine parvovirus capsid by homologous recombination in bacteria. *Virology, 293,* 26-30.

[292] Kremer, E. J.; Boutin, S.; Chillon, M. &Danos, O. (2000). Canine adenovirus vectors: an alternative for adenovirus-mediated gene transfer. *J Virol, 74,* 505-12.

[293] Loser, P.; Hofmann, C.; Both, G. W.; Uckert, W. &Hillgenberg, M. (2003). Construction, rescue, and characterization of vectors derived from ovine atadenovirus. *J Virol, 77,* 11941-51.

[294] Reddy, P. S.; Idamakanti, N.; Hyun, B. H.; Tikoo, S. K. &Babiuk, L. A. (1999). Development of porcine adenovirus-3 as an expression vector. *J Gen Virol, 80 (Pt 3),* 563-70.

[295] Zakhartchouk, A.; Zhou, Y. &Tikoo, S. K. (2003). A recombinant E1-deleted porcine adenovirus-3 as an expression vector. *Virology, 313,* 377-86.

[296] Michou, A. I.; Lehrmann, H.; Saltik, M. &Cotten, M. (1999). Mutational analysis of the avian adenovirus CELO, which provides a basis for gene delivery vectors. *J Virol, 73,* 1399-410.

[297] Francois, A.; Eterradossi, N.; Delmas, B.; Payet, V. &Langlois, P. (2001). Construction of avian adenovirus CELO recombinants in cosmids. *J Virol, 75,* 5288-301.

[298] Ferreira, T. B.; Alves, P. M.; Aunins, J. G. &Carrondo, M. J. (2005). Use of adenoviral vectors as veterinary vaccines. *Gene Ther, 12 Suppl 1,* S73-83.

[299] Bangari, D. S. &Mittal, S. K. (2006). Development of nonhuman adenoviruses as vaccine vectors. *Vaccine, 24,* 849-62.

[300] Zakhartchouk, A. N.; Pyne, C.; Mutwiri, G. K.; Papp, Z.; Baca-Estrada, M. E.; Griebel, P.; Babiuk, L. A. &Tikoo, S. K. (1999). Mucosal immunization of calves with recombinant bovine adenovirus-3: induction of protective immunity to bovine herpesvirus-1. *J Gen Virol, 80 (Pt 5),* 1263-9.

[301] Fischer, L.; Tronel, J. P.; Pardo-David, C.; Tanner, P.; Colombet, G.; Minke, J. &Audonnet, J. C. (2002). Vaccination of puppies born to immune dams with a canine adenovirus-based vaccine protects against a canine distemper virus challenge. *Vaccine, 20,* 3485-97.

[302] Hammond, J. M.; McCoy, R. J.; Jansen, E. S.; Morrissy, C. J.; Hodgson, A. L. &Johnson, M. A. (2000). Vaccination with a single dose of a recombinant porcine adenovirus expressing the classical swine fever virus gp55 (E2) gene protects pigs against classical swine fever. *Vaccine, 18,* 1040-50.

[303] Francois, A.; Chevalier, C.; Delmas, B.; Eterradossi, N.; Toquin, D.; Rivallan, G. &Langlois, P. (2004). Avian adenovirus CELO recombinants expressing VP2 of

infectious bursal disease virus induce protection against bursal disease in chickens. *Vaccine, 22,* 2351-60.

[304] Fitzgerald, J. C.; Gao, G. P.; Reyes-Sandoval, A.; Pavlakis, G. N.; Xiang, Z. Q.; Wlazlo, A. P.; Giles-Davis, W.; Wilson, J. M. &Ertl, H. C. (2003). A simian replication-defective adenoviral recombinant vaccine to HIV-1 gag. *J Immunol, 170,* 1416-22.

[305] Reyes-Sandoval, A.; Fitzgerald, J. C.; Grant, R.; Roy, S.; Xiang, Z. Q.; Li, Y.; Gao, G. P.; Wilson, J. M. &Ertl, H. C. (2004). Human immunodeficiency virus type 1-specific immune responses in primates upon sequential immunization with adenoviral vaccine carriers of human and simian serotypes. *J Virol, 78,* 7392-9.

[306] Roy, S.; Zhi, Y.; Kobinger, G. P.; Figueredo, J.; Calcedo, R.; Miller, J. R.; Feldmann, H. &Wilson, J. M. (2006). Generation of an adenoviral vaccine vector based on simian adenovirus 21. *J Gen Virol, 87,* 2477-85.

[307] Cohen, C. J.; Xiang, Z. Q.; Gao, G. P.; Ertl, H. C.; Wilson, J. M. &Bergelson, J. M. (2002). Chimpanzee adenovirus CV-68 adapted as a gene delivery vector interacts with the coxsackievirus and adenovirus receptor. *J Gen Virol, 83,* 151-5.

[308] Tatsis, N.; Blejer, A.; Lasaro, M. O.; Hensley, S. E.; Cun, A.; Tesema, L.; Li, Y.; Gao, G. P.; Xiang, Z. Q.; Zhou, D.; Wilson, J. M. &Ertl, H. C. (2007). A CD46-binding Chimpanzee Adenovirus Vector as a Vaccine Carrier. *Mol Ther, 15,* 608-17.

[309] Xiang, Z.; Gao, G.; Reyes-Sandoval, A.; Cohen, C. J.; Li, Y.; Bergelson, J. M.; Wilson, J. M. &Ertl, H. C. (2002). Novel, chimpanzee serotype 68-based adenoviral vaccine carrier for induction of antibodies to a transgene product. *J Virol, 76,* 2667-75.

[310] Kobinger, G. P.; Feldmann, H.; Zhi, Y.; Schumer, G.; Gao, G.; Feldmann, F.; Jones, S. &Wilson, J. M. (2006). Chimpanzee adenovirus vaccine protects against Zaire Ebola virus. *Virology, 346,* 394-401.

[311] Pinto, A. R.; Fitzgerald, J. C.; Giles-Davis, W.; Gao, G. P.; Wilson, J. M. &Ertl, H. C. (2003). Induction of CD8+ T cells to an HIV-1 antigen through a prime boost regimen with heterologous E1-deleted adenoviral vaccine carriers. *J Immunol, 171,* 6774-9.

[312] Rodrigues, E. G.; Claassen, J.; Lee, S.; Wilson, J. M.; Nussenzweig, R. S. &Tsuji, M. (2000). Interferon-gamma-independent CD8+ T cell-mediated protective anti-malaria immunity elicited by recombinant adenovirus. *Parasite Immunol, 22,* 157-60.

[313] Wang, D.; Raja, N. U.; Trubey, C. M.; Juompan, L. Y.; Luo, M.; Woraratanadharm, J.; Deitz, S. B.; Yu, H.; Swain, B. M.; Moore, K. M.; Pratt, W. D.; Hart, M. K. &Dong, J. Y. (2006). Development of a cAdVax-based bivalent ebola virus vaccine that induces immune responses against both the Sudan and Zaire species of Ebola virus. *J Virol, 80,* 2738-46.

[314] Wang, D.; Hevey, M.; Juompan, L. Y.; Trubey, C. M.; Raja, N. U.; Deitz, S. B.; Woraratanadharm, J.; Luo, M.; Yu, H.; Swain, B. M.; Moore, K. M. &Dong, J. Y. (2006). Complex adenovirus-vectored vaccine protects guinea pigs from three strains of Marburg virus challenges. *Virology, 353,* 324-32.

[315] Jaiswal, S.; Khanna, N. &Swaminathan, S. (2003). Replication-defective adenoviral vaccine vector for the induction of immune responses to dengue virus type 2. *J Virol, 77,* 12907-13.

[316] Khanam, S.; Khanna, N. &Swaminathan, S. (2006). Induction of neutralizing antibodies and T cell responses by dengue virus type 2 envelope domain III encoded by plasmid and adenoviral vectors. *Vaccine, 24,* 6513-25.

[317] Holman, D. H.; Wang, D.; Raviprakash, K.; Raja, N. U.; Luo, M.; Zhang, J.; Porter, K. R. &Dong, J. Y. (2007). Two complex, adenovirus-based vaccines that together induce immune responses to all four dengue virus serotypes. *Clin Vaccine Immunol, 14,* 182-9.

[318] Gao, W.; Tamin, A.; Soloff, A.; D'Aiuto, L.; Nwanegbo, E.; Robbins, P. D.; Bellini, W. J.; Barratt-Boyes, S. &Gambotto, A. (2003). Effects of a SARS-associated coronavirus vaccine in monkeys. *Lancet, 362,* 1895-6.

[319] Zakhartchouk, A. N.; Viswanathan, S.; Mahony, J. B.; Gauldie, J. &Babiuk, L. A. (2005). Severe acute respiratory syndrome coronavirus nucleocapsid protein expressed by an adenovirus vector is phosphorylated and immunogenic in mice. *J Gen Virol, 86,* 211-5.

[320] Liu, R. Y.; Wu, L. Z.; Huang, B. J.; Huang, J. L.; Zhang, Y. L.; Ke, M. L.; Wang, J. M.; Tan, W. P.; Zhang, R. H.; Chen, H. K.; Zeng, Y. X. &Huang, W. (2005). Adenoviral expression of a truncated S1 subunit of SARS-CoV spike protein results in specific humoral immune responses against SARS-CoV in rats. *Virus Res, 112,* 24-31.

[321] Arribillaga, L.; de Cerio, A. L.; Sarobe, P.; Casares, N.; Gorraiz, M.; Vales, A.; Bruna-Romero, O.; Borras-Cuesta, F.; Paranhos-Baccala, G.; Prieto, J.; Ruiz, J. &Lasarte, J. J. (2002). Vaccination with an adenoviral vector encoding hepatitis C virus (HCV) NS3 protein protects against infection with HCV-recombinant vaccinia virus. *Vaccine, 21,* 202-10.

[322] Rollier, C.; Verschoor, E. J.; Paranhos-Baccala, G.; Drexhage, J. A.; Verstrepen, B. E.; Berland, J. L.; Himoudi, N.; Barnfield, C.; Liljestrom, P.; Lasarte, J. J.; Ruiz, J.; Inchauspe, G. &Heeney, J. L. (2005). Modulation of vaccine-induced immune responses to hepatitis C virus in rhesus macaques by altering priming before adenovirus boosting. *J Infect Dis, 192,* 920-9.

[323] McConnell, M. J.; Hanna, P. C. &Imperiale, M. J. (2006). Cytokine response and survival of mice immunized with an adenovirus expressing Bacillus anthracis protective antigen domain 4. *Infect Immun, 74,* 1009-15.

[324] Casimiro, D. R.; Bett, A. J.; Fu, T. M.; Davies, M. E.; Tang, A.; Wilson, K. A.; Chen, M.; Long, R.; McKelvey, T.; Chastain, M.; Gurunathan, S.; Tartaglia, J.; Emini, E. A. &Shiver, J. (2004). Heterologous human immunodeficiency virus type 1 priming-boosting immunization strategies involving replication-defective adenovirus and poxvirus vaccine vectors. *J Virol, 78,* 11434-8.

[325] Stone, D.; Ni, S.; Li, Z. Y.; Gaggar, A.; DiPaolo, N.; Feng, Q.; Sandig, V. &Lieber, A. (2005). Development and assessment of human adenovirus type 11 as a gene transfer vector. *J Virol, 79,* 5090-104.

In: Vaccinations: Types, Potential Complications… ISBN: 978-1-60692-969-8
Editors: D. B. Steen and H. L. Dyson

Chapter VIII

Clinical Dendritic Cell Based Cancer Vaccination*

Anders Elm Pedersen[4]
Laboratory of Cellular Immunology, Department of Medical Anatomy A
Telephone 45 35327270; Fax 45 35327269
Annika Berntsen and Inge Marie Svane
Department of Oncology,
Herlev University Hospital, Denmark.

Abstract

The success of dendritic cell based cancer vaccination in animal models has resulted in a rapid transformation to human cancer trials. This has become possible by the development of methods to produce large numbers of human dendritic cells (DC) as well as protocols for antigen preparation, dendritic cell maturation and administration. Since the first clinical trial was published in 1996, more than 1000 cancer patients have received dendritic cell based cancer therapy. However, large variability of the protocols employed in the trials has made it difficult to draw firm conclusions from these studies. Here, various aspects of dendritic cell manufacturing are discussed and some of the latest clinical vaccination trials are reviewed. In addition, methods to evaluate the immunological outcome of dendritic cell based therapy are described and suggestions for future strategies will be outlined.

The immune system constantly recognizes and eliminates arising tumours based on their expression of tumour antigens (TA) (1;2). Despite this fact, effective vaccination against established cancers requires an intensive activation of the immune response to break down tolerance towards a given tumour antigen. Therefore, cancer vaccination needs to result in activation of the adaptive immune response by means of activating T cells, including tumour specific cytotoxic T lymphocytes (CTLs) and CD4+ T cells. This process is facilitated by professional antigen-presenting cells (APC), in particular dendritic cells (DCs) which express high levels of T cell costimulatory molecules and

* * A version of this chapter was also published in *Cancer Vaccines: New Research*, edited by Nathan Elliot published by Nova Science Publishers, Inc. It was submitted for appropriate modifications in an effort to encourage wider dissemination of research.

[4] E-mail address: elmpedersen@mai.ku.dk

secrete relevant T cell polarizing cytokines (3). DCs can be generated *in vitro* and pulsed with tumour antigens in order to generate a tumour-specific immune response and therefore, DCs are obvious as adjuvant cells in cancer vaccination.

Tumour Antigens

In the early 1990s, Boon and his colleagues reported the successful cloning of a tumour associated antigen (TAA), melanoma antigen-1 (4;5). This antigen (Ag) belongs to the family of cancer testis antigens which are expressed in several tumours but not in normal tissue except from spermatogonia and spermatocytes in the testis. The cancer testis antigens now include TA families such as BAGE, GAGE, SSX-2 and NY-ESO-1 among others (6-9). Other categories of TA include: 1) Differentiation antigens: MART-1, tyrosinase, gp100 and gp75 (10;11), 2) over-expressed "self antigens": HER-2/neu (12), telomerase (13) and survivin(14), 3) mutated "self antigens": p53 (15), 4) viral antigens: human papilloma virus antigens E6 and E7 (16), and 5) TA with abnormalities in their carbohydrate moieties such as MUC-1 (17;18). A detailed list of TA is available at
http://www.cancerimmunity.org/peptidedatabase/Tcellepitopes.htm

Many of the mentioned TAs have already been evaluated in cancer vaccination studies for their ability to induce CTLs (19-23). Whereas most pathogen specific vaccines are designed to elicit a protective antibody response against the three-dimensional structure of the pathogen, cancer vaccines need to evoke a powerful CTL response against the tumour, and must therefore focus on presentation of appropriate peptide T-cell epitopes. Dendritic cells are uniquely efficient in inducing such CTL responses.

Dendritic Cells

DCs are potent antigen-presenting cells with a unique capacity to take up antigens, migrate into the lymphoid tissue and interact with the cellular immune system, thereby being essential for e.g. CTL activation. By providing costimulatory molecules and cytokines during the presentation of antigen to T cells, they also determine the outcome of the T cell response in terms of e.g. Th1 or Th2 responses. Once described as "nature's adjuvant" underscore the pivotal role of these cells in initiating an adaptive immune response (24).

Biology of Natural Occurring DCs

The observation of Steinman and Cohn (25) that a subset of adherent murine splenic cells were stellate with variably arranged pseudopods and that these cells were potent stimulators of the primary mixed leukocyte reaction in mice, soon led to the designation dendritic cells and the general assumption that DCs are professional antigen presenting cells (APCs)

The understanding of dendritic cells is complexed by the existence of diverse subsets. However, the general believe is that CD34+ hematopoietic stem cells differentiate into common myeloid progenitors (CMP), which in turn differentiate into CD11c+CD14- or CD11c+CD14+ immature DC which become Langerhans DC and interstitial DC, respectively. Also, the CMP give raise to DC precursors such as monocytes and plasmacytoid cells which in the presence of relevant antigens and cytokines differentiate into monocyte-derived and plasmacytoid derived DCs (3). In human peripheral blood two major populations of immature DCs have been characterized: CD11c+ myeloid DCs and CD11c- CD123+ plasmacytoid DCs which make up 0,6% and 0,4% of PBMC, respectively (26). Myeloid DCs differentiate into Langerhans cells in the skin and interstitial DCs in other tissues, where they take up antigen and present it to T cells in the draining lymph nodes. Plasmacytoid DCs are known to produce large amounts of type I IFNs after viral infection (27;28).

DCs migrate from the bone marrow to peripheral tissue where the immature DCs take up antigen by mechanisms such as 1) constitutive macropinocytosis (29), 2) receptor-mediated phagocytosis or endocytosis by receptors for the Fc portion of various immunoglobulins (30-32), heat shock proteins (33;34), by scavenger receptors such as CD36 involved in the uptake of apoptotic bodies (35), or by C-type lectins such as macrophage-mannose receptor (MMR) and DEC-205 after carbohydrate binding (29;36).

In order to mature and subsequently initiate an antigen specific adaptive immune response, the immature DC must encounter signals indicating the presence of either an "infectious non-self" antigen or tissue "danger". "Infectious non-self" antigens are pathogen-associated molecular patterns (PAMP) such as peptidoglycan, lipoteichoic acid, LPS, CpG oligonucleotides and double-stranded RNA which lead to activation via defined Toll-like receptors (reviewed in (37)). "Danger signals" are inflammatory cytokines such as IL-1β and TNF-α, IFN-α produced by virally infected cells and heat-shock proteins such as Hsp60 and Hsp70 (reviewed in (38)). In some settings, interaction with CD4+ T cells expressing CD40L is important in the final maturation of the DC including upregulation of co-stimulatory molecules. This process is known as conditioning of the DC (39).

Maturation of DCs is associated with functional and morphologic changes; including a shift from expression of MHC class II molecules with a short half-life that are primarily abundant in endocytic compartments to MHC class II with a long half-life, which due to a boost in synthesis is up-regulated at the cell surface of mature DCs (3;40;41). Other upregulated proteins are CD80 and CD86 which is needed as co-stimulation for T cell activation, (3;42;43), adhesion molecules such as CD54 and CD58 and activation markers such as CD83.

During initiation of maturation, the DC terminate antigen uptake and commence migration towards the draining lymph node (3). This migration is made possible by a closely linked downregulation of the chemokine receptor CCR6 and upregulation of CCR7 on the maturing DC. Surface expression of CCR7 is necessary for the migration from peripheral tissue into afferent lymphatic vessels as well as for homing to the T-cell areas of the draining lymph nodes (44-47).

In the lymph node, an environment is present which favours the contact between antigen presenting DCs and antigen specific T cells. When such contact is established with the formation of an immunological synapse, a T cell mediated adaptive immune response can be initiated (3). The nature of this response is influenced by DC-released cytokines such as IL-12 and IL-10, which play a central role in Th1/Th2 differentiation. When DCs mature, they often secrete IL-12 (48), in particular the biological active form of IL-12 p70 which facilitates a Th1 response and subsequent priming of CD8+ T cells (49). Secretion of this cytokine is therefore of particular interest in DCs for therapeutic use in cancer vaccination. More recently, an additional heterodimeric cytokine, designated IL-23, was discovered. It is composed of a p19 subunit and the known IL-12 p40 subunit, and has many similarities with IL-12 (50). Both IL-12 and IL-23 are predominantly produced by activated DCs, monocytes and macrophages (51).

In Vitro Generation of Human DCs

The method to generate immature monocyte-derived DCs by plastic adherence of PBMCs and subsequent culturing of the adherent monocytes with GM-CSF and IL-4 for 5-7 days, was published by Lanzavecchias group in 1994 (52). This knowledge gave the opportunity to generate large amounts of these otherwise scarce cells (less than 0,5% of leukocytes) (53). In addition to monocytes, CD34+ hematopoietic progenitor cells from the bone marrow and peripheral blood have been used to generate DCs with various cytokine mixtures (54-56). Recently isolation techniques have also made application of plasmacytoid DCs from whole blood possible (57;58).

Culturing of peripheral blood monocytes with GM-CSF and IL-4 has been the most common way to generate dendritic cells for clinical application, and several studies have tried to improve protocols of this kind of DCs for clinical scale DC generation (59-62). However, the exact relationship of these DCs to circulating CD11c+ myeloid DCs is not known. Indeed reports have stated that they are more closely related to immature DCs resident in tissues (63).

Also, studies which demonstrate that the generated immature as well as mature and antigen preloaded DC can be frozen without significant loss of phenotype and function (64;65), have simplified the manufacturing process of DC based vaccines.

The TA of interest can be pulsed on dendritic cells in a number of ways, either as a whole protein, as DNA or RNA coding for the protein or as MHC binding peptides identified to be T-cell epitopes. However, it is important to deliver the TA in a way that facilitates correct processing and presentation of T-cell epitopes which is best obtained after maturation of dendritic cells.

Maturation of Therapeutic Dendritic Cells

Generation of mature DCs that retain capacity to secrete cytokines is important in DC based cancer vaccination(66). For clinical purposes, the *in vitro* maturation of DCs prior to injection is restricted by the requirement for reagents approved for clinical use. One commonly used maturation cocktail is TNF-α+IL-1β+IL-6+PGE_2 (67) but also polyriboinosinic polyribocytidylic acid (Poly I:C)+TNF-α (68) have been used.

IL-12 p70 secretion is generally accepted to be important for Th1 differentiation. However, in contrast to p40 production, only a narrow panel of maturation-inducing agents are able to induce IL-12 p70 production (68). On the other hand, targeting of this cytokine in generation of therapeutic DCs might suffer from the phenomenon of DC exhaustion. Strong DC maturation stimuli, such as LPS induce high but transient levels of IL-12 p70 followed by a refractory state to further stimulation (69). Also maturation with Poly I:C+TNF-α can lead to an increase in DC apoptosis (unpublished observations). Thus, "overmaturated" therapeutic DCs with high IL-12 p70 secretion might have lost their Th1 promoting cytokine secretion, once they arrive to the draining lymph node.

CCR7 expression is of pivotal importance when DCs are injected i.d. In particular, significant expression is induced by TNF-α+IL-1β+IL-6+PGE_2, and reflects that PGE_2 is a major inducer of this receptor (70). However, there is evidence that also the endothelial cells of the lymphatic vessels at the injection sight should be activated, as they only secrete CCL21, the ligand for CCR7, in response to inflammatory stimuli (71-73). This might explain why, studies in humans have indicated that only a very small proportion of i.d. injected DCs reach the draining lymph node (74). To, induce such activation of endothelial cells, treatment of the skin with adjuvant at the site of injection is a favourable step in DC based cancer vaccination (75). However, DC/T cell interaction might also occur at the injection site, as a recent study indicated that naïve and central memory T cells can be attracted to the DCs at the injection site and be activated there (76).

Maturation of Therapeutic DC and Clinical Response

In recent years, there has been an increasing concern about the tolerogenic potential of DCs in cancer vaccines. Thus, both mature plasmacytoid and monocyte-derived DCs have been reported to induce loss of cytotoxic activity in antigen specific CTLs (77;78). In particular, much concern has been given to the fact that immature DC induce IL-10 producing CD8+ regulatory T cells and suppress CTL function (79;80). These possibilities might indeed turn the potential therapeutic effect of DCs into a side-effect in terms of reinforcement of tumour tolerance and exacerbation of disease.

Only a few human cancer vaccine studies have been made, that directly compare immature and mature DCs. However, these studies clearly demonstrate that *in vitro* DC maturation is optimal for induction of a potent T cell response, also in immunotherapeutic settings (81-83), although immature DCs are also capable of inducing peptide specific CD8+ T cells (83). TNF-α is used alone or in combination with e.g. IL-1β+IL-6+PGE_2 in most clinical protocols for DC maturation, and in an evaluation of correlation between DC maturation and clinical response, it was observed that clinical response was correlated to the addition of TNF-α in any form ($p<0{,}001$) (84). Hopefully, a new maturation cocktail including TNF-α, Poly I:C, IFN-α, IL-1β and IFN-γ (85) which lead to both potent IL-12 p70 secretion and CCR7 upregulation, will also lead to improved clinical results.

Route of Delivery

The route of vaccine delivery is an important issue in DC based vaccination both regarding the point of contact with reactive T cells and the kinetics of MHC-peptide complexes (86;87). Many routes have been utilized: murine studies indicate that subcutaneous injections are superior to intravenous injection (88) which is supported by a human study of melanoma patients (89).

Subcutaneous injection have been shown to lead to rapidly migration of the DC to draining lymph nodes in chimpanzees (90), whereas migration studies in humans, indicate that only intradermal injections lead to an effective migration (91;92). Finally, intranodal injections is a time consuming technique, but does lead to effective immunization in some studies and at the same time overcomes the problem with relevant CCR7 induction of the injected DCs (93). However, data from a recent study indicated that intranodal injection induced less immune responses and clinical responses compared to intradermal injection (94).

Safety and Toxicity of DC Based Cancer Vaccination

DC based vaccination against tumour antigens that are also self-antigens can be predicted to cause autoimmunity. In accordance, it has been shown in an experimental model, that DC vaccination against glycoprotein of lymphocytic choriomeningitis virus (LCMV-GP) which induces an anti-tumour response to LCMV-GP transfected fibrosarcoma cells also induces diabetes in rat insulin promoter-GP mice (95).

In humans, however, no serious autoimmune-related events have been reported in the majority of now more than 1000 patients treated with DC based cancer vaccination in more than 100 clinical trials (55;56;81;83;96;97) (reviewed in (98-102)). Autoimmunity has been observed in malignant melanoma patients, evidenced by the hair depigmentation and vitiligo observed in melanoma patients vaccinated with DCs fused with tumour cells (103) or pulsed with melanoma tumour lysate, and this probably reflects a simultaneous anti-tumour and autoimmune response. Development of autoantibodies after DC vaccination have also been described, among others antinuclear antibodies and antithyroid antibodies but without clinical significance. In contrast, IgE antibodies to bovine serum albumin from the DC preparation have been reported to cause anaphylaxis after DC vaccination (104).

It should be mentioned that many of the initial vaccines used immature or semimature rather than mature DCs, which theoretically could reverse an immune response into a non-favourable tolerogenic response as discussed below. However, such protocols might not have induced tolerance, simply because the *in vitro* generation and manipulation of the DCs induce some degree of maturation (S Amigorena, personal communication) or the immature DCs are pulsed with MHC class II binding epitopes, that induce conditioning of the DC *in vivo* (19).

A large number of cancer vaccination studies have implicated the administration of IL-2. This is a consequence of early studies based on IL-2 administration alone, which indicated that this immunological manipulation could cause the regression of established, invasive human cancers. High-dose IL-2 can have severe acute treatment-associated toxicities, and 2-4 % of the patients have been reported to die of treatment-related adverse events in different studies (105;106). Therefore, numerous low-dose IL-2 schedules have been tested (reviewed in (107)) and it is generally found, that subcutaneous administration of lower doses primarily cause local inflammation and flue-like symptoms. However, in a recent study, that included 93 melanoma patients, autoimmune toxicities affecting several organ systems were observed in patients treated with an anti-melanoma vaccine combined with low-dose IL-2. None of these toxicities caused major long-term effects, though they contributed to treatment-related morbidity and one case was life-threatening (108). This side-effect and the possibility that IL-2 might induce CD4+CD25+ T regulatory cells (109) suggest that other γ_c-signaling cytokines such as IL-15 should be examined as an alternative choise.

Dendritic Cell Based Vaccination in Specific Malignancies

Cancer vaccines using dendritic cells is a new therapeutic approach, which has been tested in a variety of different cancers since the first study in cancer patients was published in 1996 (110). A large number of early clinical trials have been published since then: an overview can be found in Table I and selected studies are detailed below to depict major differences and the consequences central for the ongoing development of DC based cancer therapy.

Tabel 1: DC based cancer vaccination, published clinical trials

Malignancy	No of studies	No of patients	Clinical response
Malignt melanoma	27	422	18CR,30PR,4MR,36SD
Renal cell carcinoma	13	170	3CR,6PR,2MR,57SD
Mammacancer	6	49	5PR,1SD
Prostatacancer	9	291	3CR,19PR,6SD
Non small cell lung cancer and Gastrointestinal cancer	14	193	2CR, 2PR, 4MR, 18SD
Hematologic malignancies	7	60	11CR,2PR
Head and neck cancer	1	16	2PR
Urogenital cancer	4	28	1CR,2PR, 3SD
Braincancer	6	59	7PR,1MR,4SD

Malignant Melanoma

Malignant melanoma is the malignancy where the largest numbers of DC-based cancer vaccination studies have been conducted – mainly due to the sensitivity of melanoma cells to immunomodulation in general, and a lack of an effective standard treatment regime. One early study of Nestle and co-workers provided hope for a role for DC based vaccination against this disease (111). In this study, 16 patients were vaccinated with peptide or lysate pulsed DCs and 2 complete responses and 3 partial responses were observed. A more recent phase I/II melanoma study from 2003 (112) included 19 patients and utilized DCs pulsed with autologous melanoma cells. Clinical response was achieved in 6 out of 12 patients that completed the treatment with 3 patients obtaining durable complete response for 33+ to 55+ months. The best clinical effect was observed in patients with low tumour burden. In a newly published study, a DC hybride vaccine was used (113). Fusion cells were made by electrofusion of autologous tumour cells and allogeneic DCs. 20 patients with disseminated malignant melanoma were included. The major part of these patients developed an immune response against various tumour antigens and 8/17 evaluable patients had a clinical response: 1 patient had CR with regression of subcutaneous metastasis and was in CR after 58 months. 1 patient had a mixed response, while 6 patients had SD.

In melanoma patients, a larger phase III study with randomization between dacarbazine and peptide pulsed DCs was stopped prematurely last year, because an interim analysis of 108 patients did not show any significant difference in response and survival (114). However, additional explorative analyses did show an effect in the HLA-A2 positive subgroup of patients.

Breast Cancer

In breast cancer, only a few therapeutic DC vaccination studies have been published. In one study, autologous monocyte derived DCs were generated with addition of GM-CSF and IL-4, maturated with TNF-α and pulsed with HER-2/neu or MUC-1 derived peptides (115). 10 patients were vaccinated with 2-17 million DCs s.c. every 2 weeks. The vaccine elicited peptide specific CTL responses in 5 of these patients (which included both breast cancer and ovarian cancer patients) and led to epitope spreading *in vivo* in a few patients. DCs pulsed with an HER-2/neu derived peptide led to stable disease for 6 month in 1 out of 6 breast cancer patients (116). In a case report, a single woman received autologous tumour lysate-pulsed dendritic cells (DCs) leading to regression of her lymph-node metastasis (117). Other studies include DC vaccination against mucin using transfection of MUC1 cDNA (118), and fusion of DCs and tumor cells (119).

Autologous DCs pulsed with 6 different wild-type and P2 anchor modified peptides from the tumour antigen p53 have also been evaluated for treatment of HLA-A2 positive patients with progressive breast cancer. Results from the phase I/II study indicated that the treatment had no serious side effects (19) and approximately 1/3 of the 25 treated patients had clinical response, primarily as disease stabilization (up to 15 month), whereas a few had minor regressions of the tumour lesions (120).

Renal Cell Carcinoma

Renal cell carcinoma is also a tumour type known to be sensitive to immunotherapy (121). The first DC study in this group of patients was published in 1999. Since then, 13 clinical studies with metastatic renal carcinoma patients have been published and a total of 170 patients have been treated. In the largest study, 35 patients were enrolled and treated with autologous DC pulsed with autologous tumour lysate (122). 10/27 evaluable patients had a clinical response with 2 CR, 1 PR and 7 SD. Immune response to a control Ag were measured in 11 patients.

Non-small Cell Lung Cancer and Colon Cancer

Pilot studies in patients with non-small cell lung cancer have shown that CEA specific CTLs can be induced by autologous tumour RNA transfected DC, but no clinical benefit was obtained (123). A similar approach was also used for colorectal cancer patients (124). In comparison, 12 patients with advanced colon cancer or non-small cell lung carcinoma were treated with autologous DC pulsed with a CEA derived peptide or a carrierprotein (keyhole limpet hemocyanin) in a phase I study (125). 5 patients had clinical response, among these 2 CR. CEA specific CTLs were detected in 7/12 patients and correlated to clinical response.

Lymphomas

The largest study in lymphoma patients included thirty-five patients with B-cell lymphoma who were treated with autologous idiotype pulsed DC. Out of the first 10 patients treated 4 had clinical response; 2 CR, 1 PR and 1 with molecular response. Twenty-five additional patients with advanced-stage lymphoma were vaccinated after first chemotherapy, here tumour regression was observed in 4 of 18 patients with measurable disease. Induction of T cell response against the idiotype Ag were detectable in 24/33 patients (57). In a small study on cutaneous T-cell lymphomas 10 patients were treated with autologous tumour lysate and KLH pulsed DC; 1 CR and 4 PR were seen. The clinical response was associated with low tumour burden (126).

Prostatacancer

One of the first phase III studies with DC cancer vaccination was published recently (127) : a double blinded, placebo controlled study with a total number of 127 patients with progressive metastatic prostate cancer. 82 patients were randomized to treatment with autologous DC pulsed with the prostate specific Ag, prostatic acid phosphatase (PAP), while 45 patients were randomized to the control arm. In the intention to treat population there was no significant difference in time to progression between the two groups (p=0,061). However, a subgroup analysis showed, that patients with a Gleason score <7 had a significant longer time to progression (p=0,001) and increased survival (p=0,047) compared to the control arm. There was also a significant higher T cell response against the used Ag in the treated group.

Conclusions from Clinical Trials

DC based cancer vaccination is still experimental and is not a treatment option to be recommended until standard treatments such as surgery, chemotherapy and radiotherapy has been tried. Very few DC based cancer vaccinations have gone into phase III studies which makes statistic evaluation difficult. The patient populations in the clinical trials often consist of individuals with extensive metastatic disease and it is therefore an important note that relevant immune responses can be elicited even in this group of patients. This provides hope for better clinical responses in patients with less tumor burden. Some of the best results have been obtained in cancers that are known to be sensitive to immunotherapy, such as lymphoma, malignant melanoma and renal cell carcinoma. In other carcinomas, such as breast cancer only very few complete responses have been observed. A possible explanation might be the insufficient maturity of the DCs used for vaccination as well as a low expression of IL-12 p70 (128). It will therefore be of interest to await new trials that take advantage of more potent DC maturation cocktails (85). Also, new techniques for antigen pulsing, in particular transfection of DCs with tumor derived mRNA (94) need to be compared with commonly applied techniques such as peptide or tumor lysate pulsing.

Monitoring of CTL Reactivity

The establishment of reliable and quantitative assays for monitoring of vaccine specific CTLs is of crucial importance for optimizing vaccine regiments, including DC based vaccines in clinical cancer trials. A large variety of immunoassays have been used for this purpose (reviewed in (129)) comprizing structure-based assays and function based assays. Of the structure based assays peptide-MHC tetramer or dimers is most often applied but real-time PCR analysis of the hypervariable complementary-determining region 3 (CDR3) of the T-cell receptor (TCR) can also be applied if the TCR is known. The function based assays include real-time PCR analysis of antigen specific CTL cytokine secretion, intracellular cytokine or cytokine capture determined by flow cytometry and the most frequently employed ELISPOT assays. In this last assay, peptide Ag-specific T cells are detected on the basis of proximal cytokine production which is identified as visible spots on filter-bottom micro-wells. The antigen-specific T cell frequency is then calculated as the number of spots per cells initially added to the well. Because of less labour requirements compared to other assays, and a high sensitivity (1:10.000 to 1:50.000) this assay is generally applicable and is widely used in cancer vaccine studies for measuring peptide specific IFN-γ production (19). However, despite the high sensitivity of the ELISPOT assay a short *in vitro* peptide stimulation of the T cells prior to analysis is often required (130;131).

In several reports, no clear correlation between CTL responses and clinical outcome is found. CTL responses are sometimes detected in PBMC in the absence of clinical response (132-134), while evaluation of PBMC might in other cases underestimate immunogenecity (132;135;136). Indeed, response analyses of T cells at the tumour lesion, such as tumour infiltrating lymphocytes (TIL) obtained from fine needle aspirates or biopsies, may reveal data that are in better correspondence with clinical outcome. However, such biopsies are often not available, and even if biopsies are available, methodological problems have until now limited the use of this T cell source for continued close monitoring. Techniques have recently been developed to amplify RNA from sequential fine needle aspirates during a vaccination trial. With such methods, a description of the immunological scenario at the tumour lesion is a potential possibility (137-141), although this technique is primarily applicable for melanoma patients so far.

Future Strategies

It is also clear from data accumulating from phase I, II and III studies that DC based vaccination will not be able to stand alone in patients with progressive metastatic disease, even when delivery route, maturation etc. has been optimized as described above. It is therefore important to focus on relevant combinations with other treatment strategies and such studies are beginning to emerge.

Radiotherapy and chemotherapy that are routinely used in various cancer diseases are relevant options for such combination strategies. Indeed, cyklophosphamide has been demonstrated to facilitate adoptive immunotherapy of tumours (142). Rosenberg et al have demonstrated a 50% response rate including 4 complete responders in malignant melanoma patients treated with tumor-reactive lymphocyte cultures after lymphodepleting chemotherapy. Treatment with low dose cyklophosphamide has been shown to down-regulate Treg cells and a recent study of RCC patients indicated that administration of cyclophosphamide prior to DC based vaccination can augment DC-induced antitumor response (143).

The cell damage elicited by irradiation can potentially lead to the release of tumour antigens and at the same time initiate pro-inflammatory reactions that are necessary for DC migration, antigen uptake and DC differentiation/maturation (144). In line with this, animal studies have shown a beneficial effect of combining local radiotherapy with intratumoral injection of DCs (145).

Controlled immunomodulation might also be a relevant target for combination therapy. In particular, blockade of CTL-associated antigen (CTLA-4), which is generally believed to function as a negative regulator of T cell activation (146) in both CD4+ and CD8+ T cells have been promising in murine studies, and are now available for clinical use by the generation of a fully human antibody to human CTLA-4 (MDX-010). In studies with MDX-010 alone, 2 CR and one PR out of 14 patients was observed (147). Unfortunately response was accompanied by a large number of grade III/IV autoimmune manifestations, including dermatitis, enterocolitis, hepatitis and hypophysitis (147;148). Similarly, depletion of regulatory T cells such as CD4+,CD25+ T_{reg} (149) is a potent target, and it has already been shown that depletion of these cells with the fusion protein ONTAK (IL2-toxin) prior to vaccination with RNA-transfected DC elicit an increased cytotoxic immune response (150).

Finally, blockade of neo-angiogenesis might in addition to tumour growth inhibition also regulate the immune system in a beneficial direction. VEGF has a central role in the induction of angiogenesis and is highly specific for endothelial cells (151). It has a plethora of functions which include mitosis of vascular endothelial cells (152), secretion of enzymes involved in degradation of the extracellular matrix (153;154), inhibition of endothelial cell apoptosis (155), mobilization of endothelial cell precursors and endothelial cells to sites of angiogenesis (156;157) but also inhibition of DC differentiation (158) and induction of monocyte migration (159).

> To date, over 25 angiogenesis inhibitors are under study in clinical cancer trials and include monoclonal antibodies that block VEGF/VEGFR and tyrosine kinase inhibitors that block the VEGFR signalling system. It would therefore be highly relevant to test if combinations with such inhibitors could increase the effect of DC based cancer vaccination, as it has already been shown in murine models (160).

References

[1] Thomas L. Discussion of cellular and humoral aspects of the hypersensitive states. New York: Hoeber-Harper, 1959.

[2] Burnet FM. The concept of immunological surveillance. *Prog Exp Tumor Res* 1970; 13:1-27.

[3] Muriel M. Dendritic cells. In: Paul WE, editor. Fundamental Immunology. Philadelphia: Lippincott Williams & Wilkins, 2003: 455-480.

[4] van der Bruggen P, Traversari C, Chomez P, Lurquin C, De Plaen E, Van den Eynde B et al. A gene encoding an antigen recognized by cytolytic T lymphocytes on a human melanoma. *Science* 1991; 254(5038):1643-1647.

[5] Traversari C, van der Bruggen P, Van den Eynde B, Hainaut P, Lemoine C, Ohta N et al. Transfection and expression of a gene coding for a human melanoma antigen recognized by autologous cytolytic T lymphocytes. *Immunogenetics* 1992; 35(3): 145-152.

[6] Boel P, Wildmann C, Sensi ML, Brasseur R, Renauld JC, Coulie P et al. BAGE: a new gene encoding an antigen recognized on human melanomas by cytolytic T lymphocytes. *Immunity* 1995; 2(2):167-175.

[7] Chen YT, Scanlan MJ, Sahin U, Tureci O, Gure AO, Tsang S et al. A testicular antigen aberrantly expressed in human cancers detected by autologous antibody screening. *Proc Natl Acad Sci USA* 1997; 94(5):1914-1918.

[8] Sahin U, Tureci O, Schmitt H, Cochlovius B, Johannes T, Schmits R et al. Human neoplasms elicit multiple specific immune responses in the autologous host. *Proc Natl Acad Sci USA* 1995; 92(25):11810-11813.

[9] Van den Eynde B, Peeters O, De Backer O, Gaugler B, Lucas S, Boon T. A new family of genes encoding for an antigen recognized by autologous cytolytic T lymphocytes on a human melanoma. *J Exp Med* 1995; 182(3):689-698.

[10] Griffioen M, Borghi M, Schrier PI, Osanto S. Detection and quantification of CD8+ T cells specific for HLA-A*0201-binding melanoma and viral peptides by the IFNgamma-ELISPOT assay. *Int J Cancer* 2001; 93(4):549-555.

[11] Scheibenbogen C, Lee KH, Stevanovic S, Witzens M, Willhauck M, Waldmann V et al. Analysis of the T cell response to tumor and viral peptide antigens by an IFNgamma Elispot assay. *Int J Cancer* 1997; 71(6):932-936.

[12] King CR, Kraus MH, Aaronson SA. Amplification of a novel c-erB-related gene in human mammary carcinoma. *Science* 1985; 229(4717):974-976.

[13] Vonderheide RH, Hahn WC, Schultze JL, Nadler LM. The telomerase catalytic subunit is a widely expressed tumor-associated antigen recognized by cytotoxic T lymphocytes. *Immunity* 1999; 10(6):673-679.

[14] Andersen MH, Pedersen LO, Becker JC, Straten PT. Identification of a cytotoxic T lymphocyte response to the apoptosis inhibitor protein survivin in cancer patients. *Cancer Res* 2001; 61(3):869-872.

[15] Yanuck M, Carbone DP, Pendleton CD, Tsukui T, Winter SF, Minna JD et al. A mutant p53 tumor suppressor protein is a target for peptide induced CD8+ cytotoxic T cells. *Cancer Res* 1993; 53(14):3257-3261.

[16] Bontkes HJ, de Gruijl TD, van den Muysenberg AJ, Verheijen RH, Stukart MJ, Meijer CJ et al. Human papillomavirus type 16 E6/E7-specific cytotoxic T lymphocytes in women with cervical neoplasia. *Int J Cancer* 2000; 88(1):92-98.

[17] Barnd DL, Lan MS, Metzgar RS, Finn OJ. Specific major histocompatibility complex-unrestricted recognition of tumor-associated mucins by human cytotoxic T-cells. *Proc Natl Acad Sci USA* 1989; 86(18):7159-7163.

[18] Brossart P, Heinrich KS, Stuhler G, Behnke L, Reichardt VL, Stevanovic S et al. Identification of HLA-2-restricted T-cell epitopes derived from the MUC1 tumor antigen for broadly applicable vaccine therapies. *Blood* 1999; 93(12):4309-4317.

[19] Svane IM, Pedersen AE, Johnsen HE, Nielsen D, Kamby C, Gaarsdal E et al. Vaccination with p53-peptide-pulsed dendritic cells, of patients with advanced breast cancer: report from a phase I study. Cancer Immunol *Immunother* 2004; 53(7):633-641.

[20] Slingluff CL, Jr., Yamshchikov G, Neese P, Galavotti H, Eastham S, Engelhard VH et al. Phase I trial of a melanoma vaccine with gp100(280-288) peptide and tetanus helper peptide in adjuvant: immunologic and clinical outcomes. *Clin Cancer Res* 2001; 7(10):3012-3024.

[21] Sato Y, Maeda Y, Shomura H, Sasatomi T, Takahashi M, Une Y et al. A phase I trial of cytotoxic T-lymphocyte precursor-oriented peptide vaccines for colorectal carcinoma patients. *Br J Cancer* 2004; 90(7):1334-1342.

[22] Noguchi M, Itoh K, Suekane S, Yao A, Suetsugu N, Katagiri K et al. Phase I trial of patient-oriented vaccination in HLA-A2-positive patients with metastatic hormone-refractory prostate cancer. *Cancer Sci* 2004; 95(1):77-84.

[23] Andersen MH, Keikavoussi P, Brocker EB, Schuler-Thurner B, Jonassen M, Sondergaard I et al. Induction of systemic CTL responses in melanoma patients by dendritic cell vaccination: cessation of CTL responses is associated with disease progression. *Int J Cancer* 2001; 94(6):820-824.

[24] Banchereau J, Steinman RM. Dendritic cells and the control of immunity. *Nature* 1998; 392(6673):245-252.

[25] Steinman RM, Cohn ZA. Identification of a novel cell type in peripheral lymphoid organs of mice. I. Morphology, quantification, tissue distribution. *J Exp Med* 1973; 137(5):1142-1162.

[26] Pacanowski J, Kahi S, Baillet M, Lebon P, Deveau C, Goujard C et al. Reduced blood CD123+ (lymphoid) and CD11c+ (myeloid) dendritic cell numbers in primary HIV-1 infection. *Blood* 2001; 98(10):3016-3021.

[27] Siegal FPea. The nature of the principal type 1 interferon-producing cells in human blood. *Science* 1999; 284:1835-1837.

[28] Cella Mea. Plasmacytoid monocytes migrate to inflamed lymph nodes and produce high levels of type I IFN. *Nature Med* 1999; 5:919-923.

[29] Sallusto F, Cella M, Danieli C, Lanzavecchia A. Dendritic cells use macropinocytosis and the mannose receptor to concentrate macromolecules in the major histocompatibility complex class II compartment: downregulation by cytokines and bacterial products. *J Exp Med 1995*; 182(2):389-400.

[30] Fanger NA, Wardwell K, Shen L, Tedder TF, Guyre PM. Type I (CD64) and type II (CD32) Fc gamma receptor-mediated phagocytosis by human blood dendritic cells. *J Immunol* 1996; 157(2):541-548.

[31] Geissmann F, Launay P, Pasquier B, Lepelletier Y, Leborgne M, Lehuen A et al. A subset of human dendritic cells expresses IgA Fc receptor (CD89), which mediates internalization and activation upon cross-linking by IgA complexes. *J Immunol* 2001; 166(1):346-352.

[32] Jurgens M, Wollenberg A, Hanau D, de la SH, Bieber T. Activation of human epidermal Langerhans cells by engagement of the high affinity receptor for IgE, Fc epsilon RI. *J Immunol* 1995; 155(11):5184-5189.

[33] Castellino F, Boucher PE, Eichelberg K, Mayhew M, Rothman JE, Houghton AN et al. Receptor-mediated uptake of antigen/heat shock protein complexes results in major histocompatibility complex class I antigen presentation via two distinct processing pathways. *J Exp Med* 2000; 191(11):1957-1964.

[34] Arnold-Schild D, Hanau D, Spehner D, Schmid C, Rammensee HG, de la SH et al. Cutting edge: receptor-mediated endocytosis of heat shock proteins by professional antigen-presenting cells. *J Immunol* 1999; 162(7):3757-3760.

[35] Platt N, da Silva RP, Gordon S. Recognizing death: the phagocytosis of apoptotic cells. *Trends Cell Biol* 1998; 8(9):365-372.

[36] Jiang W, Swiggard WJ, Heufler C, Peng M, Mirza A, Steinman RM et al. The receptor DEC-205 expressed by dendritic cells and thymic epithelial cells is involved in antigen processing. *Nature* 1995; 375(6527):151-155.

[37] Medzhitov R. Toll-like receptors and innate immunity. *Nat Rev Immunol* 2001; 1: 135-145.

[38] Galluci S, Matzinger P. Danger signals: SOS to the immune system. *Curr Opinion Immunol* 2001; 13(1):114-119.

[39] Ridge JP, DiRosa F, Matzinger P. A conditioned dendritic cell can be a temporal bridge between a CD4+ T helper and a T-killer cell. *Nature* 1998; 393(6684):474-478.

[40] Pierre P, Mellman I. Developmental regulation of invariant chain proteolysis controls MHC class II trafficking in mouse dendritic cells. *Cell* 1998; 93(7):1135-1145.

[41] Cella M, Engering A, Pinet V, Pieters J, Lanzavecchia A. Inflammatory stimuli induce accumulation of MHC class II complexes on dendritic cells. *Nature* 1997; 388(6644):782-787.

[42] Inaba K, Witmer-Pack M, Inaba M, Hathcock KS, Sakuta H, Azuma M et al. The tissue distribution of the B7-2 costimulator in mice: abundant expression on dendritic cells in situ and during maturation in vitro. *J Exp Med* 1994; 180(5):1849-1860.

[43] Larsen CP, Ritchie SC, Pearson TC, Linsley PS, Lowry RP. Functional expression of the costimulatory molecule, B7/BB1, on murine dendritic cell populations. *J Exp Med* 1992; 176(4):1215-1220.

[44] Gunn MD, Kyuwa S, Tam C, Kakiuchi T, Matsuzawa A, Williams LT et al. Mice lacking expression of secondary lymphoid organ chemokine have defects in lymphocyte homing and dendritic cell localization. *J Exp Med* 1999; 189(3):451-460.

[45] Dieu M-C, Vanbervliet B, Vicari A, Bridon JM, Oldham E, Ait-Yahia S et al. Selective recruitment of immature and mature dendritic cells by distinct chemokines expressed in different anatomic sites. *J Exp Med* 1998; 188(2):373-386.

[46] Förster R, Schubel A, Breitfeld D, Kremmer E, Renner-Müller I, Wolf E et al. CCR7 coordinates the primary immune response by establishing functional microenvironments in secondary lymphoid organs. *Cell* 1999; 99(1):23-33.

[47] Sozzani S, Allavena P, D'Amico G, Luini W, Bianchi G, Kataura M et al. Differential regulation of chemokine receptors during dendritic cell maturation: a model for their trafficking properties. *J Immunol* 1998; 161(3):1083-1086.

[48] Trinchieri G. Interleukin-12. a cytokine produced by antigen-presenting cells with immunoregulatory functions in the generation of T-helper cells type 1 and cytotoxic lymphocytes. *Blood* 1994; 84(12):4008-4027.

[49] Bennett SR, Carbone FR, Karamelis F, Miller JF, Heath WR. Induction of a CD8+ cytotoxic T lymphocyte response by cross-priming requires cognate CD4+ T cell help. *J Exp Med 1997*; 186(1):65-70.

[50] Oppmann B, Lesley R, Blom B, Timans JC, Xu Y, Hunte B et al. Novel p19 protein engages IL-12 p40 to form a cytokine, IL-23, with biological activities similar as well as distinct from IL-12. *Immunity* 2000; 13(5):715-725.

[51] Langrish CL, McKenzie BS, Wilson NJ, Malefyt RW, Kastelein RA, Cua DJ. IL-12 and IL-23: master regulators of innate and adaptive immunity. *Immunol Rev* 2004; 202:96-105.

[52] Sallusto F, Lanzavecchia A. Efficient presentation of soluble antigen by cultured human dendritic cells is maintained by granulocyte/macrophage colony-stimulating factor plus interleukin 4 and downregulated by tumor necrosis factor alpha. *J Exp Med* 1994; 179(4):1109-1118.

[53] Bender A, Sapp M, Schuler G, Steinman RM. Improved methods for the generation of dendritic cells from nonproliferating progenitors in human blood. *J Immunol Methods* 1996; 196(2):121-125.

[54] Bernhard H, Disis ML, Heimfeld S, Hand S, Gralow JR, Cheever MA. Generation of immunostimulatory dendritic cells from human CD34+ hematopoietic progenitor cells of the bone marrow and peripheral blood. *Cancer Res* 1995; 55(5):1099-1104.

[55] Mackensen A, Herbst B, Chen JL, Kohler G, Noppen C, Herr W et al. Phase I study in melanoma patients of a vaccine with peptide-pulsed dendritic cells generated in vitro from CD34(+) hematopoietic progenitor cells. *Int J Cancer* 2000; 86(3):385-392.

[56] Banchereau J, Palucka AK, Dhodapkar M, Burkeholder S, Taquet N, Rolland A et al. Immune and clinical responses in patients with metastatic melanoma to CD34(+) progenitor-derived dendritic cell vaccine. *Cancer Res* 2001; 61(17):6451-6458.

[57] Timmerman JM, Czerwinski DK, Davis TA, Hsu FJ, Benike C, Hao ZM et al. Idiotype-pulsed dendritic cell vaccination for B-cell lymphoma: clinical and immune responses in 35 patients. *Blood* 2002; 99(5):1517-1526.

[58] Fong L, Hou Y, Rivas A, Benike C, Yuen A, Fisher GA et al. Altered peptide ligand vaccination with Flt3 ligand expanded dendritic cells for tumor immunotherapy. *Proc Natl Acad Sci U S A* 2001; 98(15):8809-8814.

[59] Guyre CA, Fisher JL, Waugh MG, Wallace PK, Tretter CG, Ernstoff MS et al. Advantages of hydrophobic culture bags over flasks for the generation of monocyte-derived dendritic cells for clinical applications. *J Immunol Methods* 2002; 262(1-2): 85-94.

[60] Morse MA, Vredenburgh JJ, Lyerly HK. A comparative study of the generation of dendritic cells from mobilized peripheral blood progenitor cells of patients undergoing high-dose chemotherapy. *J Hematother Stem Cell Res* 1999; 8(6):577-584.

[61] de Vries IJ, Eggert AA, Scharenborg NM, Vissers JL, Lesterhuis WJ, Boerman OC et al. Phenotypical and functional characterization of clinical grade dendritic cells. *J Immunother* 2002; 25(5):429-438.

[62] Thurner B, Roder C, Dieckmann D, Heuer M, Kruse M, Glaser A et al. Generation of large numbers of fully mature and stable dendritic cells from leukapheresis products for clinical application. *J Immunol Methods* 1999; 223(1):1-15.

[63] Grassi F, Dezutter-Dambuyant C, McIlroy D, Jacquet C, Yoneda K, Imamura S et al. Monocyte-derived dendritic cels have a phenotypic comparable to that of dermal dendritic cells and display ultrastructural granules distinct from Birbeck granules. *J Leukoc Biol* 1998; 64(4):484-493.

[64] Feuerstein B, Berger TG, Maczek C, Roder C, Schreiner D, Hirsch U et al. A method for the production of cryopreserved aliquots of antigen-preloaded, mature dendritic cells ready for clinical use. *J Immunol Methods* 2000; 245(1-2):15-29.

[65] Lewalle P, Rouas R, Lehmann F, Martiat P. Freezing of dendritic cells, generated from cryopreserved leukaphereses, does not influence their ability to induce antigen-specific immune responses or functionally react to maturation stimuli. *J Immunol Methods* 2000; 240(1-2):69-78.

[66] Spisek R, Bougras G, Ebstein F, Masse D, Barbieux I, Meflah K et al. Transient exposure of dendritic cells to maturation stimuli is sufficient to induce complete phenotypic maturation while preserving dendritic cell capacity to respond to subsequent restimulation. *Cancer Immunol Immunother* 2003; 52(7):445-454.

[67] Jonuleit H, Kuhn U, Muller G, Steinbrink K, Paragnik L, Scmitt E et al. Pro-inflammatory cytokines and prostaglandins induce maturation of potent immunostimulatory dendritic cells under fetal calf serum-free conditions. *Eur J Immunol* 1997; 27(12):3135-3137.

[68] Spisek R, Bretaudeau I, Barbieux I, Meflah K, Gregoire M. Standardized generation of fully mature p70 IL-12 secreting monocyte-derived dendritic cells for clinical use. *Cancer Immunol Immunother* 2001; 50(8):417-427.

[69] Langenkamp A, Messi M, Lanzavecchia A, Sallusto F. Kinetics of dendritic cell activation: impact on priming of Th1, Th2 and nonpolarized T cells. *Nat Immunol* 2000; 1(4):311-316.

[70] Scandella E, Men Y, Gillessen S, Förster R, Groettrup M. Prostaglandin E2 is a key factor for CCR7 surface expression and migration of monocyte-derived dendritic cells. *Blood* 2002; 100(4):1354-1361.

[71] Caux C, Vanbervliet B, Massacrier C, Ait-Yahia S, Vaure C, Chemin K et al. Regulation of dendritic cell recruitment by chemokines. *Tranplantation* 2002; 73((1 supplement)):7-11.

[72] Gunn MD, Tangemann K, Tam C, Cyster JG, Rosen SD, Williams LT. A chemokine expressed in lymphoid high endothelial venules promotes the adhesion and chemotaxis of naive T lymphocytes. *Proc Natl Acad Sci U S A* 1998; 95(1):258-265.

[73] Kellermann SA, Hudak S, Oldham ER, Liu YJ, McEvoy LM. The CC chemokine receptor-7 ligands 6Ckine and macrophage inflammatory protein-3 beta are potent chemoattractants for in vitro-and in vivo-derived dendritic cells. *J Immunol* 1999; 162(7):3859-3865.

[74] de Vries IJ, Krooshoop DJ, Scharenborg NM, Lesterhuis WJ, Diepstra JH, Van Muijen GN et al. Effective migration of antigen-pulsed dendritic cells to lymph nodes in

melanoma patients is determined by their maturation state. *Cancer Res* 2003; 63(1):12-17.

[75] Nair S, McLaughlin C, Weizer A, Su Z, Boczkowski D, Dannull J et al. Injection of immature dendritic cells into adjuvant-treated skin obviates the need for ex vivo maturation. *J Immunol* 2003; 171(11):6275-6282.

[76] Schrama D, Pedersen LO, Keikavoussi P, Andersen MH, Straten PT, Bröcker E-B et al. Aggregation of Antigen-specific T cells at the inoculation site of mature dendritic cells. *J Invest Dermatol* 2002; 119(6):1443-1448.

[77] Gilliet M, Liu YJ. Generation of human CD8 T regulatory cells by CD40 ligand-activated plasmacytoid dendritic cells. *J Exp Med* 2002; 195(6):695-704.

[78] Albert ML, Jegathesan M, Darnell RB. Dendritic cell maturation is required for the cross-tolerization of CD8+ T cells. *Nat Immunol* 2001; 2(11):1010-1017.

[79] Dhodapkar M, Steinman RM, Krasovsky J, Munz C, Bhardwaj N. Antigen-specific inhibition of effector T cell function in humans after injection of immature dendritic cells. *J Exp Med* 2001; 193(2):233-238.

[80] Dhodapkar M, Steinman RM. Antigen-bearing immature dendritic cells induce peptide-specific CD8+ regulatory T cells in vivo in humans. *Blood* 2002; 100(1):174-177.

[81] de Vries IJ, Lesterhuis WJ, Scharenborg NM, Engelen LP, Ruiter DJ, Gerritsen MJ et al. Maturation of dendritic cells is a prerequisite for inducing immune responses in advanced melanoma patients. *Clin Cancer Res* 2003; 9(14):5091-5100.

[82] Dhodapkar M, Krasovsky J, Steinman RM, Bhardwaj N. Mature dendritic cells boost functionally superior CD8+ T-cell in humans without foreign helper epitopes. *J Clin Invest* 2000; 105(6):R9-R14.

[83] Jonuleit H, Giesecke-Tuettenberg A, Tuting T, Thurner-Schuler B, Stuge TB, Paragnik L et al. A comparison of two types of dendritic cell as adjuvants for the induction of melanoma-specific T-cell responses in humans following intranodal injection. *Int J Cancer* 2001; 93(2):243-251.

[84] McIlroy D, Gregoire M. Optimizing dendritic cell-based anticancer immunotherapy: maturation state does have clinical impact. Cancer Immunol *Immunother* 2005; 52(10):583-591.

[85] Maillard RB, Wankowicx-K.A., Cai Q, Wesa A, Hilkens CM, Kapsenberg ML et al. alpha-type-1 polarized dendritic cells: a novel immunization tool with optimized CTL-inducing activity. *Cancer Res* 2004; 64(17):5934-5937.

[86] Kukutsch NA, Rossner S, Austyn JM, Schuler G, Lutz MB. Formation and kinetics of MHC class I-ovalbumin peptide complexes on immature and mature murine dendritic cells. *J Invest Dermatol* 2000; 115:449-453.

[87] Met O, Buus S, Claesson MH. Peptide-loaded dendritic cells prime and activate MHC-class I-restricted T cells more efficiently than protein-loaded cross-presenting DC. *Cell Immunol* 2003; 222(2):126-133.

[88] Eggert AAO, Schreurs MWJ, Boerman OC, Oyen WJC, de Boer AJ, Punt CJA. Biodistribution and vaccine efficiency of murine dendritic cells are dependent on the route of administration. *Cancer Res* 1999; 59:3340-3345.

[89] Panelli MC, Wunderlich J, Jeffries J, Wang E, Mixon A, Rosenberg SA et al. Phase 1 study in patients with metastatic melanoma of immunization with dendritic cells presenting epitopes derived from the melanoma-associated antigens MART-1 and gp100. *J Immunother* 2000; 23(4):487-498.

[90] Barratt-Boyes SM, Watkins SC, Finn OJ. In vivo migration of dendritic cells differentiated in vitro: a chimpanzee model. *J Immunol* 1997; 158:4543-4547.

[91] Morse MA, Deng Y, Coleman D, Hull S, Kitrell-Fisher E, Nair S. Phase I study of active immunotherapy with carcinoembryonic antigen peptide (CAP-1)-pulsed, autologous human cultured dendritic cells in patients with metastatic malignancies expressing carcinoembryonic antigen. *Clin Cancer Res* 1999; 5:1331-1338.

[92] Morse MA, Coleman RE, Akabani G, Niehaus N, Coleman D, Lyerly HK. Migration of human dendritic cells after injection in patients with metastatic malignancies. *Cancer Res* 1999; 59:56-58.

[93] Fong L, Brockstedt D, Benike C, Wu L, Engleman EG. Dendritic cells injected via different routes induce immunity in cancer patients. *J Immunol* 2001; 166:4254.

[94] Mu LJ, Kyte JA, Kvalheim G, Aamdal S, Dueland S, Hauser M et al. Immunotherapy with allotumour mRNA-transfected dendritic cells in androgen-resistant prostate cancer patients. *Br J Cancer* 2005;(Epub ahead of print).

[95] Ludewig B, Ochsenbein AF, Odermatt B, Paulin D, Hengartner H, Zinkernagel RM. Immunotherapy with dendritic cells directed against tumor antigens shared with normal host cells results in severe autoimmune disease. *J Exp Med* 2000; 191(5):795-803.

[96] Dhodapkar M, Steinman RM, Sapp M, Desai H, Fossella C, Krasovsky J et al. Rapid generation of broad T-cell immunity in humans after a single injection of mature dendritic cells. *J Clin Invest* 1999; 104(2):173-180.

[97] Schuler-Thurner B, Schultz ES, Berger TG, Weinlich G, Ebner S, Woerl P et al. Rapid induction of tumor-specific type 1 T helper cells in metastatic melanoma patients by vaccination with mature, cryopreserved, peptide-loaded monocyte-derived dendritic cells. *J Exp Med* 2002; 195(10):1279-1288.

[98] Cranmer LD, Trevor KT, Hersh EM. Clinical application of dendritic cell vaccination in the treatment of cancer. *Cancer Immunol Immunother* 2004; 53(4):275-306.

[99] Figdor CG, de Vries IJ, Lesterhuis WJ, Melief CJ. Dendritic cell immunotherapy: mapping the way. *Nature Medicine* 2004; 10(3):475-480.

[100] Nestle FO, Banchereau J, Hart D. Dendritic cells: On the move from bench to bedside. *Nature Medicine* 2001; 7(7):761-765.

[101] Ridgway D. The first 1000 dendritic cell vaccinees. *Cancer Invest* 2003; 21(6): 873-886.

[102] Svane IM, Soot ML, Buus S, Johnsen HE. Clinical application of dendritic cells in cancer vaccination therapy. *APMIS* 2003; 111:818-834.

[103] Krause SW, Neumann C, Soruri A, Mayer S, Peters JH, Andreesen R. The treatment of patients with disseminated malignant melanoma by vaccination with autologous cell hybrids of tumor cells and dendritic cells. *J Immunother* 2002; 25(5):421-428.

[104] Mackensen A, Drager R, Schlesier M, Mertelsmann R, Lindemann A. Presence of IgE antibodies to bovine serum albumin in a patient developing anaphylaxis after vaccination with human peptide-pulsed dendritic cells. *Cancer Immunol Immunother* 2000; 49(3):152-156.

[105] Atkins MB, Lotze MT, Dutcher JP, Fisher RI, Weiss G, Margolin K et al. High-dose recombinant interleukin 2 therapy for patients with metastatic melanoma: analysis of 270 patients treated between 1985 and 1993. *J Clin Oncol* 1999; 17(7):2105-2116.

[106] Fyfe G, Fisher RI, Rosenberg SA, Sznol M, Parkinson DR, Louie AC. Results of treatment of 255 patients with metastatic renal cell carcinoma who received high-dose recombinant interleukin-2 therapy. *J Clin Oncol* 1995; 13(3):688-696.

[107] Keilholz U, Gore ME. Biochemotherapy for advanced melanoma. *Semin Oncol* 2002; 29(5):456-461.

[108] Kimberly A, Chianese-Bullock, Woodson EMH, Tao H, Boerner SA, Smolkin M et al. Autoimmune toxicities associated with the administration of antitumor vaccines and low-dose interleukin-2. *J Immunother* 2005; 28(4):412-419.

[109] Antony PA, Restifo NP. CD4+CD25+ T regulatory cells, immunotherapy of cancer, and interleukin-2. *J Immunother* 2005; 28(2):120-128.

[110] Hsu FJ, Benike C, Fagnoni F, Liles TM, Czerwinski D, Taidi B et al. Vaccination of patients with B-cell lymphoma using autologous antigen-pulsed dendritic cells. *Nat Med* 1996; 2(1):52-58.

[111] Nestle FO, Alijagic S, Gilliet M, Sun Y, Grabbe S, Dummer R et al. Vaccination of melanoma patients with peptide- or tumor lysate-pulsed dendritic cells. *Nat Med* 1998; 4(3):328-332.

[112] O'Rourke MG, Johnson M, Lanagan C, See J, Yang J, Bell JR et al. Durable complete clinical responses in a phase I/II trial using an autologous melanoma cell/dendritic cell vaccine. *Cancer Immunol Immunother* 2003; 52(6):387-395.

[113] Trefzer U, Herberth G, Wohlan K, Milling A, Thiemann M, Sharav T et al. Tumour-dendritic hybrid cell vaccination for the treatment of patients with malignant melanoma: immunological effects and clinical results. *Vaccine* 2005; 23(17-18):2367-2373.

[114] Schadendorf D NFBE-B. Dacarbacine (DTIC) versus vaccination with autologous peptide-pulsed dendritic cells (DC) as first-line treatment of patients with metastatic melanoma: Results of a prospective-randomized phase III study. ASCO Annual Meeting Proceedings 2005; 23(18).

[115] Brossart P, Wirths S, Stuhler G, Reichardt VL, Kanz L, Brugger W. Induction of cytotoxic T-lymphocyte responses in vivo after vaccinations with peptide-pulsed dendritic cells. *Blood* 2000; 96(9):3102-3108.

[116] Morse MA, Clay TM, Colling K, Hobeika A, Grabstein K, Cheever MA et al. HER2 Dendritic Cell Vaccines. *Clin Breast Cancer* 2003; 3(Supplement 4):S164-172.

[117] Kobayashi T, Shinohara H, Toyoda M, Iwamoto S, Tanigawa N. Regression of lymph node metastases by immunotherapy using autologous breast tumor-lysate pulsed dendritic cells: report of a case. *Surg Today* 2001; 31(6):513-516.

[118] Pecher G, Haring A, Kaiser L, Thiel E. Mucin gene (MUC1) transfected dendritic cells as vaccine: results of a phase I/II clinical trial. *Cancer Immunol Immunother* 2002; 51[11-12):669-673.

[119] Avigan D. Fusions of breast cancer and dendritic cells as a novel cancer vaccine. *Clin Breast Cancer* 2003; 3 Suppl 4:S158-S163.

[120] Svane IM, Pedersen AE, Johnsen HE, Nielsen D, Kamby C, Ottesen E et al. Vaccination with wildtype p53 peptide pulsed dendritic cells in patients with advanced breast cancer. Results from a phase II study. *Breast Cancer Res Treat* 88, S246. 2004.

[121] Holtl L, Rieser C, Papesh C, Ramoner R, Bartsch G, Thurner M. CD83+ blood dendritic cells as a vaccine for immunotherapy of metastatic renal cell cancer. *Lancet* 1998; 352:1358.

[122] Holtl L, Zelle-Rieser C, Gander H, Papesh C, Ramoner R, Bartsch G et al. Immunotherapy of metastatic renal cell carcinoma with tumor lysate-pulsed autologous dendritic cells. *Clin Cancer Res* 2002; 8(11):3369-3376.

[123] Nair SK, Morse M, Boczkowski D, Cumming RI, Vasovic L, Gilboa E et al. Induction of tumor-specific cytotoxic T lymphocytes in cancer patients by autologous tumour RNA-transfected dendritic cells. *Ann Surg* 2002; 235:540.

[124] Rains N, Cannan RJ, Chen W., Stubbs RS. Development of a dendritic cell (DC)-based vaccine for patients with advanced colorectal cancer. *Hepatogastroenterology* 2001; 48:347.

[125] Fong L, Hou Y, Rivas A, Benike C, Yuen A, Fisher GA et al. Altered peptide ligand vaccination with Flt3 ligand expanded dendritic cells for tumor immunotherapy. *Proc Natl Acad Sci U S A* 2001; 98(15):8809-8814.

[126] Maier T, Tun-Kyi A, Tassis A, Jungius K-P, Burg G, Dummer R et al. Vaccination of patients with cutaneous T-cell lymphoma using intranodal injection of autologous tumor-lysate-pulsed dendritic cells. *Blood* 2003; 102:2338-2344.

[127] Schellhammer PF HR. Immunotherapy with autologous antigen presenting cells for the treatment of androgen independent prostate cancer. *World J Urol* 2005; 23:47-49.

[128] Pedersen AE, Thorn M, Gad M, Walter MR, Johnsen HE, Gaarsdal E et al. Phenotypic and Functional Characterization of Clinical Grade Dendritic Cells Generated from Patients with Advanced Breast Cancer for Therapeutic Vaccination. *Scand J Immunol* 2005; 61:147-156.

[129] Yee C, Greenberg P. Modulating T-Cell immunity to tumours: New strategies for monitoring T-cell responses. *Nature Rev Cancer* 2002; 2(6):409-419.

[130] Andersen MH, Ostergaard Pedersen L, Capeller B, Bröcker EB, Becker JC, Thor Straten P. Spontaneous cytotoxic T-cell responses against survivin-derived MHC class I restricted T-cell epitopes in situ as well as ex vivo in cancer patients. *Cancer Res* 2001; 61(16):5964-5968.

[131] Andersen MH, Gehl J, Reker S, Pedersen LO, Becker JC, Geertsen P et al. Dynamic changes of specific T cell responses to melanoma correlate with IL-2 administration. *Sem Cancer Biol* 2003; 13(6):449-459.

[132] Lee KH, Panelli MC, Kim CJ, Riker AI, Bettinotti MP, Roden MM et al. Functional dissociation between local and systemic immune response during anti-melanoma peptide vaccination. *J Immunol* 1998; 161(8):4183-4194.

[133] Nielsen M-B, Monsurro V, Migueles S, Wang E, Perez-Diaz A, Kang-Hun L et al. Status of activation of circulating vaccine-elicited CD8+ T cells. *J Immunol* 2000; 165(4):2287-2296.

[134] Rosenberg SA, Yang JC, Schwartzentruber DJ, Hwu P, Marincola FM, Topalian SL et al. Immunologic and therapeutic evaluation of a synthetic peptide vaccine for the treatment of patients with metastatic melanoma. *Nat Med* 1998; 4(3):321-327.

[135] Kammula U, Lee KH, Riker AI, Wang E, Ohnmacht GA, Rosenberg SA et al. Functional analysis of antigen-specific T lymphocytes by serial measurement of gene expression in peripheral blood mononuclear cells and tumor specimens. *J Immunol* 1999; 163(12):6867-6875.

[136] Yamshchikov GV, Barnd DL, Eastham S, Galavotti H, Patterson JW, Deacon DH et al. Evaluation of peptide vaccine immunogenicity in draining lymph nodes and peripheral blood of melanoma patients. *Int J Cancer* 2001; 92(5):703-711.

[137] Panelli MC, Riker AI, Kammula U, Wang E, Lee KH, Rosenberg SA et al. Expansion of tumor-T cell pairs from fine needle aspirates of melanoma metastases. *J Immunol* 2000; 164(1):495-504.

[138] Fetsch PA, Steinberg SM, Riker AI, Marincola FM, Abati A. Melanoma antigen expression in serial fine-needle aspiration samples in patients with metastatic malignant melanoma participating in immunotherapy clinical trials: a preliminary look. *Cancer* 2001; 93(6):409-414.

[139] Wang E, Miller LD, Ohnmacht GA, Liu ET, Marincola FM. High-fidelity mRNA amplification for gene profiling. *Nat Biotechnol* 2000; 18(4):457-459.

[140] Bittner M, Meltzer P, Chen Y, Jiang Y, Seftor E, Hendrix M et al. Molecular classification of cutaneous malignant melanoma by gene expression profiling. *Nature* 2000; 406(6795):536-540.

[141] Wang E, Marincola FM. A natural history of melanoma: serial gene expression analysis. *Immunol Today* 2000; 21(12):619-623.

[142] Eralp Y. WXWJP. Doxorubicin and paclitaxel enhance the antitumor efficacy of vaccines directed against HER 2/neu in a murine mammary carcinoma model. *Breast Cancer Res* 2004; 6:275-283.

[143] Holtl L, Ramoner R, Zelle-Rieser C. Allogeneic dendritic cell vaccination against metastatic renal cell carcinoma with or without cyclophosphamide. *Cancer Immunol Immunother* 2004.

[144] Hatfield P, Merrick A, Harrington K. Radiation-induced cell death and dendritic cells: potential for cancer immunotherapy? *Clin Oncol* 2005; 17:1-11.

[145] Chen Z, Xia D, Bi X. Combined radiation therapy and dendritic cell vaccine for treating solid tumors with liver micro-metastasis. *J Gene Med* 2005; 7:506-517.

[146] Walunas TL, Lenschow DJ, Bakker CY, Linsley PS, Freeman GJ, Green JM et al. CTLA-4 Can Function as a Negative Regulator of T Cell Activation. *Immunity* 1994; 1(5):405-413.

[147] Phan GQ, Yang JC, Sherry RM, Hwu P, Topalian SL, Schwartzentruber DJ et al. Cancer regression and autoimmunity induced by cytotoxic T lymphocyte-associated antigen 4 blockade in patients with metastatic melanoma. *Proc Natl Acad Sci U S A* 2003; 100(14):8372-8377.

[148] Sanderson K, Scotland R, Lee P, Liu D, Groshen S, Snively J et al. Autoimmunity in a Phase I Trial of a Fully Human Anti-Cytotoxic T-Lymphocyte Antigen-4 Monoclonal Antibody With Multiple Melanoma Peptides and Montanide ISA 51 for Patients With Resected Stages III and IV Melanoma. *J Clin Oncol* 2004.

[149] von Boehmer H. Mechanisms of suppression by suppressor T cells. *Nat Immunol* 2005; 6:338-345.

[150] Vieweg J, Su Z, Dannull J. Enhancement of antitumor immunity following depletion of CD4+CD25+ regulatory T cells. ASCO Annual Meeting Proceedings 2005.

[151] Cherrington JM, Strawn LM, Shawver LK. New paradigms for the treatment of cancer: The role of anti-angiogenesis agents. *Adv Cancer Res* 2000; 79:1-38.

[152] Ferrara N. Vascular endothelial growth factor as a target for anticancer therapy. *Oncologist* 2004; 9 Suppl 1:2-10.

[153] Lamoreaux WJ, Fitzgerald ME, Reiner A, Hasty KA, Charles ST. Vascular endothelial growth factor increases release of gelatinase A and decreases release of tissue inhibitor

of metalloproteinases by microvascular endothelial cells in vitro. *Microvasc Res* 1998; 55(1):29-42.

[154] Unemori EN, Ferrara N, Bauer EA, Amento EP. Vascular endothelial growth factor induces interstitial collagenase expression in human endothelial cells. *J Cell Physiol* 1992; 153(3):557-562.

[155] Alon T, Hemo I, Itin A, Pe'er J, Stone J, Keshet E. Vascular endothelial growth factor acts as a survival factor for newly formed retinal vessels and has implications for retinopathy of prematurity. *Nat Med* 1995; 1(10):1024-1028.

[156] Asahara T, Takahashi T, Masuda H, Kalka C, Chen D, Iwaguro H et al. VEGF contributes to postnatal neovascularization by mobilizing bone marrow-derived endothelial progenitor cells. *EMBO J* 1999; 18(14):3964-3972.

[157] Rousseau S, Houle F, Huot J. Integrating the VEGF signals leading to actin-based motility in vascular endothelial cells. *Trends Cardiovasc Med* 2000; 10(8):321-327.

[158] Gabrilovich D, Ishida T, Oyama T, Ran S, Kravtsov V, Nadaf S et al. Vascular endothelial growth factor inhibits the development of dendritic cells and dramatically affects the differentiation of multiple hematopoietic lineages in vivo. *Blood* 1998; 92(11):4150-4166.

[159] Barleon B, Sozzani S, Zhou D, Weich HA, Mantovani A, Marme D. Migration of human monocytes in response to vascular endothelial growth factor (VEGF) is mediated via the VEGF receptor flt-1. *Blood* 1996; 87(8):3336-3343.

[160] Pedersen AE, Buus S, Claesson MH. Treatment of transplanted CT26 tumour with dendritic cell vaccine in combination with blockade of vascular endothelial growth factor receptor 2 and CTLA-4. *Cancer Letters* 2005; May 28, Epub ahead of print.

In: Vaccinations: Types, Potential Complications…
Editors: D. B. Steen and H. L. Dyson
ISBN: 978-1-60692-969-8

Chapter IX

Nonviral Cancer Vaccines: From Free Antigens to Engineered Cells*

M. J. Herrero[1], R. Botella[2], R. Algás[3], F. Marco[4], S. Lledó[5] and S. F. Aliño[1,6]

[1]Unidad de Terapia Génica, Departmento de Farmacología, Facultad de Medicina, Universidad de Valencia, Spain;
[2]Servicio de Dermatología, Instituto Valenciano de Oncología (IVO), Valencia, Spain;
[3]Servicio de Radioterapia, Hospital Clínico Universitario, Valencia, Spain;
[4]ASAC Pharmaceutical International, Alicante, Spain;
[5]Servicio de Cirugía, Hospital clínico Universitario, Valencia, Spain;
[6]Unidad de Farmacología Clínica, Hospital Universitario La Fe, Valencia, Spain.

Abstract

In the present work we have developed several models of cancer vaccines, employing a murine melanoma and nonviral procedures for gene transfer. Many efforts have been made in relation to cancer vaccines, attempting to elucidate the best way to induce correct activation of the immune system in order to achieve proper antitumor response. Engineered cells seem to be the most successful approach, since they better reproduce the processes that occur in real patients, including events that today still escape our understanding. However, purified antigens represent an easier approach in terms of their preparation, reproducibility and facility to become a commercial medicine. This is why they continue to center attention, though their results are still not particularly satisfactory. In an attempt to establish the best approach for stimulating the immune response and also securing the simplest treatment, we have tested different preventive vaccination models such as: a) purified antigens from irradiated B16 melanoma tumor cells (Tumor Membrane Proteins, TMP); b) such antigens encapsulated in liposomes; c) lipopolyplexes

* * A version of this chapter was also published in *New Gene Therapy and Cancer Research*, edited by Wilma B. Gustafsson published by Nova Science Publishers, Inc. It was submitted for appropriate modifications in an effort to encourage wider dissemination of research.

formed by cationic liposomes bearing antigens plus the cationic polymer polyethyleneimine (PEI), carrying DNA; d) freshly transfected and irradiated B16 cells, producing cytokines; and e) a very reduced number of transfected cells, selected by means of magnetic bead procedures. The results obtained show different rates of tumor growth inhibition - performance improving when adjusting the combinations of plasmid bearing the cytokine gene and TMP antigens in the lipopolyplexes. The best inhibition (total) was obtained with freshly transfected (not selected) cells, which allowed us to perform further experiments consisting of a vaccine with only the truly transfected (cytokine-producing) cells. On this occasion, reducing the cell number to only 20% that of the prior doses, we achieved about 80% of tumor growth inhibition. All these results encourage the conduction of further studies of this kind, with the purpose of increasing accuracy and optimizing cancer vaccine procedures.

Introduction

Genetically modified tumor cells have been shown to be very efficient in various models of antitumor vaccines [1,2,3]. Still, the main problem with these models is the great difficulty of obtaining tumor cells from patients and that moreover must be kept in culture, amplified to a larger number, transfected and then returned to the same patient. This is not easy, even when employing other proposed methods - not only with tumor cells, but also with syngenic or allogenic cells [4,5]. All these efforts in the field of cancer vaccine research have converged on the idea that the best results are obtained vaccinating not only with the tumor antigens, but also with the genes that the immune system itself would use to achieve a good response: the cytokine genes. However, the functioning of the immune system is very complex, and combining these two components has not always been successful [6,7], leading to immune suppression or even anergy. Our group has also made efforts to elucidate the correct time order to supply the two signals [8]. At present, the most effective way of administering these two components is the introduction of cells, or a neoplastic nature or otherwise, that produce the cytokine themselves [8,9,10]. In this context, many studies have achieved promising results, and clinical trials have been set up [11,12]. To understand what kind of antigens work best and how they awaken a truly effective response, we also wanted to work with tumor cell antigens instead of whole cells - since they offer the advantage of being easier to prepare and standardize as commercial medicines [13]. In this sense, we have worked in a murine model of melanoma, using the two above mentioned components to develop an antitumor vaccine, antigens and cytokine genes, adopting two different approaches: purified antigens or cells. As antigens, we have used irradiated whole tumor cells (murine melanoma B16 cells) or an extract of their hydrophilic membrane antigens (tumor membrane proteins, TMP). As cytokines, we have used the m-GMCSF encoding gene (Granulocytes and Macrophages Colony Stimulating Factor), which has largely demonstrated great usefulness as an antitumor tool [1,4,6,10]. However, in later experiments, our tumor cells have also been transfected with the m-B7.2 encoding gene.

The first set of experiments is based on TMP encapsulated in liposomes or lipopolyplexes, and there we have explored the best liposome type and formulation, and the quantity of TMP and quantity of GM-CSF suitable for achieving an antitumor response.

Liposomes and lipopolyplexes also have a long trajectory in the field of vaccines, and have been shown to be good adjuvants in many different settings [14-17].

Nevertheless, being aware of the more solid results obtained with whole cells instead of purified antigens, in the second set of experiments we have worked with freshly transfected B16 cells, producing GM-CSF and B7.2.

B7.2 (also called CD86) is a costimulatory molecule of the immune system, naturally expressed only at the surface of professional Antigen Presenting Cells (APCs). This molecule has been widely employed in different antitumor approaches [18-24], as it enhances the immune response by participating in the activation of T cells: after the first signal of antigen recognition in the APC, the major histocompatibility complex (MHC) molecules present the antigenic peptides to the TCR (T Cell Receptor); however, only if the second signal (costimulation) is also present, will the T cells correctly begin sustained cell proliferation, effector or memory cell generation, and the prevention of anergy or apoptosis. It is in relation to this second signal where B7.2 plays its role by positively stimulating T cells through CD28. Our aim in employing B7.2 has been to increase the T cell response against the transfected B16 cells, but we have also taken advantage of such transfection to select and purify only the truly transfected cells from a total population of freshly transfected cells and to perform a vaccination experiment with a very reduced cell number - again attempting to define the minimum number of cells required to secure good results, and thus start with "easier to prepare" cell vaccines.

Materials and Methods

Plasmids

p2F m-gmcsf, p2F m-B7.2, p2F m-gmcsf + m-B7.2 and p2F Ø, were derived from the pVITRO2 base plasmid (Invivogen, France), with the *m-gmcsf* gene, *m-B7.2*, *m-gmcsf* plus *m-B7.2* genes or the empty plasmid, respectively. pVITRO2 allows the coexpression of two genes and contains two human ferritin composite promoters, FerH (heavy chain) and FerL (light chain), combined to the SV40 and CMV enhancers respectively, and the resistance gene to Hygromycin. To eliminate the iron regulation, their 5'UTRs have been replaced by the 5'UTR of the mouse and chimpanzee EF1α genes.

All plasmids were amplified in *Escherichia coli* DH5α, in selective LB broth (Pronadisa, Spain) and extracted with the Qiagen Giga Endofree kit (Izasa SA, Spain), quantified by spectrophotometry and tested by electrophoresis to confirm their integrity and purity.

TMP Obtainment

The mixture of hydrophilic membrane proteins from B16 cells was performed following a protocol based on the work of Bordier work [25]. Briefly, after detaching and counting the irradiated cells, their pellet is resuspended in 1 ml of extraction buffer for every 10 million cells, containing Tris 10 mM, $MgCl_2$ 2 mM, Triton X-114 0.5% (Sigma, Spain) and phenylmethylsulfonylfluoride (PMSF) 0.1 mM (Sigma, Spain), pH 7.2. The mixture is incubated in ice for 45 min., shaking gently every 10 min. Then, centrifugation is carried out at 5300 rpm, 4°C, for 15 min. The supernatant is recovered and 750 μl placed above 250 μl of centrifuge buffer (sucrose 10% in extraction buffer) in microcentrifuge tubes. After incubating 3 min. at 37°C, it is centrifuged again for 5 min. at 2100 rpm. Supernatant (750 μl) is recovered and Triton X-114 added to a final concentration of 0.5% before placing the tube in ice again over 250 μl of centrifuge buffer. After incubating for 3 min. more at 37°C and centrifuging for 5 min. more at 2100 rpm, two different phases are obtained in the microcentrifuge tube: the upper one contains the hydrophilic proteins, that will be kept in aliquots at -20°C until use.

The proteins are quantified with the CBQCA protein quantitation kit (Molecular Probes-Invitrogen, Spain), following the manufacturer's instructions.

Liposomes and Lipopolyplexes

Three different types of liposome production were tested: Multilamellar Vesicles (MLV), Dehydration-Rehydration Vesicles (DRV), and Freeze-Thawed Multilamellar Vesicles (MLV-FT), proceeding according to the literature for manufacture [26,27]. Also, four different lipidic compositions were evaluated, employing Phosphatidylcholine (PC), Sphingomyelin (SM), Cholesterol (CH) and Dicetylphosphate (DP), all from Sigma (Spain), being PC:CH and SM:CH at 6:4 molar ratio and PC:CH:DP and SM:CH:DP at 5:4:1. All were formed in Milli Q water. The liposomes chosen for lipopolyplex formation were PC:CH:DP (5:4:1), which were later coupled with PEI 25 KDa (polyethyleneimine, Sigma, Spain) linked to the plasmid in use, at a ratio of 1.41:1, PEI:DNA (polyplex, also made in Milli Q) [27,28]. To test the quantity of protein encapsulated in each type of liposome, the CBQCA protein quantitation kit (Molecular Probes-Invitrogen, Spain) was employed, following the manufacturer's instructions.

Cells and Transfection Procedures

B16 murine melanoma cells have been used in all of the experiments. These cells are syngenic with the animals used for vaccination, i.e., C57BL/6 mice (Harlan, France). B16 cells were also used as source of antigen for vaccination, either as whole cells or employed to obtain an extract of their membrane proteins (TMP). To inoculate the tumors in vaccinated and control groups of mice, 10^5 freshly detached B16 cells were injected in their usual simple culture medium into the left leg of the animals, while the vaccines were injected subcutaneously into the right leg.

B16 cells are adherent cells that are grown in flasks with DMEM (Dulbecco's modified Eagle's medium) (Sigma, Spain), supplemented with 10% heat inactivated fetal bovine serum (FBS) (Biomedia, France), Penicillin (100 U/ml) and Streptomycin (100 μg/ml). They are cultured in a humidified incubator with 5% CO_2 at 37°C, and are detached from the flasks with Trypsin-EDTA. When whole cells are used for vaccinating, they are irradiated with a 150 Gy dose, after being detached from their flasks, and are later frozen in FBS with 5% DMSO to be kept at -80 or -150°C until use.

The cells were transfected by means of a chemical procedure based on PEI 25 KDa (polyethyleneimine. Sigma, Spain) polyplexes with 20 μg/ml p2F plasmids, as previously described [8,26]. The transfection percentage with this method lies between 20-40% of total cells (data not shown), as observed using the reporter EGFP gene. Cells were transfected when more than 80% confluence was reached in their flasks, irradiated 72 hours post-transfection with 150 Gy, and then frozen in DMSO 5% in FBS and kept at -80 or -150°C until use.

Determination of m-GMCSF Production

The GM-CSF production of the transfected B16 cells is determined by Enzyme Linked Immunosorbent Assay (ELISA), performed on supernatant samples of the culture media taken 72 hours post-transfection and prior to cell detachment and irradiation, having changed the media every 24 hours. The BD OptEIA ELISA kit for m-GMCSF (Pharmingen, BD Biosciences, Spain) was used. The time-point of 72 hours was chosen on the basis of prior experimental results, assessed to study cytokine production over time, and using the referred transfection conditions [8,10,26], in order to achieve adequate production according to the literature [4].

Determination of m-B7.2 production

Flow cytometry was performed to confirm the presence of m-B7.2 in the surface of the transfected cells. At 72 h post-transfection, cells were harvested and pelleted in aliquots of 500,000 cells, washed and incubated in ice for at least 30 min. in 200 μl PBS-FBS (2.5%) - Azide (0.01%) solution of primary antibody (1 μg/million cells): Biotin-conjugated rat anti-mouse CD86 monoclonal antibody (Pharmingen, BD, Spain). Then, cells were washed twice in 1 ml PBS-Azide and incubated in ice and dark with the secondary antibody (0.5 μg/million cells): Streptavidin-Fluorescein Isothiocyanate conjugate (FITC) (Pharmingen, BD, Spain).

Finally, cells were washed twice and finally resuspended in 500 μl PBS to be passed through the cytometer (Coulter Epics, XL; Beckman Coulter, Spain) and for analysis of the fluorescence in the populations, in order to discriminate the truly transfected cells. To avoid taking autofluorescence or nonspecific binding as positive results, several controls were tested. The groups were: a) non-transfected wild type B16 cells, without any antibody; b) non-transfected wild type B16 cells incubated with both antibodies; c) B16-p2F m-gmcsf + m-B7.2 transfected cells, without any antibody; d) B16-p2F m-gmcsf + m-B7.2 transfected cells, incubated only with primary antibody; e) B16-p2F m-gmcsf + m-B7.2 transfected cells, incubated only with secondary antibody; and finally f) B16-p2F m-gmcsf + m-B7.2 transfected cells, incubated with both primary and secondary antibody.

Selection and Purification of Transfected Cells

This process is carried out by means of the Automacs device for magnetic cell separation (Miltenyi Biotec, Spain), according to the manufacturer's instructions and employing the

Automacs columns. At 72 h post-transfection, cells are harvested and incubated with the first antibody, in PBS, under the same conditions as in the flow cytometry experiments; the Streptavidin Microbeads protocol is then followed (Miltenyi Biotec, Spain), and transfected cells are separated and purified employing the "Posseld 2" program. Lastly, cells are counted and frozen until the time of the vaccination experiments.

Preventive Vaccination Procedures

C57BL/6 mice (8-10 weeks old) kept under standard laboratory conditions were housed 5 mice per cage. All the experiments were approved by the Biological Research Committee of the University of Valencia (Spain). In all cases, mice were vaccinated (right leg) with a single dose per week, in weeks -3, -1 and +1 (days –21, -7 and +7), with respect to tumor injection (day 0) in the form of 10^5 wild type B16 cells in the left leg.

For experiments with liposomes and lipopolyplexes, 100 μl of liposomes or lipopolyplexes in Milli Q water were injected at each dose, the treatment groups for the liposomes containing TMP vaccine being: a) 10 μg of TMP alone; b) PC:CH liposomes containing 10 μg of TMP; c) SM:CH liposomes containing 10 μg of TMP; and d) Control group (100 μl saline solution). For the lipopolyplexes vaccine, the complexes were prepared with 10 or 50 μg of p2F *m-gmcsf* plasmid (GM10 or GM50) and 2 or 20 μg of TMP (TMP2 or TMP20), being GM10/TMP2, GM10/TMP20, GM50/TMP2, GM50/TMP20.

For experiments with freshly transfected B16 cells (non-selected), cells were thawed and counted for $2x10^5$ B16 cells (previously transfected, irradiated and frozen) per dose (groups p2F∅, B7.2, GM, GM+B7.2/200) per mouse, in 100 μl DMEM. For p2F m-gmcsf + m-B7.2 treatment, two different cell doses were studied: one with the usual cell dose ($2x10^5$), GM+B7.2/200; and another with cells sufficient to reach the same GM-CSF production as in the GM group, according to previous ELISA experiments of GM-CSF production (data not shown), i.e., group GM+B7.2/500. In the B16* group, $2x10^5$ wild type irradiated B16cells (150 Gy) were injected in 100μl DMEM, while in the Control group only 100 μl DMEM was injected, at every three vaccination dose.

For experiments with transfected and selected B16 cells (beads selection), we chose a vaccine dose that represented only the truly transfected cells of the "non-selected cells vaccine". Thus, we had to vaccine only with 20% of the previous doses, since in this case all of the employed cells would be transfected cells. Our two groups were: Control (100 μl DMEM) and GM+B7.2/40, employing only 40,000 selected cells per mouse, per dose, in 100 μl DMEM.

In all vaccination experiments, blood samples were taken from all the animals, pooling blood from the animals from the same group at each time-point. The samples were taken on days –22 (before any manipulation of the animals, serving as base level or control in each group), -1 (the day before tumor implantation, day 0, with two vaccination doses already performed), and +15 (one week after the third and last dose was administered). Plasma was obtained by centrifugation at 3000 rpm for 5 min. and kept at –20°C until use.

Tumor Growth Measurement, Survival and Statistical Analysis

Tumor growth in mice was monitored visually and measured with a caliper in two dimensions, A, the long diameter and B, the short diameter. Tumor volume was calculated with the formula $V= (AxB^2)/2$, and expressed in mm^3. Total or partial survival was achieved in some of the treated groups; animals were collected at their death date to construct the survival curves. To statistically compare the results of the different treatment groups, a two-tailed ANOVA was used, with Bonferroni post hoc testing (95% confidence interval, 95%CI), expressing statistically significant differences on the basis of $P<0.05$, $P<0.01$ and $P<0.001$.

Specific anti-TMP IgG ELISA

Measurement of IgG and IgG subclass antibodies to TMP was performed in serum samples by specific ELISA, as previously described [13]. Plates were coated by overnight incubation of TMP at 0.8 μg/ml in carbonate buffer, pH 9.6. The next day, plates were neutralized with 1% BSA solution before addition of serum samples. For analysis, sera were diluted in dilution buffer (PBS-BSA 1%-Tween 20 0.1%) at 1/1000 for total IgG and IgG1 subclass and at 1/100 for IgG2a. Bound antibodies were detected with goat antisera to total IgG (Biocheck, USA) at 1/10000 or mouse IgG subclasses at 1/1000 (Sigma, Mouse monoclonal isotyping reagents, Spain), followed by 1/5000 dilution of biotinylated rabbit antiserum to goat IgG (Sigma, Spain) and streptavidin coupled to horseradish peroxidase (Sigma, Spain). Plates were developed with a mixture of orthophenylenediamine (OPD, Sigma, Spain) and hydrogen peroxide (Fluka, Spain), and read at 492 nm. All samples were assayed in duplicate, allowing the estimation of mean OD value and standard deviation.

Results

Efficacy of Protein Encapsulation in Liposomes

The different procedures of liposome preparation revealed a very different ability for encapsulating BSA Protein (Bovine Serum Albumin), as seen in Figure 1-A. The freeze and thaw cycles performed during the formation of MLV-FT liposomes enable these vesicles to entrap nearly 90% of the protein present in the medium. These results made us continue with this kind of liposomes, as our purpose was to use them simply as a delivery vehicle for our tumor antigens (TMP), so the more effective the better, in the sense that we would be able to deliver more antigen with less lipid.

As we wanted to simultaneously transport proteic antigens (TMP) and DNA encoding cytokine genes (GM-CSF) in two independent compartments, we prepared a lipopolyplex complex in which TMP were encapsulated in anionic liposomes, whereas DNA was prepared as a PEI/DNA polyplex. For this reason, we were interested in obtaining good encapsulation of TMP in anionic liposomes - in our case liposomes containing the anionic DP lipid. In Figure 1-B, the best encapsulation percentages are achieved with PC:CH, for the simple formulations, and are equivalent in PC:CH:DP and SM:CH:DP. The best encapsulation was achieved when liposomes incorporated 10% DP, which is why we used the more classical PC:CH:DP liposomes for the following lipopolyplex experiments.

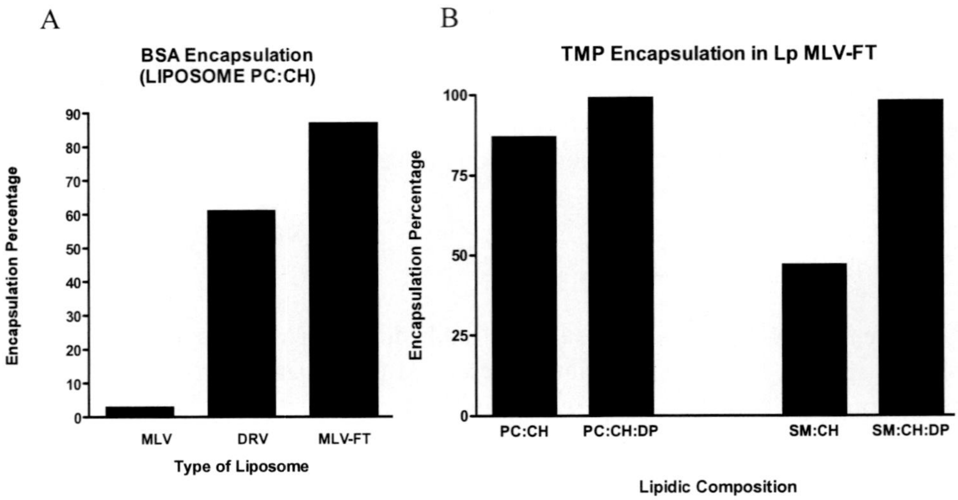

Figure 1. A- BSA protein encapsulation in liposomes. Ability for encapsulating BSA protein in different procedures of liposome preparation: Multilamellar Vesicles (MLV), Dehydration-Rehydration Vesicles (DRV) and Freeze-Thawed Multilamellar Vesicles (MLV-FT). B- TMP encapsulation in Lp MLV-FT. Percentage of TMP encapsulation in MLV-FT liposomes with different lipidic compositions: Phosphatidylcholine (PC), Sphingomyelin (SM), Cholesterol (CH) and Dicetylphosphate (DP).

Liposomes and Lipopolyplexes Vaccine

With the aim of evaluating the efficacy of TMP vaccines employing liposomes or lipopolyplexes as carriers, C57BL/6 mice (n=5 per group) were vaccinated in the right leg at a single dose per week, on weeks -3, -1 and +1 (days –21, -7 and +7), with respect to tumor injection (day 0) with 10^5 wild type B16 cells in left leg. Liposomes or lipopolyplexes (100 μl) were injected at each dose in the following groups: a) 10 μg of TMP alone; b) PC:CH liposomes containing 10 μg of TMP; c) SM:CH liposomes containing 10 μg of TMP; and d) Control group (100 μl saline solution), as seen in Figure 2. For the lipopolyplexes vaccine, in Figure 3, complexes made of 10 or 50 μg of p2F *m-gmcsf* plasmid (GM10 or GM50) and 2 or 20 μg of TMP (TMP2 or TMP20) were employed, according to the following groups: a) GM10/TMP2, b) GM10/TMP20, c) GM50/TMP2, and d) GM50/TMP20. Tumor growth was monitored in mice, measuring the long diameter (A) and the short diameter (B) with calipers. The tumor volume was calculated with the formula $V = (AxB^2)/2$, and expressed in mm^3. Statistical tests were performed by two-way ANOVA and Bonferroni post hoc testing. In Figure 2, “a” represents a statistically significant difference of $P<0.05$ regarding the TMP Lp SM group; “b” the same, but regarding the Control group; and “c” is $P<0.01$ compared also with the Control group. Tumor growth is inhibited (40-50%) with statistically significant differences on day +22 after tumor implantation (Day 0), when comparing TMP 10 μg or

TMP Lp PC versus TMP Lp SM or Control, and no differences were found within the two couples. These results led us to continue working with PC liposomes.

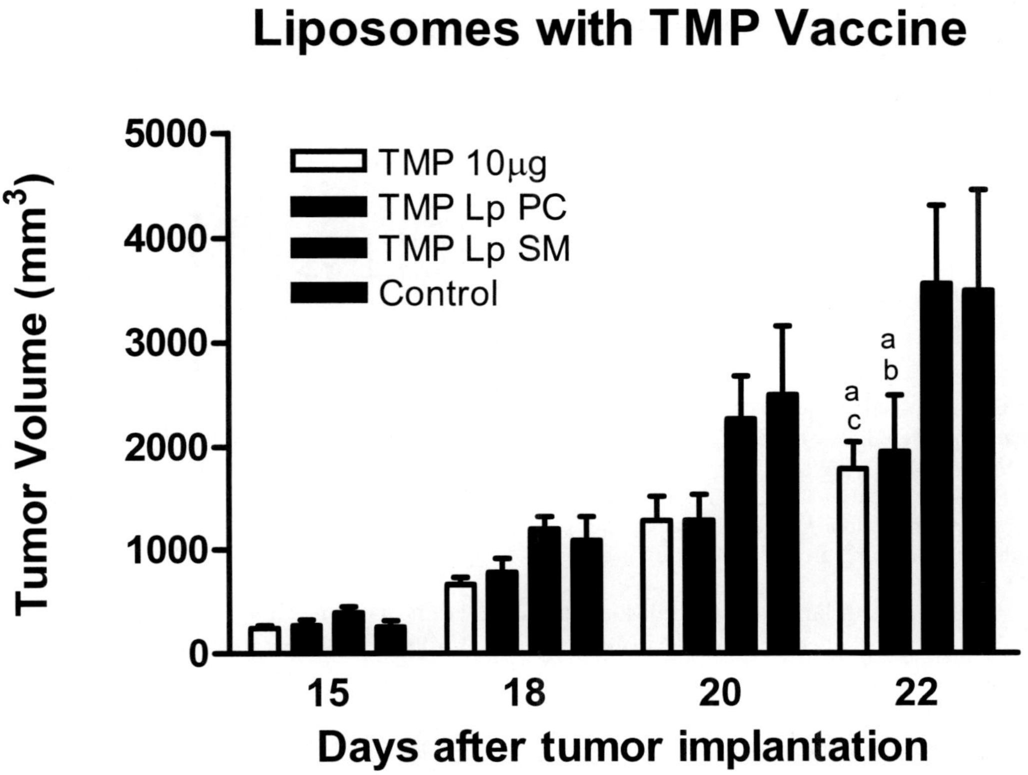

Figure 2. Liposomes with TMP vaccine. C57BL/6 mice (n=5 per group) were vaccinated in the right leg on days –21, -7 and +7 with respect to tumor injection on day 0 (10^5 wild type B16 cells) in the left leg. Treatments: a) 10 μg of TMP alone; b) PC:CH liposomes containing 10 μg of TMP; c) SM:CH liposomes containing 10 μg of TMP; d) Control group (100 μl saline solution). Tumor volume was calculated from $V = (AxB^2)/2$, where A is the long diameter and B the short diameter, with volume expression in mm^3. Statistical tests were performed by two-way ANOVA and Bonferroni post hoc testing. Statistically significant difference of $P<0.05$ regarding TMP Lp SM group = a, b is the same but regarding Control group, and c is $P<0.01$ likewise versus the Control group.

In Figure 3, "a, b, c, d" represent a statistically significant difference of $P<0.001$ comparing GM10/TMP20 with each following group in the figure, respectively. The figure shows statistically significant differences in tumor growth inhibition on days +20 and +23, regarding tumor implantation, achieved only by group GM10/TMP20 (40-50%) when compared with all other treatments, and reaching the maximum degree of significance. The other groups did not show any difference between each other. Thus, the best combination in this experiment was vaccinating with a lipopolyplex that contained the lowest DNA and the highest antigen quantities.

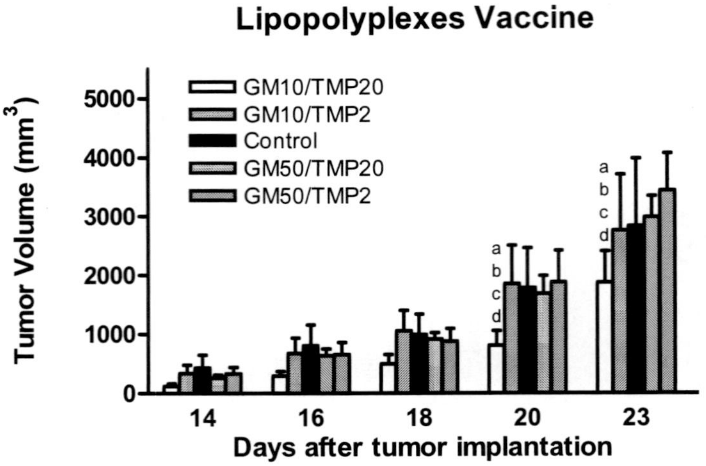

Figure 3. Lipopolyplexes vaccine. The same vaccination pattern as in Fig. 2 was followed, but treatments were lipopolyplexes prepared with 10 or 50 μg of p2F *m-gmcsf* plasmid: PEI polyplexes (GM10 or GM50) linked with 2 or 20 μg of TMP (TMP2 or TMP20) in PC:CH:DP liposomes, being GM10/TMP2, GM10/TMP20, GM50/TMP2, GM50/TMP20. Volume formula and statistical analysis were the same as in Fig. 2. Statistically significant difference of $P<0.001$ comparing GM10/TMP20 with each following group in the figure is represented by a, b, c and d, respectively.

Although similar growth inhibition was achieved in liposomes and lipopolyplex vaccines, differences were observed in the survival results. While in the Liposome Vaccine experiment we did not observe any differential survival between treated and control groups (data not shown), better survival results were observed in the Lipopolyplex Vaccine experiment (Figures 4-A and B). In Fig. 4-A, the groups with the lower DNA doses are represented, both of them achieving longer survival periods than the control group. According to the results of tumor growth inhibition, the longest survival was reached with 10 DNA μg of GM-CSF, while the groups treated with higher than 50 μg DNA doses (Figure 4-B) performed worse than the control group.

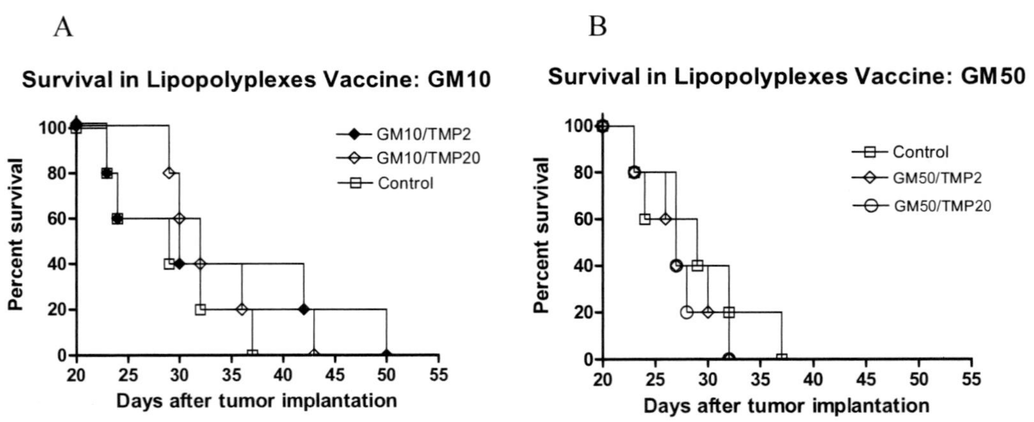

Figure 4. Survival in lipopolyplexes vaccine. Animal death dates were collected to construct survival curves. A- Results of Control and groups treated with lipopolyplexes containing 10 μg p2F *m-gmcsf*. B- Results of Control and groups treated with lipopolyplexes containing 50 μg p2F *m-gmcsf*.

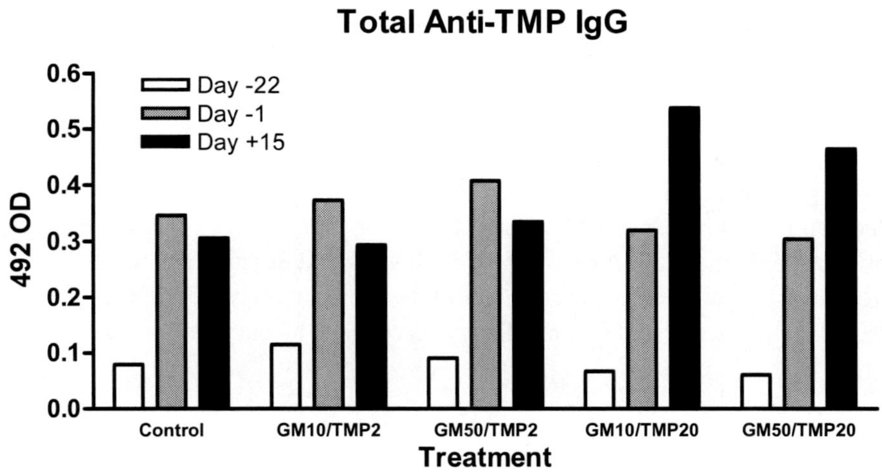

Figure 5. Total Anti-TMP IgG in lipopolyplex vaccine. Blood samples were taken from all the animals on days -22, -1 and +15, pooling the blood of the animals from the same group at each time-point, with respect to the tumor transplant day (day 0). Plasma was obtained by blood centrifugation at 3000 rpm during 5 min. Specific anti-TMP IgG were measured in plasma by ELISA: Plates were coated by overnight incubation of TMP at 0.8 μg/ml in carbonate buffer, pH 9.6. The next day, plates were neutralized with 1% BSA solution before addition of serum samples. For analysis, sera were diluted in dilution buffer (PBS-BSA 1%-Tween 20 0.1%) at 1/1000 for total IgG and IgG1 subclass and at 1/100 for IgG2a. Bound antibodies were detected with goat antisera to total IgG (Biocheck, USA) at 1/10000 or mouse IgG subclasses at 1/1000 (Sigma, mouse monoclonal isotyping reagents, Spain), followed by 1/5000 dilution of biotinylated rabbit antiserum to goat IgG (Sigma, Spain) and streptavidin coupled to horseradish peroxidase (Sigma, Spain). Plates were developed with a mixture of orthophenylenediamine (OPD, Sigma, Spain) and hydrogen peroxide (Fluka, Spain), and read at 492 nm. All samples were assayed in duplicate, allowing the estimation of mean OD value and standard deviation.

Blood samples were taken from all the animals during the experiment, pooling blood from the animals from the same group at each time-point, with respect to the tumor transplant day (day 0). The samples were taken on days –22 (before any manipulation of the animals, which serves as base level or control in each group), day -1 and day +15. The total anti-TMP IgG found by ELISA in the vaccinated mice and control group is shown in Figure 5. The measurements were made in duplicate, and means and standard deviations (SD) were calculated and represented, although SD is inappreciable, since it was less than 5% of the mean value, which also happened in the rest of the vaccine experiments in this work. In this figure, the treatments with higher antigen doses (20 μg TMP) show the maximum IgG response on day +15, whereas the two groups with the lower TMP dose (2 μg), show their maximums on day -1, and these levels are always lower than those recorded for the other two groups. In order to know the immunoglobulin switch induced by vaccination, specific subtypes IgG1 and IgG2a were also studied, and the results were summarized in Figures 6-A and B, respectively. The same pattern as for total IgG is observed, with more relevant differences between the two TMP conditions in IgG1. On the other hand, optimal responses in IgG2a are achieved when 20 μg TMP and 10 μg DNA GM-CSF were employed, since higher DNA doses did not offer any advantages. Also, GM50/TMP2 increased IgG2a response, but mainly limited to day-1.

Determination of m-B7.2 Production

The efficiency of m-B7.2 expression on B16 cell surface 72 h after transfection was evaluated by flow cytometry. The results are summarized in Figure 7, which plots counts versus F1 Log, and where we can identify specific surface expression of m-B7.2 in the right peak of the figure, whereas the middle and left peaks correspond to the transfected and non-transfected control cells, respectively. The intersection area between the middle peak and the right peak represents the proportion of transfected cells that are also fluorescent, i.e., the cells that express m-B7.2 at their surface. This area is approximately 20-40% of the right peak, which was our expected transfection efficacy, according to our previous experiments (data not shown).

A

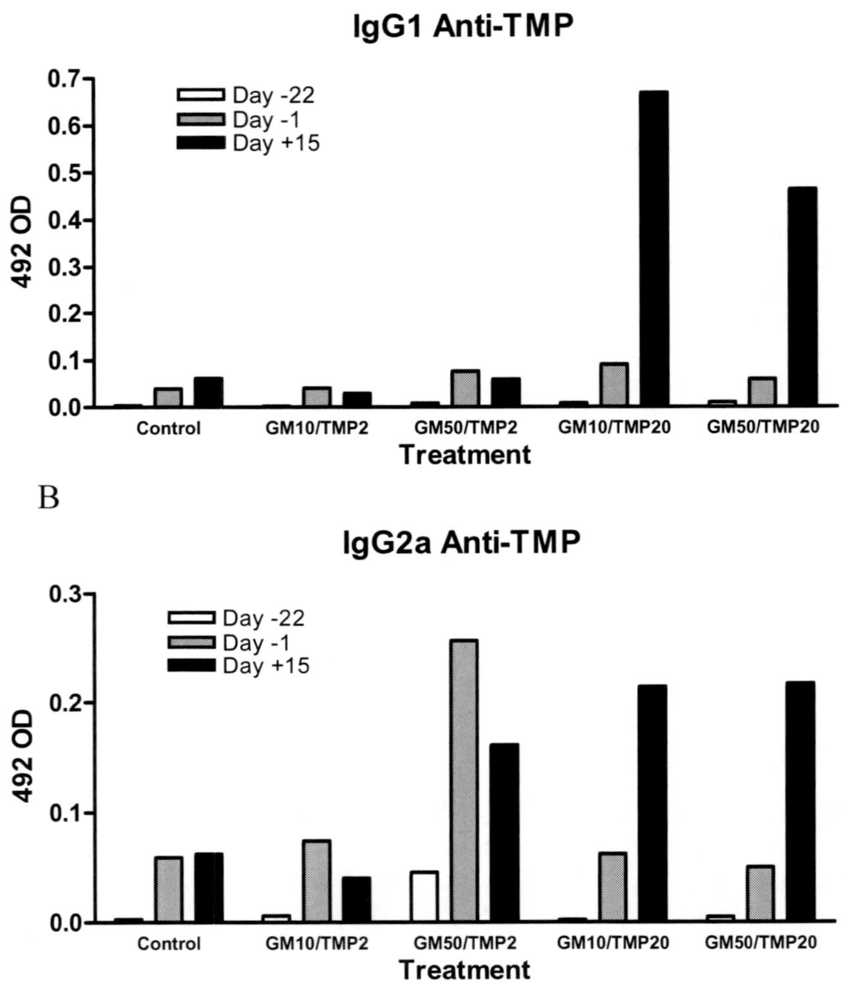

Figure 6. Specific anti-TMP IgG subclasses in lipopolyplexes vaccine. The same protocol as described in Fig. 5 was used, this time for IgG1 subclass (A) and IgG2a subclass (B).

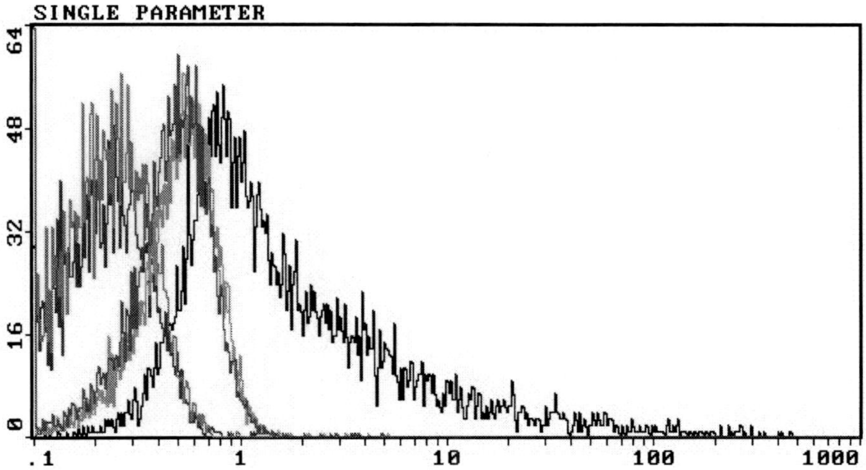

Figure 7. Flow cytometry of p2F m-gmcsf+mB7.2 transfected B16 cells. Groups of B16 cells were passed through the cytometer: a) non-transfected wild type B16 cells, without antibodies; and b) non-transfected wild type B16 cells incubated with both antibodies, both corresponding to the left peaks. Corresponding to the middle peak: c) B16-p2F m-gmcsf + m-B7.2 transfected cells, without antibodies, d) B16-p2F m-gmcsf + m-B7.2 transfected cells, only with primary antibody, e) B16-p2F m-gmcsf + m-B7.2 transfected cells, only with secondary antibody. Finally, f) B16-p2F m-gmcsf + m-B7.2 transfected cells, with both primary and secondary antibody, corresponding to the right peak. The figure plots counts versus FL1 log.

Cell Vaccine Employing Non-Selected Freshly Transfected Cells

The aim of this experiment was to evaluate the efficacy of the antitumor vaccine with genetically engineered tumor cells, expressing cytokines such as mGM-CSF and mB7.2. Thus, $2x10^5$ B16 cells previously transfected (p2F∅, B7.2, GM, GM+B7.2/200), irradiated (150 Gy) and frozen, were injected on days -21, -7 and +15 with 100 μl DMEM. For p2F m-gmcsf + m-B7.2 treatments, two different cell doses were studied: one with the usual cell dose ($2x10^5$), GM+B7.2/200; and another with cells sufficient to reach the same GM-CSF production as in the GM group, according to the ELISA experiments of GM-CSF production (data not shown), i.e., group GM+B7.2/500 ($5x10^5$ cells). In the B16* group, $2x10^5$ irradiated wild type B16 cells (150 Gy) were injected, and in the Control group, only DMEM was injected for each dose. The best results (Figure 8) were obtained employing GM+B7.2/200 and GM alone groups, since no tumor development was observed (marked with arrows in the figure) in any of the animals with those treatments 23 days after tumor implantation, when animals from other groups had started to die. In the figure,"a" corresponds to the maximum statistically significant difference, P= 0.001, and "b" represents P= 0.01, both versus the Control group. The survival curves of these groups are shown in Figure 9, and were consistent with the tumor inhibition results. In group GM, 100% mice survival was observed more than three months after tumor transplant. The GM+B7.2/200, GM+B7.2/500 and B7.2 groups achieved 80, 40 and 20% survival, respectively. Groups B16* and p2F Ø failed to increase survival versus the control group.

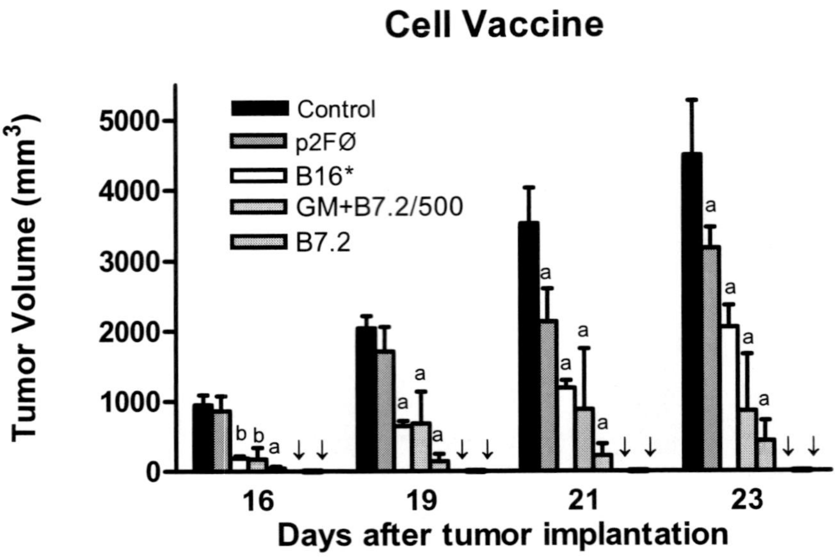

Figure 8. Cell vaccine. The freshly transfected (non-selected) cell vaccine followed the same pattern as in Fig. 2. Treatment groups were $2x10^5$ B16 cells (previously transfected, irradiated and frozen, then thawed and counted) per dose (groups p2F∅, B7.2, GM, GM+B7.2/200) per mouse, in 100μl DMEM. For p2F m-gmcsf + m-B7.2 treatment, two different cell doses were studied: one with the usual cell dose ($2x10^5$), GM+B7.2/200; and the other with cells sufficient to reach the same GM-CSF production as in group GM, i.e., GM+B7.2/500. In the B16* group, $2x10^5$ wild type irradiated B16 cells (150 Gy) were injected in 100 μl DMEM, while in the Control group only 100 μl DMEM, at every three vaccination dose. Arrows show the position in the figure of groups GM, GM+B7.2/200, which developed no tumors at all. The symbol "a" represents P<0.001, and "b" P<0.01, statistically significant difference versus the Control group.

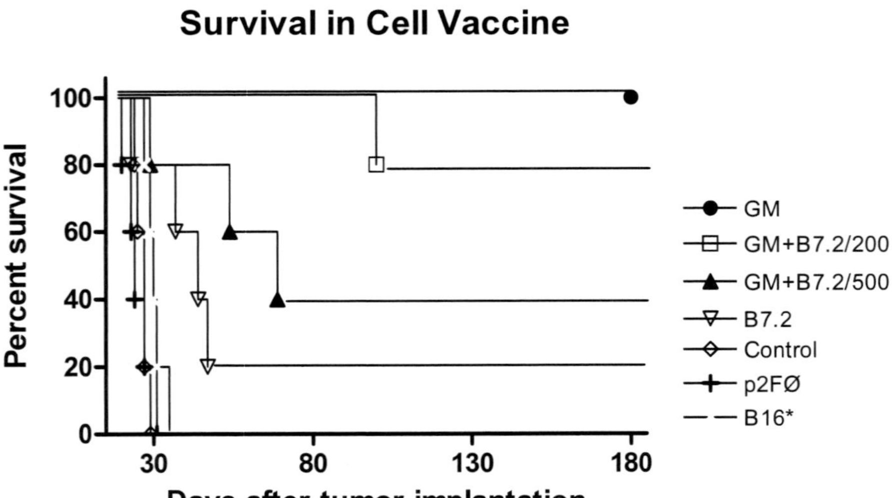

Figure 9. Survival in cell vaccine. As in Fig. 4, the figure plots the survival curves of mice from the Cell Vaccine experiment. In group GM, 100% mice survival was observed more than 3 months after tumor transplant. The GM+B7.2/200, GM+B7.2/500 and B7.2 groups achieved 80, 40 and 20% survival, respectively. The groups B16* and p2F Ø failed to increase survival versus the Control group.

Figure 10 shows the total specific IgG found in the plasma of the animals from this experiment, as explained also for Figure 5. All the groups showed the highest production on day +15, the best performance corresponding to the groups containing GM-CSF in the transfection. In addition, the study of IgG1 and IgG2a subtypes supports the same idea. GM-CSF transfection must contribute to the efficacy of the antitumor response in a significant way, while B7.2 exerts a more limited effect, and no synergistic effect was observed with GM-CSF gene.

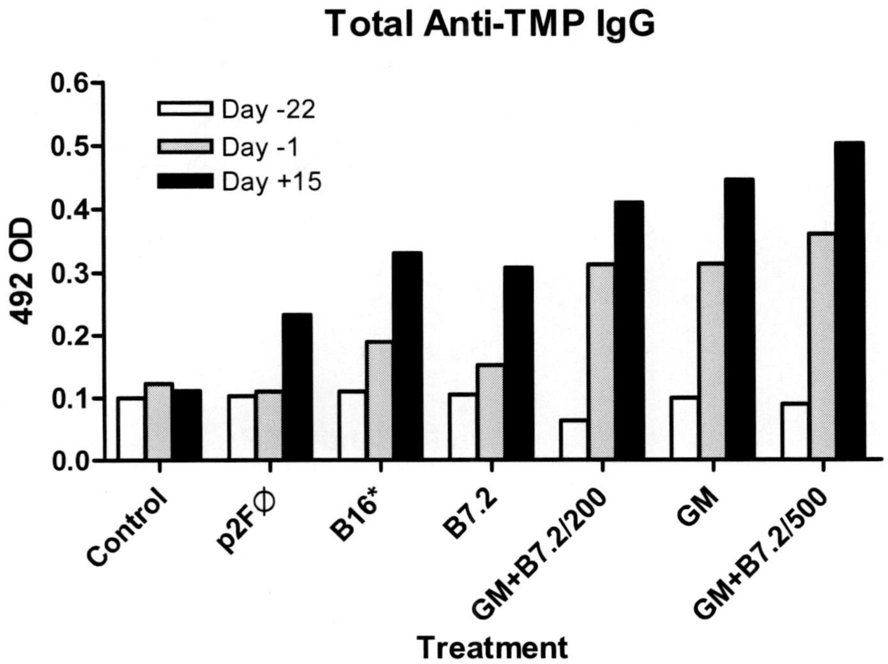

Figure 10. Total anti-TMP IgG production in cell vaccine. As in Fig. 5, this figure shows the specific anti-TMP total IgG from the different groups. Data were obtained from ELISA made with the plasma obtained on days -21, -1 and +15, with respect to tumor injection (day 0).

Expression-Selected Cell Vaccine

Since the maximal efficacy of our non-viral transfection procedure was 20-40% of the cells, we must expect that the non-transfected cells (80-60%) contribute poorly to vaccine efficacy. Therefore, we thought that our previous procedure, employing non-selected transfected cells, could be improved if only the cytokine-expressing cells, selected by magnetic beads purification, were used in the vaccine. For this purpose, we designed the experiments employing both GM-CSF and B7.2, due to their contribution to antitumor vaccine success and the B7.2 protein membrane location serving for cell magnetic selection. Thus, two groups were established: Control (100 μl DMEM) and GM+B7.2/40, employing only 40,000 selected cells per dose, in 100 μl DMEM.

A

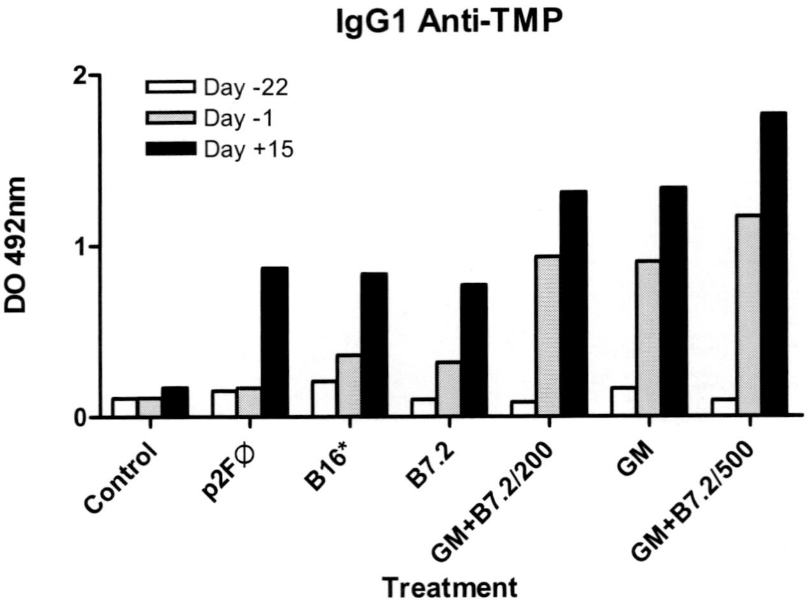

B

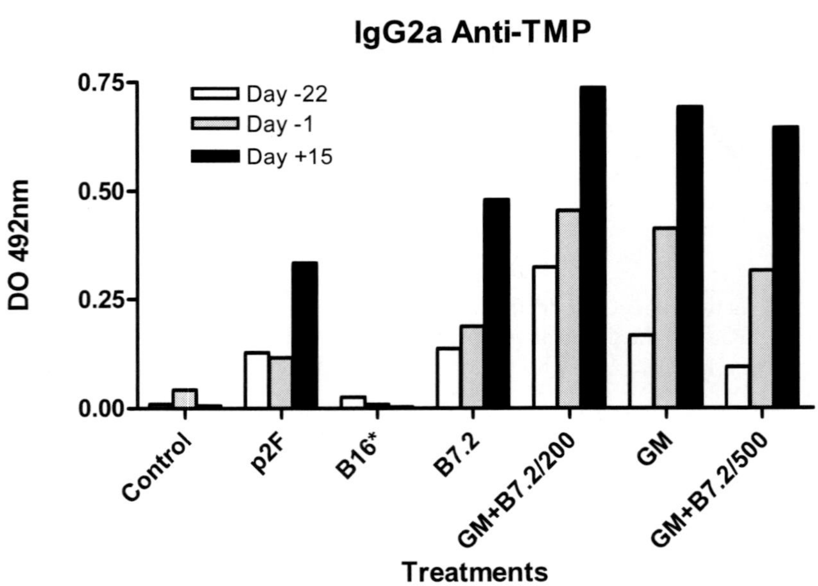

Figure 11. Specific anti-TMP IgG subclasses in cell vaccine. Following the same protocol as in Fig. 5, IgG1 analysis (A) and IgG2a (B) were performed.

The tumor growth inhibition results of the Selected Cells Vaccine are shown in Figure 12. The results on each measurement day were maximally significant (a= $P<0.001$), achieving reductions of more than 80% in tumor volume. These results are consistent with increased survival (Figure 13) in the GM+B7.2/40 group.

The total specific anti-TMP IgG and the IgG1 and IgG2a subtypes are shown in Figures 14-A and B, respectively. The immunoglobulin levels are again consistent with the tumor growth inhibition and survival data.

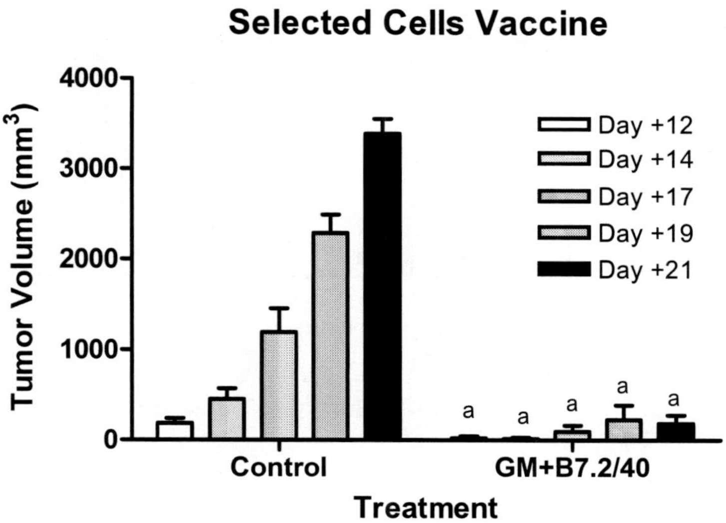

Figure 12. Selected cells vaccine. The tumor growth inhibition obtained in this vaccine is represented. Control and GM+B7.2/40 group, which is 40,000 selected by expression transfected B16 cells. The selection is made by Streptavidin microbeads, thanks to m-B7.2 surface expression. The symbol "a" represents P<0.001, statistically significant difference versus the Control group, where only DMEM was injected at each dose.

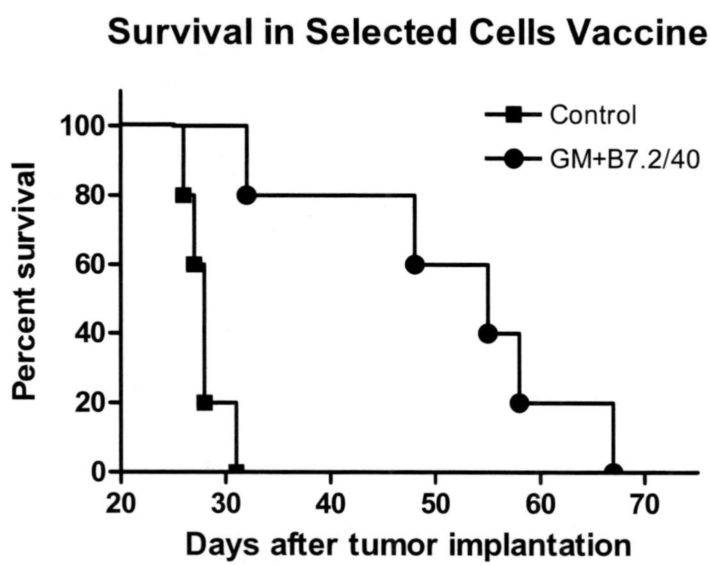

Figure 13. Survival in selected cells vaccine. As in Fig. 4, the survival curves are plotted.

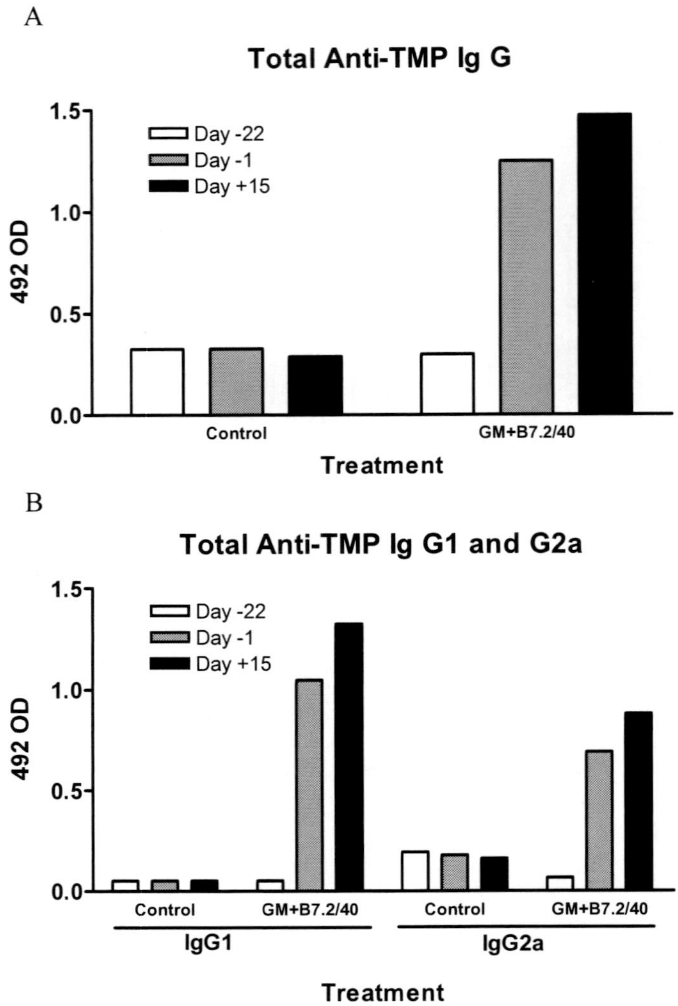

Figure 14. Specific anti-TMP IgG in selected cells vaccine. As in Fig. 5, the total IgG production (A) and the subclasses IgG1 and IgG2a (B) are represented in the graphs.

Conclusion

The aim of this work has been to try to improve the antitumor vaccine methods in order to establish the easiest and most efficient protocol. Engineered cells secreting cytokines have been widely demonstrated to be the most effective vaccines [1-7,9,11], as we have also seen [8,10,12], though we are aware of the great difficulty of working with this approach in actual clinical practice. In effect, taking cells from the patients that also must be kept in culture, amplified to a larger number, transfected and then returned to the same patient, guaranteeing sterility, no contamination, an acceptable number of cells, as well as cytokine production, is not an easy task. This is why we decided to focus effort on two different fronts. The first involved an attempt to reduce the cell number required to start a proper immune response against the tumor, thus avoiding very complex cell work in future patients. The second front focusing our effort is more difficult, because not so good results have been achieved with this kind of procedure to date [13,16], i.e., forgetting about cells and returning to the origins: vaccines made only of components supposed to be necessary, i.e., tumor antigens derived from cell membrane proteins (TMP) and plasmids containing the *gm-csf and B7.2* genes.

For the antigens approach, we studied the antitumor efficacy of several models: TMP alone, TMP encapsulated in liposomes, and finally lipopolyplexes bearing both TMP antigens and the GM-CSF cytokine gene. After choosing the best liposome type, we performed two vaccination experiments and conclude that although the tumor growth inhibitions were similar in the best groups from the three models, the best survival results were obtained with the lipopolyplexes comprising liposomes PC:CH:DP and polyplex PEI:p2F *m-gmcsf*, containing 20 μg TMP and 10 μg of the plasmid per dose. These results were also reflected in mice IgG production, not only in terms of total production but also in terms of the IgG1 and IgG2a subtypes. It should be noted that the groups with the higher TMP dose in the lipopolyplexes showed a later maximum production of IgG2a (day +15), while the groups with the lower TMP dose peaked earlier (day-1). However, this difference is apparently not correlated to survival. In contrast, high and low GM-CSF doses, which discriminated between better or worse survival results, did not have significant effect upon IgG2a plasma levels, suggesting that while IgG switching should be interesting for cell memory induction and antitumor response activation, this effect must be limited and other mechanisms must be involved in a negative regulation [7].

The best results were obtained with the cell vaccine approach on vaccinating with $2x10^5$ transfected cells, 100% and 80% survival levels were achieved in GM and GM+B7.2/200 groups, respectively. This cell vaccine also confirms the idea that higher amounts of GM-CSF production are not necessarily better [4,6,7]; on the contrary, GM+B7.2/500 induced poorer survival results than GM+B7.2/200, which had half the GM-CSF production. However, we think that synergistic effects between GM-CSF and B7.2 must exist, due to the good survival response promoted by the GM+B7.2/200 group. Again, the GM-CSF transfected cell groups showed the highest IgG productions. In this vaccine, a good correlation was observed between IgG response and survival, mainly in relation to the IgG2a subtype. Finally, from all these experiments, we must consider that in some cases the humoral response may not show a good correlation to survival, probably due to other phenomena such as regulatory T cell immune suppression.

Since the survival results suggest that cell vaccines achieve significant antitumor effects, we made additional efforts to improve the efficacy of the procedure by reducing the cell number required for each vaccine dose. In this respect, we knew that only 20-40% of the cells that we had employed in cell vaccination were transfected, and for this reason we designed new vaccine experiments employing only the cytokine-expressing cells. Thus, we made use of the B7.2 surface membrane expression strategy because it has been shown in our experiments and in the literature [18-24] to be helpful and even synergistic with GM-CSF in some cases. Moreover, its location in the cell could help us select the cells expressing the protein on their membranes, i.e., only the transfected cells. The aim of the experiment was to determine whether only the transfected cells (20% of $2x10^5$ = 40,000 cells) were able to mediate the same successful results as those obtained in nonselected-cell vaccines. The selected cells vaccine showed a very significant tumor growth reduction employing only 40,000 cells, and this reduction correlated to a longer survival and good IgG response of the treated mice. Although the results were not as good as those with the non-selected cells vaccine, no conclusions can be drawn before a dose-dependent study is made. It remains to be elucidated how synergistic effects between antigens, GM-CSF and costimulatory B7.2 molecules cooperate in the generation of efficient antitumor response or toxicity. We cannot exclude a lack of net antigen contribution due to the reduction in cell number or, contrarily, an excess in GM-CSF production which could result in a loss of vaccine efficacy. These experiments will focus our future attention, and will contribute to clarify the exact need of each component in a cell vaccine that could become suitable for use in clinical practice.

Acknowledgments

This work has been partially supported by the *Ministerio de Educación y Ciencia* SAF 2004-08161 and SAF 2007-64492 and the *Generalitat Valenciana* GVACOMP 2006-217.

References

[1] Dunussi-Joannopoulos K, Dranoff G, Weinstein HJ, Ferrara JLM, Bierer BE, Croop JM. Gene immunotherapy in murine acute myeloid leukemia: granulocyte-macrophage colony-stimulating factor tumor cell vaccines elicit more potent antitumor immunity compared with B7 family and other cytokine vaccines. *Blood*, 1998, Vol 91, No 1, 222-230.

[2] Mastrangelo MJ & Lattime EC. Virotherapy clinical trials for regionale disease: *in situ* immune modulation using recombinant poxvirus vectors. *Cancer Gene Therapy*, 2002, 9, 1013-1021.

[3] Se-Heon K, Carew JF, Kooby DA, Shields J, Entwisle C, Patel S, Shah JP, Fong Y. *Cancer Gene Therapy*, 2000, Vol 7, No 9, 1279-1285.

[4] Borrello I & Pardoll D. *Cytokine and Growth Factor Reviews*, 2002, 13, 185-193.

[5] Jaffee EM, Abrams R, Cameron J et al. A phase I clinical trial of lethally irradiated allogeneic pancreatic tumor cells transfected with the GM-CSF gene for the treatment of pancreatic adenocarcinoma. *Human Gene Therapy*, 1998, 9, 1951-1971.

[6] Serafini P, Carbley R, Noonan KA, Tan G, Bronte V, Borrello I. High-dose granulocyte-macrophage colony-stimulating factor-producing vaccines impair the immune response through the recruitment of myeloid suppressor cells. *Cancer Research*, 2004, 64, 6337-6343.

[7] Rodríguez-Lecompte JC, Kruth S et al. Cell-based cancer gene therapy: breaking tolerante or inducing autoimmunity? *Anim Health Res Rev.*, 2004, Dec; 5(2), 227-234.

[8] Herrero MJ, Botella R, Dasí F, Algás R, Sánchez M, Aliño SF. Antigens and cytokine genesin antitumor vaccines: the importance of teh temporal delivery sequence in antitumor signals. *Ann. N.Y. Acad. Sci.*, 2006, 1091, 412-424.

[9] Shi FS, Weber S, Gan J, Rakhmilevich A, Mahvi DM. Granulocyte-macrophage colony-stimulating factor (GM-CSF) secreted by cDNA-transfected tumor cells induces a more potent antitumor response than exogenous GM-CSF. *Cancer Gene Therapy*, 1999, Vol 6, 81-88.

[10] Moret-Tatay I, Diaz J, Marco FM, Crespo A, Aliño SF. Complete tumor prevention by engineered tumor cell vaccines employing nonviral vactors. *Cancer Gene therapy*, 2003, 10, 887-897.

[11] Wiley, J and sons, Ltd. Gene Therapy Clinical Trials Worldwide. 2007. Available from: www.wiley.co.uk/genmed/clinical

[12] Moret-Tatay I, Sanmartín I, Marco FM, Díaz J, Aliño SF. Nonviral therapeutic cell vaccine mediates potent antitumor effects. *Vaccine*. 2006, 24, 3937-3945.

[13] Aliño SF, Lejarreta M et al. Antimetastatic effect of immunization with liposome-encapsualted tumor cell-membrane proteins obtained from experimental tumors. *Immunopharmacology and immunotoxicology*, 1995, 17 (3), 419-436.

[14] Guillem VM, Tormo M, et al. Targeted oligonucleotide delivery in human lymphoma cell lines using a polyethileneimine based immunopolyplex. *Journal of controlled release*, 2002, 83, 133-146.

[15] Guillem VM, Tormo M, et al. Polyethyleneimine-based immunopolyplex for targeted gene transfer in human lymphoma cell lines. *The Journal of Gene Medicine*, 2002, 4, 170-182.

[16] Massó O, Aliño SF et al. Specific serological response by active immunization with GD3-bearing liposomes. *The Journal of Pharmacology and Experimental Therapeutics*, 1996, 278(3), 1114-1120.

[17] Garcia L, Bunuales M, Duzgunes N, Tros de Ilarduya C. Serum-resistant lipopolyplexes for gene delivery to liver tumor cells. *Eur J Pharm Biopharm*, 2007.

[18] Zajac P, Oertli W at al. Phase I/II Clinical trial of a nonreplicative vaccinia virus expressing multiple HLA-A0201-restricted tumor-associated epitopoes and costimulatory molecules in metastatic melanoma patients. *Human Gene Therapy*, 2003, 14, 1497-1510.

[19] Chong H, Todryk S et al. Tumor cell expression of B7 costimulatory molecules and interleukin-12 or granulocyte-macrophage colony-stimulating factor induces a local antitumor response and may generate systemis protective immunity. 1998, *Gene Therapy*, 5, 223-232.

[20] Pizzoferrato E. B7-2 expression above a threshold elicits anti-tumor immunity as effective as interleukin-12 and prolongs survival in murine B-cell lymphoma. *Int J Cancer*, 2004, 110, 61-69.

[21] Kim k-Y, Kang M-A, Nam M-J. Enhancement of natural killer cell-mediated cytotoxicity by coexpression of GM-CSF/B70 in hepatoma. *Cancer Letters*, 2001, 166, 33-40.

[22] Grosenbach DW, Barrientos JC, et al. Synergy of vaccine strategies to amplify antigen-specific immune responses and antitumor effects. *Cancer Research*, 2001, 61, 4497-4505.

[23] Parney IF, Farr-Jones MA et al. Human autologous in vitro models of glioma immunogene therapy using B7-2, GM-CSF and IL-12. *Can J Neurol Sci*, 2002, 29(3), 267-275.

[24] Mukherjee S, Nelson D, et al. The immune anti-tumor effects of GM-CSF and B7-1 gene transfection are enhanced by surgical debulking of tumor. *Cancer Gene Therapy*, 2001, 8, 580-588.

[25] Bordier C. Phase separation of integral membrane proteins in Triton X-114 solution. *J Biol Chem*. 1981, 25, 1604-1607.

[26] Guillem VM & Aliño SF. Transfection pathways of nonspecific and targeted PEI-polyplexes. *Gene Therapy and Molecular Biology*, 2004, Vol 8, 369-384.

[27] Walde P & Ichikawa S. Enzymes inside lipid vesicles: preparation, reactivity and applications. *Biomolecular Engineering*, 2001, 18, 143-177.

[28] Moret I, Peris JE, Guillem VM, Benet M, Revert F, Dasí F, Crespo A, Aliño SF. Stability of PEI-DNA and DOTAP-DNA complexes: effect of alkaline pH, heparin and serum. *Journal of controlled Release,* 2001, 76, 169-181.

In: Vaccinations: Types, Potential Complications...
Editors: D. B. Steen and H. L. Dyson
ISBN: 978-1-60692-969-8

Chapter X

New Vaccination Strategies for the Improvement of DNA Vaccines Against Virus in Fish*

***Carolina Tafalla*[1,*]*, Amparo Estepa*[2] *and Julio Coll*[3]**
[1.]Centro de Investigación en Sanidad Animal (CISA-INIA). Carretera de Algete a El Casar km. 8,1. Valdeolmos 28130. Madrid, Spain
[2.]Instituto de Biología Molecular y Celular (IBMC). Universidad Miguel Hernández. Elche. Alicante, Spain
[3].SGIT, INIA, Biotecnología, Carretera de La Coruña km. 7. 28040 Madrid, Spain

Abstract

Vaccination seems like the most adequate method to control viral diseases in aquacultured fish. Up to date, very few viral vaccines are commercialised, since it has been a difficult task to obtain effective vaccines in fish that are both safe and cost-effective. In the past years, DNA vaccination has been proven as a very effective method to control some rhabdoviral infections, such as those caused by infectious hematopoietic necrosis virus (IHNV) and viral hemorrhagic septicemia virus (VHSV), responsible for great losses in aquaculture production. These vaccines consisting in a plasmid in which the viral glycoprotein gene is expressed under the control of the citomegalovirus (CMV) promoter, are able to confer protection in fish after intramuscular injection. Even though the protection conferred is high and long-lasting, these vaccines are still not being used worldwide due to safety issues concerning the viral promoter, to difficulties in the administration of the vaccine at a large scale, and to high vaccination costs. Up to date, only an IHNV DNA vaccine has been licensed for use in Canada.

* * A version of this chapter was also published in *Aquaculture Research Trends*, edited by Stephen H. Schwartz published by Nova Science Publishers, Inc. It was submitted for appropriate modifications in an effort to encourage wider dissemination of research.

* Correspomding author : Tel. +34-91-6202300 / Fax +34-91-6202247 Email: tafalla@inia.es

Moreover, the immune mechanism through which they confer protection is still unknown, and this is a major restriction for the optimisation of DNA vaccines for other viral pathogens also of great importance in fish, such as for example nodavirus, for which DNA vaccines as formulated for rhabdovirus are not effective.
In this chapter, we discuss the trends in research dealing with DNA vaccination in fish, that will hopefully allow the improvement and finally the routine use of these vaccines in aquaculture. These will include the possible use of molecular adjuvants; the use of attenuated mutant glycoprotein genes and studies dealing with conformation versus lineal epitopes; the substitution of the CMV promoter for promoters of a non-viral origin; the use of induced plasmids or fish transposons, the study of new mass vaccination methods, or the inclusion of specific siRNA sequences within the plasmid. As well, we will review the most recent advances in studies related to the immune response towards these vaccines, some of them based on microarray technologies, that may help elucidate the immune mechanisms responsible for protection.

Introduction

One of the major problems for aquaculture is the impact that infectious diseases have on production. Among the different infectious agents, viruses are the major concern for the aquaculture industry since they usually produce very high mortalities upon infection and there are no effective treatments available such as antibiotics for bacterial infections.

Rhabdoviruses constitute one of the largest groups of viruses isolated from teleost fish, and include viruses such as infectious hematopoietic necrosis virus (IHNV) that affects different salmonid species like rainbow trout *Oncorhynchus mykiss*, Atlantic salmon *Salmo salar* or sockeye salmon *Oncorhynchus nerka* among others; and viral hemorrhagic septicemia virus (VHSV) that affects many salmonid (rainbow trout, Atlantic salmon, sockeye salmon, etc…), as well as many other non-salmonid and / or marine species (turbot *Scophthalmus maximus*, Atlantic cod *Gadus morhua*, etc…) [1]. Both IHNV and VHSV are responsible for great losses in aquaculture production, and even though IHNV was initially confined to America and VHSV was restricted to Europe, at the moment they are both spread worldwide. Moreover, rhabdoviruses not only affect fish at the early stages of development as most other viruses that infect fish, but can also produce a high percentage of mortality in adult fish of high economic value. Among other viruses affecting fish, infectious pancreatic necrosis virus (IPNV), a member of the *Birnaviridae* family, is also responsible for high mortalities, specially in salmonid fry [2], although it can also infect many other fresh water and marine species [3, 4]. Infectious salmon anaemia virus (ISAV), an orthomyxovirus, is a great problem for the salmon industry as well [5]. Regarding marine species, especially those held in moderate-warm water temperatures, nodavirus are nowadays a major concern [6-8]. Other virus belonging to the Togavirus, Aquareovirus, Iridovirus and Retrovirus families can also infect different fish species, but are a much lesser problem at a global scale [3].

There are no specific agents for the treatment of any of these diseases, consequently, the use of preventive measures such as vaccination seems as the most adequate method to control these viral agents in aquacultured fish [6]. Despite extensive research over many years, very few anti-viral vaccines are available. For instance, in China and Japan, an inactivated vaccine against spring viremia of the carp virus (SVCV), another fish rhabdovirus and a recombinant protein vaccine against red seabream iridovirus have been respectively licensed. In both Chile and Norway, different variants of a polyvalent vaccine against IPNV consisting in the recombinant VP2 viral protein are commercialised by different companies. One live attenuated VHSV vaccine is licensed in Germany, although its effectiveness is really limited. Most recently, the first DNA vaccine has been approved for use in Canada against IHNV (APEX-IHN, Vical Inc. San Diego CA).

In fact, the most efficient vaccines developed against viral diseases in fish to date are DNA vaccines against rhabdoviruses [9]. These vaccines are based on a naked DNA plasmid coding for the rhabdoviral G glycoprotein gene under the control of the cytomegalovirus promoter (CMV). After intramuscular injection, plasmids are taken by muscle cells, and the viral G glycoprotein is expressed on the surface of muscle cells [9-12]. The gene encoding the G protein was chosen for rhabdovirus DNA vaccines because this is the protein against which protective neutralizing host antibodies are directed [13]. Accordingly, efficient vaccination upon intramuscular injection was only observed with the inclusion glycoprotein G gene and other rhabdoviral genes failed to induce protection [14]. Protection levels of more than 95 % have been obtained with these DNA vaccines [9, 11, 15-21], while the injection of trout with recombinant rhabdoviral G proteins produced in *Escherichia coli* [22, 23], yeast [23] or baculovirus [24] have not been able to confer good protection levels. Furthermore, DNA vaccines have been proved effective not only for VHSV and IHNV, but for all fish rhabdovirus tested: SVCV [25] and other more exotic rhabdovirus such as hirame rhabdovirus (HIRRV) [26] and snakehead rhabdovirus (SHRV) [25].

Although DNA vaccines have also been assayed for some other fish viruses, their effectiveness and the state of knowledge of their mechanism of action are actually very limited. For instance, for IPNV, five different plasmids coding for different regions of the segment A of the viral genome were tested [27], finding that the full segment A had to be included in the plasmid in order to obtain some protection. For ISAV, a DNA vaccine coding for the viral hemagglutinin-esterase gene only showed moderate protection [28]. Different open reading frames (ORFs) for early and late genes of channel catfish herpesvirus (IHV-1) were also tested with two of them inducing some protection [29]. For nodavirus, the recombinant capsid protein conferred protection while a plasmid coding for this same protein was not effective [30]. This last result is surprising, since even rhabdoviral DNA vaccines conferred protection against nodavirus at early times post-vaccination [8].

Even though, in the case of rhabdovirus, the protection conferred is high and relatively long-lasting, these vaccines are still not being used worldwide due to safety issues, mostly concerning the viral regulatory sequences present in plasmids, to difficulties in the administration of the vaccine at a large scale (mass vaccination methods) and to relatively high vaccination costs for fingerlings. In this chapter, we discuss the new trends in research dealing with DNA vaccination in fish, which might hopefully improve and finally allow their routine use in aquaculture. We have included possible improvements in the DNA vaccine formulations which might contribute to an increased effectiveness such as the potential use of molecular adjuvants, attenuated pathogen mutant genes, new non-viral promoters, inducible plasmid vectors, fish transposons or the inclusion of specific siRNA sequences as hairpin DNA, as well as trends in the possible search for new mass vaccination methods (Figure 1). Moreover, we have reviewed the most recent studies related to the early and late immune response towards these vaccines which may help elucidate the immune mechanisms responsible for protection and produce new ideas to improve DNA vaccination for rhabdovirus as well as for other fish viruses.

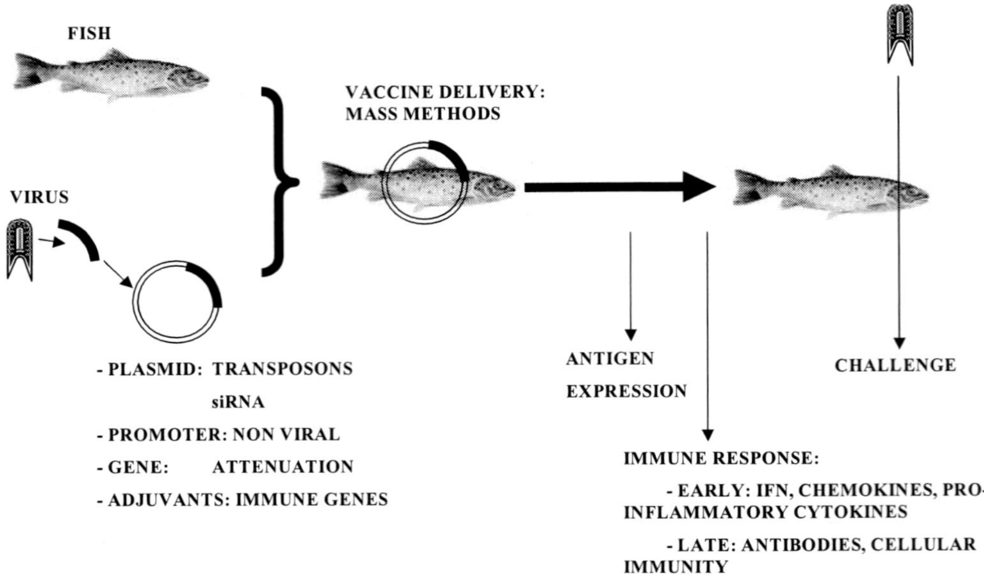

Figure 1. Research areas to be explored concerning fish DNA vaccination. The main elements to be taken into account for improvement of fish DNA vaccines include the vaccine plasmid (possible modifications in the type of promoter; use of adjuvants; attenuation of viral genes, possible use of transposons, siRNA etc.). Concerning the vaccine delivery, new mass delivery systems need to be optimised (oral or bath administration seem as the most suitable methods). From studies concerning the immune response to vaccination, new adjuvants might be elucidated.

Immune Response to DNA Vaccination

At the moment, the immune mechanism(s) responsible for the protection conferred by injected DNA vaccines are still unknown. Moreover, DNA vaccines seem to be more effective in fish, that in other mammalian models [6], making difficult that studies performed in mammals may serve as a guide for what might be happening in fish. It seems however, that DNA vaccines are to some extent able to mimic the natural infection and thus produce high levels of protection [9, 11, 15-21].

Antigen-specific immune responses induced by DNA vaccines are elicited by the intramuscular inoculation of a plasmid containing foreign DNA expressed under the control of a viral promoter [31]. Because the inoculated genes (the antigens) are expressed intracellularly, epitope peptides are presented on MHC class I molecules, and are therefore capable of stimulating $CD8^+$ T cells. These gene products expressed by muscle cells are also phagocytosed by antigen presenting cells (APCs) and are either cross-presented on MHC class I molecules or presented by MHC class II molecules, inducing $CD4^+$ T cell responses [32]. DNA vaccines also induce the expression of co-stimulatory molecules on APCs, probably because the vaccine plasmids are recognised as bacterial DNA through the presence of specific "danger" motifs, leading to the initiation of a strong immune response [33]. Whether immunogenic plasmids directly transfect APCs or only muscle cells which then present the antigen to APCs has been the subject of considerable debate [32].

Non-Specific Early Stage of Protection

DNA vaccines against salmonid rhabdoviruses once intramuscularly injected induce an early stage of protection as soon as 4-7 days post-vaccination. During this period, protection is not only observed against the virus against which fish were vaccinated, but also against heterologous viruses [17], even to virus from families different than rhabdovirus, such as nodavirus [8] although not against bacterial pathogens [12]. No cross-protection was observed however, when fish were vaccinated with a plasmid coding for the G protein of rabies virus, a mammalian rhabdovirus [17]. All these results suggest that a non-specific but exclusively viral immune mechanism is responsible for protection at this early stage, because specific antibodies (Abs) and / or cellular responses are not developed in most fish species until at least two weeks post-immunization [34].

Type I interferon (IFN) seems like a solid candidate for being responsible for most if not all of the early protection induced by DNA vaccines. Since IFN genes were not identified in fish up until recently, most studies performed with DNA vaccines so far involved the analysis of the IFN-induced Mx gene expression. It has been demonstrated that Mx was induced in response to DNA vaccination [20, 35, 36] and correlation between the levels of Mx expression and the levels of trout early protection was observed by using a VHSV DNA vaccine [20]. However, in a further study Mx synthesis was not detectable until day 7 and its higher level of expression was reached 14 days post-vaccination [36]. In most species various isoforms of Mx proteins are present. In fish, three isoforms have been identified in rainbow trout [37] or Atlantic salmon [38], but studies concerning the differential regulation have not been approached for most of them, although differential antiviral activity has been demonstrated for human, murine and rat isoforms [39]. Moreover, some Mx isoforms do not seem to have antiviral activity, such as human MxB that exclusively plays a role in the control of the cell cycle [40]. In rainbow trout, we have recently demonstrated differential regulation of the three trout Mx isoforms depending on the cell or tissue cell type rather than to the stimuli used [41], however no antiviral activity against viruses has been demonstrated yet for any of the Mx isoforms [37]. Polymorphisms (variations of amino acid sequences) should also be taken into account when studying these immune early genes, and specially Mx, since differences in activity among polymorphisms have been observed in other species, with some polymorphisms having high and some low or even absent antiviral activity [42-44].

To date, it has been demonstrated that IFN is induced in response to DNA vaccines as expected from Mx studies [45], but as for Mx, different genes have identified for most fish species [46, 47], and studies concerning the role of each of the forms in protection have not been performed and should be carried out. In rainbow trout, for example, one of the IFN genes identified does not have an apparent antiviral activity [47]. Moreover, there are many other genes different than Mx with a direct antiviral role that are induced in response to IFN. In fact, more than 1000 genes are induced in a cell in response to IFN [48]. Therefore, in order to establish whether the protection conferred by DNA vaccination at this early stage is dependent of the IFN expression system at some point, much more work needs to be performed involving functional studies of Mx and IFN genes taking into account polymorphisms, as well as studies concerning other IFN-induced genes.

Specific Late Stage of Protection

After this stage of early non-specific immune protection, there is a later stage at which fish are specifically protected only against the virus they were DNA vaccinated for. The switching time from early (non-specific) to late (specific) immune response varies depending on the size of the trout, the dosage of challenge, the dosage of vaccine and the temperature [20, 49, 50]. It has been demonstrated that at this later stage, both humoral (Abs) [15] and cellular [51, 52] immune responses are induced. However, at this late stage again the mechanisms responsible for the protection are still unknown, since induced neutralizing Ab titers as estimated by *in vitro* assays did not always correlate with *in vivo* protection levels. For example, *in vitro* neutralizing Abs induced by injection of the G gene of VHSV could only be detected for up to 6 months after immunization, whereas protection lasted longer than 9 months [20]. Possible explanations for this lack of correlation could be that: i) the *in vitro* techniques used do not detect all induced neutralizing Abs with enough sensitivity; ii) some non-neutralizing Abs *in vitro* could be neutralizing *in vivo,* as it happened with some monoclonal Abs [53] or iii) there are other specific mechanisms mediating the protection such as cellular mechanisms. Not enough evidences are yet available in favour of any of these possible hypotheses.

Studies previously performed with VHSV revealed that it is not so simple to correlate neutralization titers *in vitro* with protection. Even though immunity to VHSV could be transferred by injection of the immunoglobulin M (IgM) fraction of the serum from survivors [54], contradictions still appear in the results. The *in vitro* neutralization assays of trout Abs are restricted to the detection of G conformational-dependent Abs [22, 55, 56], not detectable by immunoblotting [22, 57, 58]. Confirming these results, most G epitopes recognized by neutralizing monoclonal Abs are also conformation-dependent and some of them are even discontinuous in their sequence [59-61]. Attempts to map the B-cell epitopes on the VHSV G by the use of overlapping 15-mer synthetic peptides confirmed that none of the neutralizing monoclonal Abs could be mapped to lineal epitopes [62]. On the other hand, non-neutralizing Abs (those directed towards lineal epitopes) could also induce *in vivo* protection and persist longer than neutralizing Abs [53]. Furthermore, *in vitro* neutralizing Abs do not always correlate with its VHSV protection properties *in vivo* [53, 56, 63] and their *in vitro* neutralization was highly dependent on the VHSV isolate used [64]. Therefore, assays to detect trout Abs directed towards lineal epitopes on the G of VHSV (such as ELISA) or injection of fingerlings for *in vivo* protection assays should be also developed and conducted in vaccinated fish, as a complement to the *in vitro* neutralizing Ab assays.

Moreover, up until recently, teleost Igs were thought to be only of isotype IgM, whereas, we now know that IgD is also produced in fish [65, 66] and that a new exclusive isotype (IgT) is present at least in rainbow trout [67]. No studies have been yet performed on the possible significance of these new molecular species of fish Ig isotypes on the Ab response in vaccination or infection. To make these studies possible, however, more specific monoclonal Abs against the new fish Igs would be required.

Specific late protection to rhabdoviral infections can also be mediated by a delayed cellular memory consisting in both helper and/or cytotoxic activities (T-like cell responses). Up-regulation of MHC class II expression (a sign of T-cell activation) was observed in trout immunized with the G gene [51] and proliferation of kidney cells in response to the antigen encoded by the DNA vaccine was also demonstrated [50]. Recently, it has been shown that immunization of rainbow trout with both DNA encoding the glycoprotein G and the nucleocapsid protein N of VHSV provoked the activation of antiviral cytotoxic cells [68]. Since both VHSV-infected MHC class I mismatched (xenogeneic) and matched target cells were killed, cytotoxicity was probably executed by both cytotoxic cells of the adaptive (CTLs) and innate (NK cells) immune systems. As expected, the VHSV G protein was more potent in the triggering of cell-mediated immune responses than the VHSV N protein. Despite these studies, much more efforts on research in this area need to be made to elucidate the role of cellular immunity on antiviral protection.

With the use of microarrays, a technology is now available to study new genes involved in immune response induced by DNA vaccines. To design which fish sequences could be included in the microarrays, orthologous immune-related genes mapped in other species might be first selected and compared with fish EST (expressed sequence tags). This compared analysis will help identify the existence of possible candidate sequences not yet identified or mapped in the selected genome, but present in the genome maps of other fish or mammalian species. The cDNA obtained from tissue mRNA (transcriptomes) and / or oligo probes defined from EST fish sequences could be also used in microarrays. There are only a few examples where cDNA microarrays were used to compare transcriptomes obtained from DNA vaccinated and non-vaccinated samples [69-71]. As an example of the information that the use of microarrays gives concerning DNA vaccination [69, 70], by vaccinating Japanese flounder with a rhaddoviral G gene DNA vaccine and comparing it to fish vaccinated with the empty plasmid, using a cDNA chip with a total of 779 flounder sequences consisting in 228 known immune-related genes and 551 unknown genes, they observed that the greatest number of genes (16.6 %) with changed expression levels was observed at 3 days after injection. Of those 91.4 % were up-regulated (31 % known and 60.4 % unknown). Up-regulated genes include genes related to the non-specific immune response such as Kupffer cell receptor, TNF-α, MIP1α, IL-1 receptor, coagulation factor XIII, CC chemokine receptor, Mx, transcription factors such as IF-induced protein, TAP2 protein, caspase-10d, and even a few genes related to the late specific Ab response such as the CD20 receptor and B cell adhesion molecule. A great number of unknown genes were also up-regulated, in particular one gene was up-regulated 56-fold in vaccinated fish, pointing it as an interesting gene for future research. Even though microarray studies show a great amount of information, all these results will not be of relevance to future applications in vaccine technology if they are not taken as a first step to identify potential genes involved and if no functional studies are performed with the proteins that these genes encode. Moreover, up to date, all the studies performed to study genes regulated upon vaccination have only been performed at early stages post-vaccination. It would be also of great importance to perform these kind of studies after a viral challenge in vaccinated fish at later stages post-vaccination, in order to further studies genes that are involved in the specific immune response. The comparison of the gene response to a virus in vaccinated fish compared to fish susceptible to the disease would be of great importance in determining which genes are relevant in protection.

Possible New Adjuvants for DNA Vaccination

Adjuvants (from the Latin *adjuvare,* to help) are agents capable of increasing the immunogenicity of a vaccine, and thus increasing its effectiveness. Usually they act by increasing the presentation of the antigen to the immune system, or by inducing a slight inflammatory process that activates immune cells, specially antigen presenting cells. For many adjuvants, the mechanism of action remains unclear, and in some cases their discovery has been a matter of trial and error for many years, explaining why alum, an aluminium salt developed in the early 1920s, is still one of the most widely used adjuvant for traditional vaccines. Consequently, there is a major need for safer and more effective adjuvants suitable for human and animal use, and this constitutes a wide field of research that is being explored in different animal models. Moreover, an adjuvant that might be suitable for a vaccination model against one virus, does not necessarily have to be suitable for vaccination against another virus in the same host, since the pathogenesis of the virus has also to be taken into account. Therefore, each new adjuvant should be tested independently for each host, type of vaccine and virus. In this chapter, we review some of the trends in the current search for adjuvants that would be useful for DNA vaccination in fish.

Cytokines

In mammals, different cytokines have been proved to be successful adjuvants for DNA vaccination, while others expected to have positive effects according to their biological activity decreased the protection conferred by the DNA vaccine. For example, co-administration of interleukin 12 (IL-12) within a DNA vaccine resulted in an inhibition of the Ab response, whereas the co-injection of granulocyte-macrophage colony stimulating factor (GM-CSF) enhanced it [72]. Among cytokine adjuvants, chemokines (cytokines with chemoattractant capacity) are those more widely studied for vaccination against viruses in mammals [73-75], since they are not only capable of recruiting more specific cell types to the site of immunization, but they can also drive the immune system to a more favourable response.

In fish, almost no studies on the adjuvant capacity of cytokines have been performed to date, since the state of knowledge of cytokine and chemokine functionality is still scarce compared to mammals, and this is essential for the right choice of genes to be used as adjuvants. The co-administration of mouse GM-CSF had a marked effect on cytotoxic T-cell-like activity in fish by reducing the average number of myocites expressing the antigen [52]. In rainbow trout, our laboratory has studied the effects of the chemokine IL-8 as a potential adjuvant for DNA vaccination against VHSV. We have found that the co-administration of a plasmid coding for rainbow trout IL-8 with a DNA vaccine, increases the expression of pro-inflammatory cytokines such as IL-1β and TNF-α [76]. Moreover, an increase in the levels of expression of other chemokines was also observed [77], suggesting that IL-8 might be an efficient molecular adjuvant for DNA vaccination in fish. However, whether these effects on the immune response to the vaccine correlate with a higher protection still has not been demonstrated (ongoing experiments). A close attention must be given to the doses used, since the optimal dose for immunostimulation may not be the optimal dose for adjuvant activity, as an exaggerated inflammatory response can also be detrimental for the immunization, something widely demonstrated in mammals.

TLR Ligands

Toll-like receptors (TLRs) are a family of invariant pathogen-specific molecular pattern (PAMPS) recognition receptors, that initiate the immune response against a pathogen upon activation [78]. Examples of PAMPs that trigger TLR pathways are lipopolysaccharides (LPS; recognized by TLR4), lipopeptides (by cooperation of TLR2 with TLR1 or TLR6), viral single- or double-stranded RNA (by TLR7 with TLR8 and by TLR3, respectively), bacterial DNA containing CpG motifs (by TLR9) or flagellin (by TLR5). In addition, recent investigations have demonstrated that TLRs are the critical in the linkage between innate and adaptive immunity.

The involvement of TLRs in vaccine responses is explained by the control they exert over the activation of adaptive immunity. This control is mediated through several mechanisms, including maturation of DCs, induction of expression of cytokines and co-stimulatory proteins, and reversal of tolerance [79]. Although the importance of TLR signalling for vaccine response in humans has been demonstrated conclusively only for the OspA vaccine against [80], many promising experimental vaccine strategies for infectious diseases include the use of TLR ligands as adjuvants.

Among TLR ligands, those that have been more thoroughly studied in mammalian systems are the oligodeoxynucleotides containing CpG motifs. These CpG motifs enable the vertebrate immune system to recognise bacterial DNA via TLR 9 since while methylation of bacterial CpG sequences is rare, vertebrates usually methylate most CpG sequences at the 5´position of the cytosine [81]. It has been demonstrated that some of these CpG motifs in the plasmid backbone of DNA vaccines play an important role in the induction of immunity [82], and that the inclusion of additional CpG motifs increase the effectiveness of DNA vaccination [83]. In fish, activation of lymphocyte proliferation [84] and production of immunostimulatory [85, 86] or antiviral [87] factors have been demonstrated by CpG motifs, but few more studies have been performed to test their possible adjuvant activity, except for a study in which a CpG motif known to stimulate mice, increased the Ab response to an antigen in fish when included in the plasmid vector [88]. No other TLR ligands have been assayed in fish so far since fish TLR are poorly characterized to date. In mammalian systems, successful adjuvant activities have also been obtained by using other TLR ligands such as flagellin (as DNA encoding format) [89] as well as TLR adaptor molecules, particularly TRIF [90] and MyD88 [91]. Recently, there have been several studies on fish that have identified many fish orthologs of mammalian TLRs [78, 92-94], that appear to be functionally analogous, therefore, future studies should determine whether or not TLR signalling has a significant role in fish responses to DNA vaccines, and which TLR ligands are the most effective adjuvants.

Possible Attenuation of the Viral Gene(S)

One of the possibilities to reduce present concerns about the potential risks of introducing fish pathogen virulent genes into the wild through the use of DNA vaccines, could be the use of artificially attenuated mutant genes with low possibilities of reversion to wild type, such as multiple mutants. The desired mutant genes can be easily obtained by site directed mutagenesis once established that the mutations do not interfere with the induction of protective immune responses within the host. One of the few examples of this strategy is the collection of sixteen VHSV G gene mutants (two of them double mutants) that were recently obtained in our laboratory [95]. When susceptible cells are transfected with a plasmid coding for the wild type G protein, the transfected cells form syncitia equivalent to those formed upon infection. According to the sequences that affect fusion previously identified in the G protein [96, 97] and confirmed by the elucidation of the tridimensional structure of the G of other rhabdovirus [98, 99], these mutants were affected in fusion and conformation but nevertheless they were recognized by polyclonal as well as for some neutralizing mouse Abs. It remains to be demonstrated whether polyclonal trout Abs still recognize these mutants and if DNA vaccination using these mutant genes induces equivalent rates of protection.

Substitution of the Cmv Promoter by New Promoters

A main concern for the efficiency and safety of fish DNA vaccines is the promoter and regulatory sequences responsible for the transcription of the pathogen gene within the plasmid. To date, all DNA vaccines use the immediate early cytomegalovirus promoter (CMV). When used for gene expression, it acts as a very strong promoter capable of transcribing most genes assayed in a wide range of eukaryotic cells [100, 101], including fish cells [102]. For example, with this system and after intramuscular injection of 1 μg of a VHSV vaccine plasmid, the relative percent of survival (RPS) values were 98% [18].

Despite the effectiveness of this system, CMV is a viral promoter responsible for the regulation of eukaryotic transcription, and this is an impairment to the license and commercialisation of these vaccines worldwide, for example in Europe. Therefore, a search for alternative promoters seems necessary, although the efficiency and price of the vaccine should not be compromised. Various promoters from salmonid genes have already been tested to control gene expression in fish, such as the rainbow trout metallothionein-A promoter [103], the Atlantic salmon histone H3 promoter [104] and the sockeye salmon histone, metallothionein and protamine promoters [105] without very promising results. However the optimisation of β-actine promoters seems as a good alternative, since β-actine promoters of different species have proved to be almost as effective as CMV [106]. We have recently demonstrated that whereas the carp β-actine promoter induced levels of expression of the VHSV G protein lower than those of the CMV promoter at very early times, it then increased and reached levels higher than those induced by CMV at later times. This was assayed both *in vitro* after transfection of fish cell lines and *in vivo* after intramuscular injection, where we found an increase in the Ab titers induced when the β-actine carp promoter was used instead of that of CMV (unpublished data).

Much more research needs to be performed in the search for new fish promoters among those existing in fish or from synthetic and/or semi-synthetic sources, in order to optimise vaccination systems that are both safe and efficient.

Possible Use of Inducible Plasmids

Regulating the control of recombinant protein expression by inducible systems could some day help obtain vectors that induce stronger immune responses that are long-lasting. Further technical complications arise from the fact that the inducible constructs should be inserted into the genome of some of the somatic cells to obtain a long lasting capacity of response rather than a temporary response. In the inducible approach, the switching on / off of the target gene depends on a specific inducer acting over a control protein that binds the target promoter [107, 108]. The constitutive expression of genes is thus avoided and the most adequate time and place of the expression could be controlled, for instance upon a risk of infection. One prerequisite for a useful inducible system is that the inducer / controller must be innocuous and that the possible activation of other gene loci would be inconsequential. The ideal inducible system should also allow the switching of gene expression on and off, rapidly, reversibly, in a dose-dependent manner and only in the desired time and tissue [109]. Limitations that have arisen during the use of these systems in mammals include leaky expression, cellular toxicity, unstable transcripts and insensitivity to the inducer. In the targeted gene approach, the introduction of genes into cells is generally made by homologous recombination by incorporating long genomic inserts or specific recombination sequences. The combination of gene targeting with inducible gene systems constitutes the highest possible control of gene expression available today [109]. At the moment, no inducible systems have been yet tested as possible DNA vaccines, but the development of this technology could be useful in the future for fish vaccination uses.

Fish Transposon Technology Applied to DNA Vaccines

DNA-based active transposons are repetitive DNA sequences found in the genomes of animals and plants that move from one genome locus to another. Although active transposons have been difficult to detect in most vertebrates including fish [110], due to the fact that most of their existing copies are inactivated through deletions, frameshift mutations or premature termination codons in their transposase genes, the enzymes controlling transposon mobilization [111], expression systems based in transposons have been developed and widely studied for applications, such as the improvement of the efficiency of vaccine plasmids and / or the increase of the duration of protection in mammalian systems [112-115]. For example, a decade ago, an active transposase named *Sleeping Beauty* (SB) was artificially reconstructed from trout and salmon genome sequences [116] which recognized sequences flanked by inverted terminal repeats (ITR) of 225 bp. Dual transposition systems consisting in two independent plasmids were designed to transform mammalian cells. One plasmid contained an expression cassette flanked by left and right SB ITRs whereas the other plasmid contained the SB transposase (pSB) under the control of a constitutive promoter like CMV.

Concerning fish, complete SB transposase sequences suggesting their active transposition have been demonstrated in *Salvelinus namaycush* and *Pleuronectes platessa* [117, 118] and active transposition has been detected in zebrafish [119]. In addition, we have demonstrated that active transposases are present in fish cells such as RTG-2 from rainbow trout or EPC from carp and that the *in vitro* temporal expression of genes included in a transposon expression system is notably increased if compared to a plasmid in which the gene is not flanked by ITRs (unpublished data). A *priori* the integration in the genome would not be a problem for the commercialisation of transposon system-based vaccines, and the inclusion of transposon sequences within the plasmid would increase the efficiency and favour the integration with consequent effects of duration of protection. Thus, expectations now might be high for possible new applications of this technology to fish DNA vaccination.

Possible Use of Sirna Generating Sequences

During the last years, double stranded RNAs of 19-25-nucleotides (silencer RNA or siRNA) have been shown to inhibit specifically the translation of complementary mRNAs into proteins. This technology is being applied to specifically knockdown gene expression. Some examples of viral replication inhibition by using dsRNAs that are complementary in sequence to some viral proteins include respiratory synthitial virus [120], hepatitis virus [121, 122] and the mammalian rhabdovirus, vesicular stomatitis [123]. In most mammalian cells, transfected siRNAs that target different viral proteins can inhibit the synthesis of virus at nM concentrations without inducing IFN synthesis or other cellular genes [123]. However, in fish cells such as EPC cells, the transfection of siRNAs targeting the G glycoprotein was shown to induce IFN, being this IFN at least in part responsible for the inhibition of VHSV infection [124]. Many different possibilities of other siRNAs targeting other viral genes need to be explored to elucidate the mechanism of action of the interference in viral replication of these siRNAs in fish cells. In any case, a method including the injection of complexes of siRNAs with DOTAP has been described to delay VHSV *in vivo* infection during 4-5 days [125]. The siRNA can not only be delivered as synthetic RNAs but also through the use plasmids that include the corresponding hairpin DNA sequences (two complementary sequences of 21 nucleotides separated by a loop of 9 nucleotides) under the control of a strong promoter [126]. When transcribed, these sequences form a dsRNA forming an hairpin which behaves as a siRNA, and this could be the system through which this technology could be incorporated into DNA vaccines in fish.

In our laboratory, several potential targets to VHSV L polymerase sequences were designed, chemically synthesized and tested by Q-PCR and microneutralization. Some of them gave inhibitory results and were cloned into commercial plasmids codifying both siRNA and puromicin resistance genes (data not published). EPC transfected cell lines were derived for each of them to demonstrate that some clones acquired the capacity to inhibit VHSV replication. At the moment however, we still do not know whether the inhibition of replication is only due to IFN synthesis or to as in mammals to an interference with the translation of the targeted gene.

The use of siRNAs opens the possibility to interfere with one of the early steps of VHSV infection such as those affected by the polymerase L, thus offering possibilities to potentiate

DNA vaccines. For example, the delay seen in the effects of VHSV infection seen after the injection of complexes of siRNAs with DOTAP [125] might be useful to protect the fish from viral infection until the early immune response induced by the vaccine four days post-vaccination is established.

Moreover, in the future, as advances are available in the understanding of the immune mechanisms responsible for the protection conferred by DNA vaccines, the siRNA technology could be used to block the action of immune factors that interfere with the immune response. For example, the incorporation in a vaccine of siRNAs that target apoptotic proteins, prolonged the life of transfected dendritic cells and thus increased the T cell responses induced by a vaccine [127].

New Mass Vaccination Strategies

A suitable delivery of DNA vaccines allowing mass vaccination of fingerling fish should substitute the actual muscular injection, if DNA vaccines are to be of practical use in those most desirable sizes. Probably, the optimal route for the administration of a vaccine in aquaculture fish would be through bath administration, however, the only route that so far has proved effective for the administration of DNA vaccines has been the intramuscular injection, a very laborious methodology that almost makes impossible a mass vaccination method of small fish of low economic value. Through the use of low frequency ultrasounds [21] or hiperosmotic shock [128], the protection levels after bath DNA vaccination were significantly improved in comparison to the protection levels obtained after a regular bath vaccination, but were still far from the results obtained by intramuscular injection. The bombardment of fish muscle with gold particles covered with DNA [129] proved as an efficient delivery method and the antigen expression lasted for at least 60 days post-bombardment. This method, however, remains expensive and no further optimisation was yet reported. When different routes of administration of a plasmid DNA coding for luciferase coupled to liposomes or chitosan were tested, acceptable levels of luciferase expression were obtained after intraperitoneal, intramuscular or intravenous injection of these complexes, but no detectable luciferase levels were obtained after oral or bath administration [130]. In any case, there are many different possible formulations and improvements that could be tested for liposomes, that have been studied in different mammalian systems, therefore, the area of mass delivery still offers a wide room for further research to make fish DNA vaccines more suitable from a practical point of view.

Conclusion

Vaccination is the most adequate method to control viral diseases, specially in animals of relatively low economic value such as fish. With the efficacy of DNA vaccination against rhabdovirus seen in fish, we have a great opportunity to finally obtain efficient vaccines that are easy to produce, safe, cheap, and provide long-lasting immunity. We only need to continue our research efforts to solve some of the problems they still offer, which still impair their routine use worldwide. In this chapter, we have tried to outline some of the most important lines of research along which the improvement of these vaccines may be achieved.

It seems obvious that concerning vaccines, one of the most important fields of research is the study of immune mechanisms responsible for protection. Previous experience in mammals has demonstrated that from immunological studies, many new ideas can be obtained for the optimisation of vaccine systems to produce more successful and long-lasting fish DNA vaccines. Moreover, this will be a critical point for the development of efficient DNA vaccines against other viral pathogens in fish, that are still not as efficient as those against rhabdovirus.

Acknowledgments

This work was supported by INIA strategic project CPE03-016-C4 and Spanish MEC projects AGL2004-07404-CO2/ACU and AGL05 00339-ACU.

References

[1] Coll, J. M. (2001). Fish Rhabdoviruses. *Recent Research Developmental Virology, 3*, 229-241.

[2] Smail, D. A., Bruno, D. W., Dear, G., McFarlane, L. A. and Ross, K. (1992). Infectious pancreatic necrosis (IPN) virus sp serotype in farmed Atlantic salmon, *Salmo salar* L. post-smolt associated with mortality and clinical disease. *Journal of Fish Diseases, 15*, 77-83.

[3] Bernard, J. and Bremont, M. (1995). Molecular biology of fish viruses: a review. *Veterinary Research, 26*, 341-51.

[4] Macdonald, R. D. and Gower, D. A. (1981). Genomic and phenotypic divergence among three serotypes of aquatic birnaviruses (infectious pancreatic necrosis virus). *Virology, 114*, 187-95.

[5] Gregory, A. (2002). Detection of infectious salmon anaemia virus (ISAV) by *in situ* hybridisation. *Diseases of Aquatic Organisms, 50*, 105-110.

[6] Biering, E., Villoing, S., Sommerset, I. and Christie, K. E. (2005). Update on viral vaccines for fish. *Developmental Biology, 121*, 97-113.

[7] Frerichs, G. N., Rodger, H. D.and Peric, Z. (1996). Cell culture isolation of piscine neuropathy nodavirus from juvenile sea bass, *Dicentrarchus labrax*. *Journal of General Virology, 77*, 2067-2071.

[8] Sommerset, I., Lorenzen, E., Lorenzen, N., Bleie, H. and Nerland, A. H. (2003). A DNA vaccine directed against a rainbow trout rhabdovirus induces early protection against a nodavirus challenge in trout. *Vaccine, 21*, 4661-4667.

[9] Lorenzen, N. and LaPatra, S. E. (2005). DNA vaccines for aquacultured fish. *Reviews Science Technology Office International Epizooties, 24*, 201-213.

[10] Leong, J. A. and Munn, C. B. (1991). Potencial uses of recombinant DNA in development of fish vaccines. *Bulletin of the European Association Fish Pathologists, 11*, 30-40.

[11] Anderson, E. D., Mourich, D. V., Fahrenkrug, S. C., LaPatra, S. C., Shepherd, J. and Leong, J. C. (1996). Genetic immunization of rainbow trout (*Oncorhynchus mykiss*) against infectious hematopoietic necrosis virus. *Molecular Marine Biology and Biotechnology, 5*, 114-122.

[12] Lorenzen, N., Lorenzen, E.,Einer-Jensen, K.and LaPatra, S. E. (2002). Immunity induced shortly after DNA vaccination of rainbow trout against rhabdoviruses protects against heterologous virus but not against bacterial pathogens. *Developmental and Comparative Immunology, 26*, 173-179.

[13] Huang, C. J., Chien, M. S., Landolt, M.,Batts, W. and Winton, J. (1996). Mapping the neutralizing epitopes on the glycoprotein of infectious haematopoietic necrosis virus, a fish rhabdovirus. *Journal of General Virology, 77*, 3033-3040.

[14] Corbeil, S., LaPatra, S. E., Anderson, E. D., Jones, J., Vincent, B., Hsu, Y. L. and Kurath, G. (1999). Evaluation of the protective immunogenicity of the N, P, M, NV and G proteins of infectious hematopoietic necrosis virus in rainbow trout *Oncorhynchus mykiss* using DNA vaccines. *Diseases of Aquatic Organisms, 39*, 29-36.

[15] Anderson, E. D., Mourich, D. V. and Leong, J. C. (1996). Gene expression in rainbow trout (*Onchorynchus mykiss*) following intramuscular injection of DNA. *Molecular Marine Biology and Biotechnology, 5*, 105-113.

[16] Lorenzen, E., Einer-Jensen, K., Martinussen, T., LaPatra, S. E. and Lorenzen, N. (2000). DNA vaccination of rainbow trout against viral hemorrhagic septicemia virus: A dose-response and time-course study. *Journal of Aquatic Animal Health, 12*, 167-180.

[17] LaPatra, S. E., Corbeil, S., Jones, G. R., Shewmaker, W. D., Lorenzen, N., Anderson, E. D. and Kurath, G. (2001). Protection of rainbow trout against infectious hematopoietic necrosis virus four days after specific or semi-specific DNA vaccination. *Vaccine, 19*, 4011-4019.

[18] Lorenzen, N., Lorenzen, E. and Einer-Jensen, K. (2001). Immunity to viral haemorrhagic septicaemia (VHS) following DNA vaccination of rainbow trout at an early life-stage. *Fish and Shellfish Immunology, 11*, 585-591.

[19] Lorenzen, N., Lorenzen, E., Einer-Jensen, K., Heppell, J., Wu, T. and Davis, H. (1998). Protective immunity to VHS in rainbow trout (*Oncorhynchus mykiss*, Walbaum) following DNA vaccination. *Fish and Shellfish Immunology, 8*, 261-270.

[20] McLauchlan, P. E., Collet, B., Ingerslev, E., Secombes, C. J., Lorenzen, N. and Ellis, A. E. (2003). DNA vaccination against viral haemorrhagic septicaemia (VHS) in rainbow trout: size, dose, route of injection and duration of protection-early protection correlates with Mx expression. *Fish and Shellfish Immunology, 15*, 39-50.

[21] Fernandez-Alonso, M., Rocha, A. and Coll, J. M. (2001). DNA vaccination by immersion and ultrasound to trout viral haemorrhagic septicaemia virus. *Vaccine, 19*, 3067-3075.

[22] Lorenzen, N., Olesen, N. J. and Jorgensen, P. E. V. (1993). Antibody response in rainbow trout to VHS virus proteins. *Fish and Shellfish Immunology, 3*, 461-473.

[23] Estepa, A., Thiry, M. and Coll, J. M. (1994). Recombinant protein fragments from haemorrhagic septicaemia rhabdovirus stimulate trout leucocyte anamnestic *in vitro* responses. *Journal of General Virology, 75*, 1329-1338.

[24] Koener, J. F. and Leong, J. A. (1990). Expression of the glycoprotein gene from a fish rhabdovirus by using baculovirus vectors. *Journal of Virology, 64*, 428-30.

[25] Kim, C. H., Johnson, M. C., Drennan, J. D., Simon, B. E., Thomann, E. and Leong, J. A. (2000). DNA vaccines encoding viral glycoproteins induce nonspecific immunity and Mx protein synthesis in fish. *Journal of Virology, 74*, 7048-7054.

[26] Takano, T., Iwahori, A., Hirono, I. and Aoki, T. (2004). Development of a DNA vaccine against hirame rhabdovirus and analysis of the expression of immune-related genes after vaccination. *Fish and Shellfish Immunology, 17*, 367-374.

[27] Mikalsen, A. B., Torgersen, J., Alestrom, P., Hellemann, A. L., Koppang, E. O. and Rimstad, E. (2004). Protection of Atlantic salmon *Salmo salar* against infectious pancreatic necrosis after DNA vaccination. *Diseases of Aquatic Organisms, 60*, 11-20.

[28] Mikalsen, A. B., Sindre, H., Torgersen, J. and Rimstad, E. (2005). Protective effects of a DNA vaccine expressing the infectious salmon anemia virus hemagglutinin-esterase in Atlantic salmon. *Vaccine, 23*, 4895-905.

[29] Nusbaum, K. E., Smith, B. F., DeInnocentes, P. and Bird, R. C. (2002). Protective immunity induced by DNA vaccination of channel catfish with early and late transcripts of the channel catfish herpesvirus (IHV-1). *Veterinary Immunology and Immunopathology, 84*, 151-168.

[30] Sommerset, I., Skern, R., Biering, E., Bleie, H., Fiksdal, I. U., Grove, S. and Nerland, A. H. (2005). Protection against Atlantic halibut nodavirus in turbot is induced by recombinant capsid protein vaccination but not following DNA vaccination. *Fish and Shellfish Immunology, 18*, 13-29.

[31] Wolff, J. A., Malone, R. W., Williams, P., Chong, W., Acsadi, G., Jani, A. and Felgner, P. L. (1990). Direct gene transfer into mouse muscle *in vivo*. *Science, 247*, 1465-1468.

[32] Greenland, J. R. and Letvin, N. L. (2007). Chemical adjuvants for plasmid DNA vaccines. *Vaccine, 25*, 3731-41.

[33] Krieg, A. M. (1999). Direct immunologic activities of CpG DNA and implications for gene therapy. *Journal of General Medicine, 1*, 56-63.

[34] Chiller, J. M., Hodgins, H. O. and Weiser, R. S. (1969). Antibody response in rainbow trout (*Salmo gairdneri*). II. Studies of the kinetics of development of antibody-producing cells and on complement and natural haemolysin. *Immunology, 102*, 1202-1207.

[35] Purcell, M. K., Kurath, G., Garver, K. A., Herwig, R. P. and Winton, J. R. (2004). Quantitative expression profiling of imune response genes in rainbow trout following infectious haematopoietic necrosis virus (IHNV) infection or DNA vaccination. *Fish and Shellfish Immunology, 17*, 447-462.

[36] Acosta, F., Petrie, A., Lockhart, K., Lorenzen, N. and Ellis, A. E. (2005). Kinetics of Mx expression in rainbow trout (*Oncorhynchus mykiss*) and Atlantic salmon (*Salmo salar* L.) parr in response to VHS-DNA vaccination. *Fish and Shellfish Immunology, 18*, 81-89.

[37] Trobridge, G. D., Chiou, P. P. and Leong, J. C. (1997). Cloning of the rainbow trout (*Oncorhynchus mykiss*) Mx2 and Mx3 cDNAs and characterization of trout Mx protein expression in salmon cells. *Journal of Virology, 71*, 5304-5311.

[38] Robertsen, B., Trobridge, G. and Leong, J. A. (1997). Molecular cloning of double-stranded RNA inducible Mx genes from Atlantic salmon (*Salmo salar* L.). *Developmental and Comparative Immunology, 21*, 397-412.

[39] Staeheli, P., Pitossi, F. and Pavlovic, J. (1993). Mx proteins: GTPases with antiviral activity. *Trends Cell Biology, 3*, 268-72.

[40] King, M. C., Raposo, G. and Lemmon, M. A. (2004). Inhibition of nuclear import and cell-cycle progression by mutated forms of the dynamin-like GTPase MxB. *Proceedings of the National Academy of Sciences of the United States of America, 101*, 8957-62.

[41] Tafalla, C., Chico, V., Pérez, L., Coll, J. and Estepa, A. (2007). In vitro and in vivo differential expression of rainbow trout (*Oncorhynchus mykiss*) Mx isoforms in response to viral hemorrhagic septicemia virus (VHSV) G gene, Poly I:C and VHSV. *Fish and Shellfish Immunology, 23*, 210-21.

[42] Zurcher, T., Pavlovic, J. andStaeheli, P. (1992). Mechanism of human MxA protein action: variants with changed antiviral properties. *The EMBO Journal, 11*, 1657-61.

[43] Nakajima, E., Morozumi, T., Tsukamoto, K., Watanabe, T., Plastow, G. and Mitsuhashi, T. (2007). A naturally occurring variant of porcine Mx1 associated with increased susceptibility to influenza virus *in vitro*. *Biochemical Genetics, 45*, 11-24.

[44] Palm, M., Leroy, M., Thomas, A., Linden, A. and Desmecht, D. (2007). Differential anti-influenza activity among allelic variants at the *Sus scrofa* Mx1 locus. *Journal of Interferon and Cytokine Research, 27*, 147-55.

[45] Purcell, M. K., Nichols, K. M., Winton, J. R., Kurath, G., Thorgaard, G. H., Wheeler, P., Hansen, J. D., Herwig, R. P. and Park, L. K. (2006). Comprehensive gene expression profiling following DNA vaccination of rainbow trout against infectious hematopoietic necrosis virus. *Molecular Immunology, 43*, 2089-2106.

[46] Robertsen, B., Bergan, V., Rokenes, T., Larsen, R. and Albuquerque, A. (2003). Atlantic salmon interferon genes: cloning, sequence analysis, expression, and biological activity. *Journal of Interferon and Cytokine Research, 23*, 601-12.

[47] Zou, J., Tafalla, C., Truckle, J. and Secombes, C. (2007). Identification of a second group of type I interferons in fish sheds light on interferon evolution in vertebrates. *Journal of Immunology, In press*.

[48] Der, S. D., Zhou, A., Williams, B. R. and Silverman, R. H. (1998). Identification of genes differentially regulated by interferon alpha, beta, or gamma using oligonucleotide arrays. *Proceedings of the National Academy of Sciences of the United States of America, 95*, 15623-8.

[49] Traxler, G. S., Anderson, E., LaPatra, S. E., Richard, J., Shewmaker, B. and Kurath, G. (1999). Naked DNA vaccination of Atlantic salmon *Salmo salar* against IHNV. *Diseases of Aquatic Organisms, 38*, 183-190.

[50] Kanellos, T., Sylvester, I. D., Ambali, A. G., Howard, C. R. and Russell, P. H. (1999). The safety and longevity of DNA vaccines for fish. *Immunology, 96*, 307-13.

[51] Boudinot, P., Blanco, M., de Kinkelin, P. and Benmansour, A. (1998). Combined DNA immunization with the glycoprotein gene of viral hemorrhagic septicemia virus and infectious hematopoietic necrosis virus induces double-specific protective immunity and nonspecific response in rainbow trout. *Virology, 249*, 297-306.

[52] Kanellos, T., Sylvester, I. D., Howard, C. R. and Rusell, P. H. (1999). DNA is as effective as protein at inducing antibody in fish. *Vaccine, 17*, 965-972.

[53] Lorenzen, N., Olesen, N. J. and Vestergaard-Jorgensen, P. E. (1990). Neutralization of Egtved virus pathogenicity to cell cultures and fish by monoclonal antibodies to the viral G protein. *Journal of General Virology, 71*, 561-567.

[54] DeKinkelin, P., Geraed, J. P., Dorson, M. and Le Berre, M. (1977). Viral Haemorrhagic Septicemia: Demonstration of a protective immune response following natural infection. *Fish Health News, 6*, 43-45.

[55] Estepa, A., Fernandez-Alonso, M. and Coll, J. M. (1999). Structure, binding and neutralization of VHSV with synthetic peptides. *Virus Research, 63*, 27-34.

[56] Lorenzen, N. and LaPatra, S. E. (1999). Immunity to rhabdoviruses in rainbow trout: the antibody response. *Fish and Shellfish Immunology, 9*, 345-360.

[57] Ristow, S., Avila, J., La Patra, S. and Lauda, K. (1993). Detection and characterization of rainbow trout antibody against infectious hematopoietic necrosis virus. *Diseases of Aquatic Organism, 15*, 109-114.

[58] Lapatra, S. E., Fryer, J. L. and Rohovec, J. S. (1993). Virulence cmparison of different electrophero-types of infectious hematopoietic necrosis virus. *Diseases of Aquatic Organisms, 16*, 115-120.

[59] [59] Olesen, N. J., Lorenzen, N. and Jorgensen, P. E. V. (1993). Serological differences among isolates of viral haemorrhagic septicemia virus detected by neutralizing monoclonal and polyclonal antibodies. *Diseases of Aquatic Organisms, 16*, 163-170.

[60] Huang, C. J., Chien, M. S., Landolt, M. and Winton, J. (1994). Characterization of the infectious hematopoietic necrosis virus glycoprotein using neutralizing monoclonal-antibodies. *Diseases of Aquatic Organisms, 18*, 29-35.

[61] Bearzotti, M., Monnier, A. F., Vende, P., Grosclaude, J., DeKinkelin, P. and Benmansour, A. (1995). The glycoprotein of viral hemorrhagic septicemia virus (VHSV): antigenicity and role in virulence. *Veterinary Research, 26*, 413-422.

[62] Fernandez-Alonso, M., Lorenzo, G., Perez, L., Bullido, R., Estepa, A., Lorenzen, N. and Coll, J. M. (1998). Mapping of the lineal antibody epitopes of the glycoprotein of VHSV, a salmonid rhabdovirus. *Diseases of Aquatic Organisms, 34*, 167-176.

[63] Lefrancois, L. (1984). Protection against lethal viral infection by neutralizing and nonneutralizing monoclonal antibodies: distinct mechanisms of action *in vivo*. *Journal of Virology, 51*, 208-14.

[64] Fregeneda-Grandes, J. M. and Olesen, N. J. (2007). Detection of rainbow trout antibodies against viral haemorrhagic septicaemia virus (VHSV) by neutralisation test is highly dependent on the virus isolate used. *Diseases of Aquatic Organisms, 74*, 151-8.

[65] Wilson, M., Bengten, E., Miller, N. W., Clem, L. W., Du Pasquier, L. and Warr, G. W. (1997). A novel chimeric Ig heavy chain from a teleost fish shares similarities to IgD. *Proceedings of the National Academy of Sciences of the United States of America, 94*, 4593-7.

[66] Hordvik, I. (2002). Identification of a novel immunoglobulin delta transcript and comparative analysis of the genes encoding IgD in Atlantic salmon and Atlantic halibut. *Molecular Immunology, 39*, 85-91.

[67] Hansen, J. D., Landis, E. D. and Phillips, R. B. (2005). Discovery of a unique Ig heavy-chain isotype (IgT) in rainbow trout: Implications for a distinctive B cell developmental pathway in teleost fish. *Proceedings of the National Academy of Sciences of the United States of America, 102*, 6919-24.

[68] Utke, K., Kock, H., Schuetze, H., Bergmann, S. M., Lorenzen, N., Einer-Jensen, K., Kollner, B., Dalmo, R. A., Vesely, T., Ototake, M. and Fischer, U. (2007). Cell-

mediated immune responses in rainbow trout after DNA immunization against the viral hemorrhagic septicemia virus. *Developmental and Comparative Immunol*ogy. In press.

[69] Byon, J. Y., Ohira, T., Hirono, I. and Aoki, T. (2005). Use of a cDNA microarray to study immunity against viral hemorrhagic septicemia (VHS) in Japanese flounder (*Paralichthys olivaceus*) following DNA vaccination. *Fish and Shellfish Immunology, 18*, 135-147.

[70] Byon, J. Y., Ohira, T., Hirono, I. and Aoki, T. (2006). Comparative immune responses in Japanese flounder, *Paralichthys olivaceus* after vaccination with viral hemorrhagic septicemia virus (VHSV) recombinant glycoprotein and DNA vaccine using a microarray analysis. *Vaccine, 24*, 921-30.

[71] Yasuike, M., Kondo, H., Hirono, I. and Aoki, T. (2007). Difference in Japanese flounder, *Paralichthys olivaceus* gene expression profile following hirame rhabdovirus (HIRRV) G and N protein DNA vaccination. *Fish and Shellfish Immunology, 23*, 531-41.

[72] Kim, J. J., Bagarazzi, M. L., Trivedi, N., Hu, Y., Kazahaya, K., Wilson, D. M., Ciccarelli, R., Chattergoon, M. A., Dang, K., Mahalingam, S., Chalian, A. A., Agadjanyan, M. G., Boyer, J. D., Wang, B. and Weiner, D. B. (1997). Engineering of *in vivo* immune responses to DNA immunization via codelivery of costimulatory molecule genes. *Nature biotechnology, 15*, 641-6.

[73] Kim, J. J., Yang, J. S., Dentchev, T., Dang, K. and Weiner, D. B. (2000). Chemokine gene adjuvants can modulate immune responses induced by DNA vaccines. *Journal of Interferon and Cytokine Research, 20*, 487-498.

[74] Eo, S. K., Lee, S., Kumaraguru, U. and Rouse, B. T. (2001). Immunopotentiation of DNA vaccine against herpes simplex virus via co-delivery of plasmid DNA expressing CCR7 ligands. *Vaccine, 19*, 4685-4693.

[75] Lusso, P. (2002). HIV and chemokines: implications for therapy and vaccine. *Vaccine, 20*, 1964-1967.

[76] Jimenez, N., Coll, J., Salguero, F. J. and Tafalla, C. (2006). Co-injection of interleukin 8 with the glycoprotein gene from viral haemorrhagic septicemia virus (VHSV) modulates the cytokine response in rainbow trout (*Oncorhynchus mykiss*). *Vaccine, 24*, 5615-26.

[77] Sanchez, E., Coll, J. and Tafalla, C. (2007). Expression of inducible CC chemokines in rainbow trout (*Oncorhynchus mykiss*) in response to a viral haemorrhagic septicemia virus (VHSV) DNA vaccine and interleukin 8. *Developmental and Comparative Immunology, 31*, 916-26.

[78] Purcell, M. K., Smith, K. D., Hood, L., Winton, J. R. and Roach, J. C. (2006). Conservation of toll-like receptor signalling pathways in teleost fish. *Comparative Biochemistry and Physiology Part D: Genomics Proteomics, 1*, 77-88.

[79] van Duin, D., Medzhitov, R. and Shaw, A. C. (2006). Triggering TLR signalling in vaccination. *Trends in Immunology, 27*, 49-55.

[80] Steere, A. C., Sikand, V. K., Meurice, F., Parenti, D. L., Fikrig, E., Schoen, R. T., Nowakowski, J., Schmid, C. H., Laukamp, S., Buscarino, C. and Krause, D. S. (1998). Vaccination against Lyme disease with recombinant *Borrelia burgdorferi* outer-surface lipoprotein A with adjuvant. Lyme Disease Vaccine Study Group. *The New England journal of medicine, 339*, 209-15.

[81] Krieg, A. M. (2000). The role of CpG motifs in innate immunity. *Current Opinion in Immunology, 12*, 35-43.

[82] Klinman, D. M., Yamshchikov, G. and Ishigatsubo, Y. (1997). Contribution of CpG motifs to the immunogenicity of DNA vaccines. *Journal of Immunology, 158*, 3635-9.

[83] Sato, Y., Roman, M., Tighe, H., Lee, D., Corr, M., Nguyen, M. D., Silverman, G. J., Lotz, M., Carson, D. A. and Raz, E. (1996). Immunostimulatory DNA sequences necessary for effective intradermal gene immunization. *Science, 273*, 352-354.

[84] Carrington, A. C., Collet, B., Holland, J. W. and Secombes, C. J. (2004). CpG oligodeoxynucleotides stimulate immune cell proliferation but not specific antibody production in rainbow trout (*Oncorhynchus mykiss*). *Veterinary Immunology and Immunopathology, 101*, 211-22.

[85] Jorgensen, J. B., Zou, J., Johansen, A. and Secombes, C. J. (2001). Immunostimulatory CpG oligodeoxynucleotides stimulate expression of IL-1 beta and interferon-like cytokines in rainbow trout macrophages via a chloroquine-sensitive mechanism. *Fish and Shellfish Immunology, 11*, 673-682.

[86] Shen, K. Y., Hogstrand, C. and Davies, D. H. (2006). A newly identified CpG oligodeoxynucleotide motif that stimulates rainbow trout (*Oncorhynchus mykiss*) immune cells to produce immunomodulatory factors. *Developmental and Comparative Immunology, 30*, 311-24.

[87] Jorgensen, J. B., Johansen, A., Stenersen, B. and Sommer, A. I. (2001). CpG oligodeoxynucleotides and plasmid DNA stimulate Atlantic salmon (*Salmo salar* L.) leucocytes to produce supernatants with antiviral activity. *Developmental and Comparative Immunology, 25*, 313-321.

[88] Kanellos, T. S., Sylvester, I. D., Butler, V. L., Ambali, A. G., Partidos, C. D., Hamblin, A. S. and Russell, P. H. (1999). Mammalian granulocyte-macrophage colony-stimulating factor and some CpG motifs have an effect on the immunogenicity of DNA and subunit vaccines in fish. *Immunology, 96*, 507-10.

[89] Applequist, S. E., Rollman, E., Wareing, M. D., Liden, M., Rozell, B., Hinkula, J. and Ljunggren, H. G. (2005). Activation of innate immunity, inflammation, and potentiation of DNA vaccination through mammalian expression of the TLR5 agonist flagellin. *Journal of Immunolology, 175*, 3882-91.

[90] Takeshita, F., Tanaka, T., Matsuda, T., Tozuka, M., Kobiyama, K., Saha, S., Matsui, K., Ishii, K. J., Coban, C., Akira, S., Ishii, N., Suzuki, K., Klinman, D. M., Okuda, K. and Sasaki, S. (2006). Toll-like receptor adaptor molecules enhance DNA-raised adaptive immune responses against influenza and tumors through activation of innate immunity. *Journal of Virology, 80*, 6218-24.

[91] Zhu, J., Huang, X. and Yang, Y. (2007). Innate immune response to adenoviral vectors is mediated by both Toll-like receptor-dependent and -independent pathways. *Journal of Virology, 81*, 3170-80.

[92] Oshiumi, H., Tsujita, T., Shida, K., Matsumoto, M., Ikeo, K. and Seya, T. (2003). Prediction of the prototype of the human Toll-like receptor gene family from the pufferfish, *Fugu rubripes*, genome. *Immunogenetics, 54*, 791-800.

[93] Jault, C., Pichon, L. and Chluba, J. (2004). Toll-like receptor gene family and TIR-domain adapters in *Danio rerio*. *Molecular Immunology, 40*, 759-71.

[94] Tsujita, T., Tsukada, H., Nakao, M., Oshiumi, H., Matsumoto, M. and Seya, T. (2004). Sensing bacterial flagellin by membrane and soluble orthologs of Toll-like receptor 5 in

rainbow trout (*Onchorhynchus mykiss*). *Journal of Biological Chemistry, 279*, 48588-97.

[95] Rocha, A., Ruiz, S., Tafalla, C. and Coll, J. M. (2004). Conformation and fusion defective mutants in the hypothetical phospholipid-binding and fusion peptides of the protein G of viral haemorrhagic septicemia salmonid rhabdovirus. *Journal of Virology, 78*, 9115-9122.

[96] Nuñez, E., Fernandez, A. M., Estepa, A., Gonzalez-Ros, J. M., Gavilanes, F. and Coll, J. M. (1998). Phospholipid interactions of a peptide from the fusion-related domain of the glycoprotein of VHSV, a fish rhabdovirus. *Virology, 243*, 322-330.

[97] Estepa, A., Rocha, A., Pérez, L., Encinar, J. A., Nuñez, E., Fernandez, A., Gonzalez Ros, J. M., Gavilanes, F. and Coll, J. M. (2001). A protein fragment from the salmonid VHS rhabdovirus induces cell-to-cell fusion and membrane phosphatidylserine translocation at low pH. *Journal of Biological Chemistry, 276*, 46268-46275.

[98] Roche, S., Bressanelli, S., Rey, F. A. and Gaudin, Y. (2006). Crystal structure of the low-pH form of the vesicular stomatitis virus glycoprotein G. *Science, 313*, 187-91.

[99] Roche, S., Rey, F. A., Gaudin, Y. and Bressanelli, S. (2007). Structure of the prefusion form of the vesicular stomatitis virus glycoprotein G. *Science, 315*, 843-8.

[100] Ramesh, N., Shin, Y. K., Lau, S. and Osborne, W. R. (1995). High-level expression from a cytomegalovirus promoter in macrophage cells. *Human gene therapy, 6*, 1323-7.

[101] Artuc, M., Nurnberg, W., Czarnetzki, B. M. and Schadendorf, D. (1995). Characterization of gene regulatory elements for selective gene expression in human melanoma cells. *Biochemical and biophysical research communications, 213*, 699-705.

[102] Heppell, J., Lorenzen, N., Armstrong, N. K., Wu, T., Lorenzen, E., Einer-Jensen, K., Ahrens, P., Schorr, J. and Davis, H. L. (1998). Development of DNA vaccines for fish: vector design, intramuscular injection and antigen expression using viral haemorrhagic septicemia virus genes as model. *Fish and Shellfish Immunology, 8*, 271-287.

[103] Mayer, G. D., Leach, A., Kling, P., Olsson, P. E. and Hogstrand, C. (2003). Activation of the rainbow trout metallothionein-A promoter by silver and zinc. *Comparative Biochemistry and Physiology Part B: Biochemistry and Molecular Biology, 134*, 181-8.

[104] Hanley, S., Smith, T. J., Muller, F., Maclean, N., Uzbekova, S., Prunet, P. and Breton, B. (1998). Isolation and functional analysis of the histone H3 promoter from Atlantic salmon (*Salmo salar* L.). *Molecular marine biology and biotechnology, 7*, 165-72.

[105] Chan, W. K. and Devlin, R. H. (1993). Polymerase chain reaction amplification and functional characterization of sockeye salmon histone H3, metallothionein-B, and protamine promoters. *Molecular marine biology and biotechnology, 2*, 308-18.

[106] Hwang, G. L., Rahman, A., Razak, S. A., Sohm, F., Farahmand, H., Smith, A., Brooks, C. and Maclean, N. (2003). Isolation and characterisation of tilapia ß-actin promoter comparison of its activity with carp ß-actin promoter. *Biochimica and Biophysica Acta, 1625*, 11-18.

[107] Lewandoski, M. (2001). Conditional control of gene expression in the mouse. *Nature Review Genetics, 2*, 743-755.

[108] Ristevski, S. (2001). Transgenic studies in the mouse. Improving the technology towards a conditional temporal and spatial approach. *Methods in Molecular Biology, 158*, 319-334.

[109] Gao, X., Kemper, A. and Popko, B. (1999). Advanced transgenic and gene-targeting approaches. *Neurochemical Research, 24*, 1181-1188.

[110] Tafalla, C., Estepa, A. and Coll, J. M. (2006). Fish transposons and their potential use in aquaculture. *Journal of Biotechnology, 123*, 397-412.

[111] Ivics, Z., Kaufman, C. D., Zayed, H., Miskey, C., Wallsko, O. and Izsvak, Z. (2004). The sleeping beauty transposable element: evolution, regulation and genetic applications. *Current Issues in Molecular Biology, 6*, 43-56.

[112] Izsvak, Z.,Ivics, Z.andPlasterk, R. H. (2000). Sleeping beauty, a wide host-range transposon vector for genetic transformation in vertebrates. *Journal of Molecular Biology, 302*, 93-102.

[113] Dupuy, A. J., Clark, K., Carlson, C. M., Fritz, S., Davidson, A. E., Markley, K. M., Finley, K., Fletcher, C. F., Ekker, S. C., Hackett, P. B., Hom, S. and Largaespeda, D. A. (2002). Mammalian germ-line transgenesis by transposition. *Proceedings of the National Academy of Sciences of the United States of America, 99*, 4495-4499.

[114] Horie, K., Yusa, K., Yae, K., Odajima, J., Fisher, S. E., Keng, V. W., Hayakawa, T., Mizuno, A., Kondoh, G., Ijiri, T., Matsuda, Y., Plasterk, R. H. and Takeda, J. (2003). Characterization of sleeping beauty transposition and its application to genetic screening in mice. *Molecular Cell Biology, 23*, 9189-9207.

[115] Masuda, K.,Yamamoto, S.,Endoh, M.andKaneda, Y. (2004). Transposon-independent increase of transcription by the sleeping beauty transposase. *Biochemical and Biophysical Research Communications, 317*, 796-800.

[116] Ivics, Z., Izsvak, Z. and Hackett, P. B. (1997). Molecular reconstruction of sleeping beauty, a Tc1-like transposon system from fish and its transposition in human cells. *Cell, 91*, 501-510.

[117] Reed, K. M. (1999). Tc1-like transposable elements in the genome of lake trout (*Salvelinus namycush*). *Marine Biotechnology, 1*, 60-67.

[118] Leaver, M. J. (2001). A family of Tc1-like transposons from the genomes of fishes and frogs: evidence for horizontal transmission. *Gene, 271*, 203-214.

[119] Lam, W. L., Lee, T. S. and Gilbert, W. (1996). Active transposition in zebrafish. *Proceedings of the National Academy of Sciences of the United States of America, 93*, 10870-10875.

[120] Li, T., Zhang, Y., Fu, L., Yu, C., Li, X., Li, Y., Zhang, X., Rong, Z., Wang, Y., Ning, H., Liang, R., Chen, W., Babiuk, L. A. and Chang, Z. (2005). siRNA targeting the Leader sequence of SARS-CoV inhibits virus replication. *Gene Therapy, 12*, 751-761.

[121] Baltayiannis, G., Filis, S., Tsianos, E. and Karayiannis, P. (2005). Small interfering RNA(siRNA)-mediated inhibition of hepatitis C virus replication using bicistronic vector *in vivo* (cell line Huh-7) and *in vitro*. *Journal of Hepatology, 42*, 154-154.

[122] Korf, M., Jarczak, D., Beger, C., Manns, M. P. and Kruger, M. (2005). Inhibition of hepatitis C virus translation and subgenomic replication by siRNAs directed against highly conserved HCV sequence and cellular HCV cofactors. *Journal of Hepatology, 43*, 225-234.

[123] Barik, S. (2004). Control of nonsegmented negative-strand RNA virus replication by siRNA. *Virus Research, 102*, 27-35.

[124] Schyth, B. D., Lorenzen, N. and Pedersen, F. S. (2006). Antiviral activity of small interfering RNAs: specificity testing using heterologous virus reveals interferon-related effects overlooked by conventional mismatch controls. *Virology, 349*, 134-41.

[125] Schyth, B. D., Lorenzen, N. and Pedersen, F. S. (2007). A High throughput in vivo model for testing delivery and antiviral effects of siRNAs in vertebrates. *Molecular Ther*apy

[126] Wang, E., Sun, X., Qian, Y., Zhao, L., Tien, P. and Gao, G. F. (2003). Both heptad repeats of human respiratory syncytial virus fusion protein are potent inhibitors of viral fusion. *Biochemical and biophysical research communications, 302*, 469-75.

[127] Kang, T. H., Lee, J. H., Noh, K. H., Han, H. D., Shin, B. C., Choi, E. Y., Peng, S., Hung, C. F., Wu, T. C. and Kim, T. W. (2007). Enhancing dendritic cell vaccine potency by combining a BAK/BAX siRNA-mediated antiapoptotic strategy to prolong dendritic cell life with an intracellular strategy to target antigen to lysosomal compartments. *Internation Journal of Cancer, 120*, 1696-703.

[128] Huising, M. O., Guichelaar, T., Hoek, C., Verburg-vanKemenade, B. M., Flik, G., Savelkoul, H. F. J. and Rombout, J. H. W. M. (2003). Increased efficacy of immersion vaccination in fish with hyperosmotic pretreatment. *Vaccine, 21*, 4178-4193.

[129] Tucker, C., Endo, M., Hirono, I. and Aoki, T. (2000). Assessment of DNA vaccine potential for juvenile Japanese flounder *Paralichthys olivaceus*, through the introduction of reporter genes by particle bombardment and histopathology. *Vaccine, 19*, 801-9.

[130] Romoren, K., Thu, B. J. and Evensen, O. (2002). Immersion delivery of plasmid DNA II. A study of the potentials of a chitosan based delivery system in rainbow trout (*Oncorhynchus mykiss*) fry. *Journal of Controlled Release, 85*, 215-225.

Index

E

F

G

H

I

J

K

L

M

N

O

P

Q

R

S

T

U

V

W

X

Y

Z